T3-BHN-497

POCKET GUIDE TO

Intravenous Therapy

POCKET GUIDE TO

Intravenous Therapy

Joanne C. LaRocca, MN, RN, FNPC

Assistant Nursing Director
Olive View–UCLA Medical Center
Los Angeles, California

Shirley E. Otto, MSN, CRNI, AOCN

Clinical Nurse Specialist
Via Christi Regional Medical Center
St. Francis Campus
Wichita, Kansas

Third Edition

with 84 illustrations

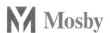 Mosby

St. Louis Baltimore Boston Carlsbad Chicago Naples New York
Philadelphia Portland London Madrid Mexico City Singapore
Sydney Tokyo Toronto Wiesbaden

Vice President and Publisher: Nancy L. Coon
Editor: Robin Carter
Developmental Editor: Jeanne Allison
Project Manager: Patricia Tannian
Project Specialist: Ann E. Rogers
Production: Graphic World Publishing Services
Book Design Manager: Gail Morey Hudson
Manufacturing Supervisor: Karen Lewis
Cover Designer: Teresa Breckwoldt
Cover Image: Abbott Laboratories

Third Edition

Copyright © 1997 by Mosby–Year Book, Inc.

Previous editions copyrighted 1989, 1993.

All rights reserved. No part of this publication may be reproduced, stored in a retrieval system, or transmitted, in any form or by any means, electronic, mechanical, photocopying, recording, or otherwise, without written permission from the publisher.

Permission to photocopy or reproduce solely for internal or personal use is permitted for libraries or other users registered with the Copyright Clearance Center, provided that the base fee of $4.00 per chapter plus $.10 per page is paid directly to the Copyright Clearance Center, 27 Congress Street, Salem, MA 01970. This consent does not extend to other kinds of copying, such as copying for general distribution, for advertising or promotional purposes, for creating new collected works, or for resale.

Printed in the United States of America.
Composition by Graphic World, Inc.
Printing/binding by RR Donnelley and Sons Company.

Mosby–Year Book, Inc.
11830 Westline Industrial Drive
St. Louis, Missouri 63146

Library of Congress Cataloging in Publication Data

LaRocca, Joanne C.
    Pocket guide to intravenous therapy/Joanne C. LaRocca, Shirley
  E. Otto—3rd ed.
       p.   cm.
    Includes bibliographical references and index.
    ISBN 0-8151-5298-1
    1. Intravenous therapy—Handbooks, manuals, etc. 2. Nursing—
  Handbooks, manuals, etc.   I. Otto, Shirley E.   II. Title.
    [DNLM: 1. Infusions, Intravenous—handbooks. 2. Infusions,
  Intravenous—nurses' instruction. 3. Parenteral Nutrition—
  handbooks. WB 39 L326p 1997]
  RM170.L37 1997
  615.8′55—dc20
  DNLM/DLC
  for Library of Congress   96-14139
                                                                        CIP
  96 97 98 99 00 / 9 8 7 6 5 4 3 2 1

To staff nurses everywhere
who have generously shared their hints along the way

Contributors

Kimberly A. McAlpine, BSN, RN
Infusion Liaison
Comfort Care Home Medical
Troy, Michigan

Pediatric IV Therapy

Susan Newsom, MSN, RN, CCRN
Clinical Nurse Specialist, Surgical Nursing
Olive View–UCLA Medical Center
Los Angeles, California

Vascular Access in Adult Critical Care

Stacey L. Prieur, BSN, RN
Infusion Liaison
Comfort Care Home Medical
Troy, Michigan

Pediatric IV Therapy

Consultants

Lyn A. Tepper, MSN, RN
University of Illinois at Chicago
Chicago, Illinois

Emily Yale, MSN, RN
Missouri Baptist Medical Center and
St. Louis Community College at Meramec
St. Louis, Missouri

Preface

All health-care professionals are practicing in a rapidly changing, highly complicated environment in which IV therapy is a major treatment modality. Tremendous technological and reimbursement changes have necessitated proficiency in not only clinical skills but also in documentation, patient teaching, and demonstration of quality improvement and risk management. Implantable ports, peripherally inserted central venous catheters, state-of-the-art pain management, and complex home/clinic IV medication regimens have challenged the nurse's practice climate. Increasingly, greater numbers of patients with serious illnesses—for example, AIDS, cancer, and end-stage organ diseases—require astute, long-term IV medication management. *Pocket Guide to Intravenous Therapy* has been designed to give nurses working in diverse patient care settings and with varying clinical preparation an easily accessible, accurate, and concise reference based on recognized national standards of practice. This book is an ideal study guide for those entering IV therapy practice and/or reviewing for the Intravenous Nurse's Society certification examination.

The advent and increased use of multiple and diverse IV products and equipment in all settings have added a new dimension of complexity to the demands on the busy nurse. Now more than ever, advanced IV skills are sought by all nurses. For the nurse entering practice, returning to practice, or changing areas, learning these skills can be intimidating, and therefore a quick reference is needed. Home IV therapy, integration of nursing diagnoses into the care plan, and third-party documentation demands may be new or changing concepts in some areas. This book features practical strategies and tools for patient teaching, sample documentation using nursing diagnoses, and nursing practice audits that can be readily adapted to all settings.

Each chapter discusses a major aspect of IV therapy. All chapters contain pertinent information, clinical alerts to clarify topics, tables for convenient reference, documentation recommendations, nursing diagnoses, patient/family teaching for self-management, home care considerations, and geriatric considerations. The content of the book has been organized in the manner in which nurses think and perform while providing care.

Chapter 1: *Infusion Guidelines* presents an overview of IV therapy principles.

Chapter 2: *Venipuncture* examines skills, product selection, and infection control issues.

Chapter 3: *Central Venous Catheters* contrasts and compares all of the central venous catheters and provides step-by-step procedures for each device.

Chapter 4: *Peripherally Inserted Central Catheters* provides guidelines on catheter placement, indications, contraindications, products, maintenance procedures, trouble shooting tips, and potential complications.

Chapter 5: *IV Fluids* reviews the assessments and interventions required for the basic electrolytes. A table of replacement fluids is included.

Chapter 6: *IV Medication Administration* describes all modalities of IV medication administration. Information of all the most frequently administered IV medications is included, as is a discussion of state-of-the-art pain medication administration.

Chapter 7: *Blood and Blood Component Administration* presents all components and transfusion reactions in readily available tables. Guidelines for home administration of blood products are included.

Chapter 8: *Chemotherapy Administration* explains theoretical information and nursing management for preparation, delivery, and disposal of cytotoxic drugs in the hospital or outpatient setting.

Chapter 9: *Parenteral Nutrition* explains assessment parameters and nursing interventions and emphasizes teaching needs for self-management.

Chapter 10: *Vascular Access in Adult Critical Care* discusses aspects of IV therapy for the patient receiving varied multimodality infusion therapy; specifics on drug/infusion dose calculations, compatibilities, and therapeutic monitoring guidelines are provided.

Chapter 11: *Pediatric Intravenous Therapy* provides multiple IV topics: fluid and electrolyte balance, IV site access, central venous catheters, intraosseous infusion, and IV medication, blood product, chemotherapy, and parenteral nutrition administration for the pediatric patient.

Chapter 12: *Calculations for IV Therapy* illustrates the use of all formulas required for accurate administration of IV therapy.

Appendixes:

A: *Adult Infusion Therapies*

B: *Use of Nursing Diagnoses with Sample Charting*

C: *Risk Management Considerations in IV Therapy*

D: *Basic IV Therapy Course Objectives*

Bibliography: each chapter has suggested readings for those desiring more information.

Pocket Guide to Intravenous Therapy continues to be an excellent clinical resource for many nurses in all practice settings. The authors have responded to the many requests to "please include more IV therapy information for critical care and pediatric patients" and "expand the information on the peripherally inserted central catheter." This edition contains separate chapters on peripherally inserted central catheters, critical care issues, and the pediatric patient. **Additional features** include study questions with answers for each chapter, as well as Appendix A, which contains a very "user friendly" Adult Infusion Therapy Table for biotherapy drugs, anticoagulants, antifungals, antimicrobials, antivirals, bronchodilators, hypoglycemics, immunosuppressants, and cardiovascular drugs. We continue to strive for excellence in all aspects of intravenous therapy.

The authors are indebted to the following persons: our families for consistent encouragement and support; representatives of the manufacturers of IV supplies and equipment for information and assistance; and Robin Carter, Jeanne Allison, Trish Tannian, Gail Hudson, and Ann Rogers at Mosby for guidance.

Joanne C. LaRocca
Shirley E. Otto

Contents

Infusion Guidelines

1

Objectives

1. List the factors that interfere with the delivery of accurate intravenous (IV) flow rates by gravity infusion and the measures that will promote accurate fluid delivery.

2. Identify nursing interventions shown to prevent IV therapy–related problems.

3. Describe safety considerations that reduce exposure to needle-stick injuries and exposure to patient body fluids during IV therapy.

4. Identify requirements for documentation of IV infusions.

IV therapy has seen dramatically increasing use because of improving catheter and pump technology and increasing numbers of patients receiving therapies. Administrators' desire to shorten inpatient hospital stays by placing patients who require IV therapy in outpatient settings has required nurses in all settings to expand their IV therapy skills. Technological improvements have moved complex therapies to outpatient settings, requiring astute management and specialized skills in home, clinic, and long-term care settings.

This chapter focuses on observations required when administering IV infusions and on supplies and equipment commonly required for delivering IV infusion therapy.

Accurate Flow Rates

Achieving accurate flow rates is always an important concern in IV therapy because accuracy decreases the incidence of complications. Complications may include infiltration, phlebitis, loss of patency, metabolic alterations, and circulatory overload. When gravity is the force for fluid delivery, a combination of factors causes fluctuations in flow rates. Time-taping fluid containers (Fig. 1-1), using flow control regulators and volumetric chambers, and selecting tubing

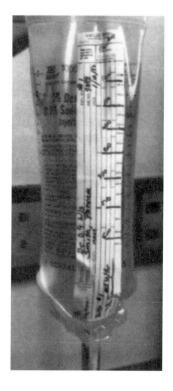

Fig. 1-1

Infusion bag with time strip.

From Perry AG, Potter PA: *Clinical nursing skills and techniques,* ed 3, St. Louis, 1994, Mosby.

with the appropriate drop size all aid in establishing accurate fluid delivery by gravity. IV pumps provide the greatest accuracy of fluid delivery.

Observations

Nursing observations required to maintain an accurate flow rate include determining whether any mechanical factors interfere with fluid delivery, evaluating patient factors that can alter the flow rate, and observing the patient for complications at the venipuncture site. The following mechanical factors may interfere with gravity flow rate:

1. Positioning the fluid container less than 36 inches above the IV site does not allow gravity to overcome vascular pressure and thus prevents the infusion of IV fluids.
2. Kinks in either IV tubing or catheter tubing do not allow fluids to flow.
3. Taping at the catheter site can obstruct the catheter lumen, particularly if a piece of tape is tightly placed directly over the bevel of the catheter.
4. Small-gauge catheters can slow fluid delivery and may require the use of a positive-pressure infusion device or replacement with a larger gauge catheter.
5. IV catheters placed near joints may occlude when the patient moves.

Patient factors such as the presence of tortuous veins and venous spasm can alter flow rates. Infiltration, phlebitis, and loss of patency may all occur at the IV site and terminate infusion.

Infusion System Evaluation

The following points should be confirmed during periodic evaluations of the entire infusion system:

1. IV is infusing at the prescribed rate.
2. All connections are intact.
3. The correct fluid is being infused.
4. IV tubing is placed correctly—not hooked on siderails or kinked.
5. The drop chamber contains the correct fluid level.
6. The IV catheter is securely taped.
7. The tubing is checked and its replacement is considered.

CLINICAL ALERT: Tubing needs to be changed according to the manufacturer's recommendations and in the following situations that reflect guidelines of the Centers for Disease Control and the Intravenous Nurses Society:

1. Routinely every 72 hours and when the IV catheter is changed
2. If the tip becomes contaminated from touch
3. If blood backs up in the tubing and is not immediately flushed out
4. Following piggyback administration of blood or lipid products

When the flow stops in tubing equipped with an in-line filter and no other cause can be found, the filter may need replacement.

Problems During IV Therapy

Most patients are able to assist with problems encountered during IV therapy if provided with the necessary information. Infiltration is the most common problem. Infiltration occurs when fluid infuses into tissue surrounding the venipuncture because the following occurs:

- The IV catheter passes through the wall of the vessel.
- The catheter slips out of the vein.
- The tip of the catheter remains in the vein, and the vessel wall allows some fluid to infuse into the vein and some to infiltrate the tissue.

When the catheter passes through the vein wall or slips completely out of the vein, a blood return does not occur. It is possible to obtain a blood return if the catheter tip remains in the vein. Swelling is due to fluid leakage into the tissue and is most likely to occur proximal to the insertion site. Leakage from the insertion site may be caused by puncturing the vein wall. A narrowing of the vessel wall may also cause a buildup of pressure in the vein, forcing the IV fluid out at the venipuncture site.

Common ways to assess for infiltration include asking patients about their level of discomfort, observing the site for swelling, checking for coolness of the tissues surrounding the IV site, and checking for a blood return. If the patient experiences pain, the IV should be restarted even if other symptoms are absent.

Early identification of problems reduces the severity of most adverse outcomes. The following list provides troubleshooting tips and preventive measures for common IV problems.

Nursing Assessment	Nursing Intervention
Infiltration Infusion slows or stops Infusion device sounds occlusion alarm Tissue induration or swelling with cool tissue	Relocate IV site to other arm or above area of infiltration; if infiltration is severe, apply warm compress and elevate the arm *Prevention:* Observe site hourly during continuous infusions, especially if using a positive-pressure pump
Phlebitis Two or more of the following present: pain, redness, swelling, induration, cord	Relocate catheter to other arm or above area of phlebitis; if infiltration is severe, apply warm compress *Prevention:* Filter solutions; rotate sites on a planned basis every 48 to 72 hours; secure catheter to prevent motion in vein; flush catheter after each medication
Runaway IV Dry IV or greater amount infused than scheduled	Notify physician and observe patient for signs of fluid overload and effects of IV additives *Prevention:* Recheck flow rate after tubing changes; time-tape all infusions; use electronic pumps, controllers, or volumetric chambers for patients at greatest risk of developing complications
Sluggish IV Amount to be infused behind schedule	Observe entire system for mechanical or patient factors, such as kinked tubing or patient lying on IV tubing; reposition or relocate IV device *Prevention:* Verify gauge of catheter is appropriate for type of infusion

Nursing Assessment	Nursing Intervention
Tubing disconnection Dampness from leaking fluid	Replace tubing if contamination occurs *Prevention:* Tape all connections or use locking devices for piggyback connections; use Luer-Lok connections for central venous catheters and other high-risk situations, such as for a human immuno-deficiency virus (HIV) sero-positive patient
Blood backup in tubing	Flush tubing with normal saline if blood backed up only briefly; change tubing if backup time is unknown *Prevention:* Place arm restraints below a venipuncture site; avoid dry IVs; keep fluid container 36 inches above site; teach patient not to raise arm above heart
IV line obstruction Resistance met when flushing attempted	Remove catheter or needle; do not force flush; relocate IV *Prevention:* Flush IV locks at least twice daily; in active children flush every 4 hours; change IV container before infusion runs dry

Systemic Complications of IV Infusions

Although the majority of IV-related problems are localized to the infusion system or the catheter site, the following systemic complications can occur: circulatory overload, air embolism, foreign-body embolism, and septicemia.

Circulatory overload

Symptoms: Dyspnea, cough, pitting edema in dependent areas, puffy eyelids, weight increase during the past 24 hours
Treatment: Decrease IV rate, elevate the patient's head, dangle the patient's feet if possible, check vital signs frequently, assess

breath sounds for presence of moist crackles, and contact the physician

Complications: Congestive heart failure and pulmonary edema

Possible cause: The patient has a history of compromised cardiac or renal condition, liver disease, or cerebral damage; an IV solution was inadvertently infused at a rapid rate; or the patient has received saline solution in excessive amounts, especially at night when renal function is normally reduced

Air embolism

Symptoms: Chest pain, shoulder pain, shortness of breath, cyanosis, low back pain, hypotension, weak pulse, loss of consciousness

Treatment: Immediately place the patient on left side in Trendelenburg position and contact the physician; stay with the patient, take vital signs, and consider oxygen administration; keep the IV site open

Complications: Shock and death

Possible cause: Inadvertent entry of air into the venous system, a greater problem with central lines than peripheral IVs; use Luer-Lok connections for all central lines

Foreign-body embolism

Symptoms: Same as for air embolism; this is a rare complication

Treatment: Immediately place the patient on left side in Trendelenburg position and contact the physician; take vital signs; apply tourniquet to extremity above the venipuncture site to confine embolus to the effected extremity; stay with the patient

Complications: Occlusion of blood flow to a body part; shock and death

Possible cause: Portion of the IV catheter was severed or another foreign body such as hair or a needle fragment inadvertently entered the IV catheter

Septicemia

Symptoms: Sudden or gradual rise in temperature, chills and shaking; increased pulse and respiratory rate, headache, nausea and vomiting, diarrhea

Treatment: Symptomatic as ordered by the physician. Save IV catheter, tubing, and solution for possible culture; if IV supply is suspect, follow steps for alerting manufacturer of need for a product recall; establish another IV site for administration of drugs

Complications: Septic shock and death

Possible cause: Contamination of IV product(s), break in aseptic technique, especially in immunocompromised patients

Common Infusion-Related Supplies and Equipment

Supplies and equipment commonly required for IV therapy include IV poles, labels for the infusion container and IV tubing, tape, armboards, administration sets, filters, and flow regulation devices. Each IV admixture needs a label listing the following information: patient's name and identification number; additives, strengths, and amounts; primary solution and total volume; flow rate; preparation and expiration dates; storage requirements (when applicable); and identification of the person preparing and hanging the infusion. Each tubing should also be labeled with information on the date and time hung and the initials of the person hanging the tubing.

Selecting an Administration Set

Because many options are available in IV tubings, the choice of IV set depends on the needs of the particular situation. Some important considerations follow.

Drop size

Drop chambers deliver either microdrops (60 drops/ml) or macrodrops (10 to 15 drops/ml). A macrodrop system should be selected when large quantities of solution or fast rates are required.

Vents

Vents permit air to enter the vacuum in the bottle and to displace the solution as it flows out. Unlike rigid glass containers, flexible IV containers do not require vents. The tubing that is appropriate for either the flexible or rigid IV container should be selected.

IV ports

Ports are required to administer secondary infusions and medications. Continuous-flow sets are designed with a back-check valve that allows a piggyback to run and the solution to begin infusing again after the piggyback is completed.

Volumetric chamber

Volumetric chamber IV sets are used to deliver small doses of medication or fluid over an extended period. They are used frequently with children and in intensive care settings to reduce the risk of infusing large amounts of fluids too rapidly.

IV Filter Considerations

Infusion-related phlebitis is a common occurrence and may result from particulates and microbes in the IV system or irritation caused by the IV catheter. IV filters are designed to remove particulates and microbes from IV infusions. However, filters are designed to complement IV therapy and not to replace aseptic technique.

Filtering may be done in a pharmacy area before delivery to the patient care area or with a filter attached to the IV tubing. Filter sizes range from 5 μm to 0.22 μm. The 0.45 μm filter may have an air-eliminating capacity, but like the 0.5 μm to 5 μm filters, it retains particulate matter. However, the 0.22 μm filter removes all particulate matter, fungi, and bacteria and is also air eliminating. The benefits of in-line filters and add-on filters have not been universally supported. However, no studies have contraindicated filter uses, and many strongly encourage it. Problems associated with filters include clogging that may slow or stop the flow rate when debris accumulates on the filter surface; drug binding to the surface of the filter that may occur with some drugs, such as insulin and amphotericin B; and unnecessary cost increases for basic IV systems when filters may not be indicated for short-term infusions.

Flow Control Devices

Flow rates can be regulated with clamps, accessory devices, and IV pumps and controllers.

Clamps

Every IV administration set has one or more clamps to regulate flow. Roller clamps adjust tubing diameter and restrict or increase the flow rate. A slide clamp either stops or starts IV flow and should not be used in conjunction with a roller clamp.

Accessory devices

Small accessory flow-regulation devices may be added to administration sets to control the drop rate more precisely than a roller clamp. Most of these devices depress a larger area of tubing than do roller clamps, although they are less precise than electronic pumps and controllers.

IV pumps and controllers

Electronic devices deliver fluids with the highest degree of accuracy. Their ability to sound an alarm when an occlusion occurs may assist with early identification of flow problems. A pump has the ability to add pressure to an infusion under conditions of restricted flow. Controllers do not add pressure to the line to overcome resistance. (Pumps and controllers are discussed more completely in Chapter 6.)

Infection Control Practices

Patient Protection

Patients may be exposed to IV-related infections in a variety of ways. Nosocomial infections are best prevented by ensuring that nurses wash their hands before making contact with any part of IV systems. Product and equipment contamination can occur during manufacture, storage, or therapy. If a break occurs in aseptic technique during the course of therapy, tubing should be changed immediately, because the patient is at risk of developing a systemic infection. Potential sources of patient infection are summarized in the following list.

Source of Contamination	Protective Measures
Manufacture or storage	Verify integrity of all packaging before use; discard a cracked bottle; check IV solutions against a light and a dark background for particulate matter; check expiration dates on packaging
Break in aseptic technique during therapy	Avoid touch contamination when spiking bags, priming tubing, or adding medications; change tubings if touch contamination occurs; *do not* reconnect disconnected equipment

Source of Contamination	Protective Measures
Blood in tubing	Flush IV immediately when blood backs up or change tubing if the time since backed up unknown; teach patients not to raise arm with IV above heart; *do not* use IV for routine blood drawing

Nurse Protection from IV-Related Infection

Needlestick injuries are a compelling issue for all nurses and are a special concern for nurses working with IV therapy. Despite an increased awareness of the dangers involved with handling sharps and the incorporation of universal blood and body precautions into practice, injuries involving needlesticks remain unacceptably frequent occurrences in health care settings.

Needlesticks can occur anytime a needle is used, particularly if a patient moves unexpectedly, or if a caregiver recaps needle. When starting an IV on active patients, one practitioner might accidently stick another.

Many believe that up to 80% of needlestick injuries can be prevented with improved product safety design. Ideally, devices should eliminate hazards without sacrificing efficiency or requiring special training. A wide variety of products that eliminate sharps exposure is available. Blunt needles and the substitution of plastic cannulas for needles reduce needlestick injuries. Some shield or recess needles are designed for use with IV piggyback medications.

Besides using new products, everyone working in patient care has a responsibility to reduce sharps use whenever possible. Seek non-needle alternatives for an IV procedure. Sometimes a traditional approach can eliminate or reduce needle use; e.g., the practitioner can connect IV tubing directly to the venous access device.

Other important needlestick prevention strategies include awareness and avoidance of unsafe practices such as recapping needles (responsible for about 25% of all needlestick injuries) and disposal of needles in containers that are not puncture resistant. In the event that a procedure is interrupted and a needle must be recapped, cover the needle using a scoop technique. Position the cap on its side on a table and scoop up the cap with the tip of the needle. When a rigid container is not available at the bedside, place

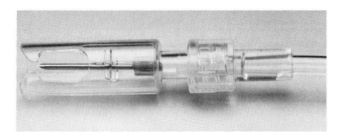

Protected needle.
Courtesy McGaw, Inc.

needles in a plastic cup or other small container for transporting to the rigid container. Finally, clean up after a procedure methodically. Account for all sharps that were brought into the area.

Documentation Recommendations
Records
Records are maintained to provide an accurate and easily retrievable account of patient care and treatment. Complete records are a principal means of communication among health care team members. Increasingly, records are used by insurers to justify supply and equipment costs, by review organizations to evaluate quality of care, and by courts for malpractice claims. Therefore, IV therapy must be accurately and completely documented. Efficient chart forms can facilitate complete, concise documentation. IV therapy easily lends itself to flow sheet documentation.

Documentation Elements of Infusion Therapy
- Date and time of tubing changes; list of all accessory tubings
- Date, time, and contents of IV fluids
- IV flow rate, including subsequent rate changes
- Electronic equipment used to regulate the flow
- Regular site assessments
- Presence of any complications and action taken to correct the problem
- Time IV therapy was discontinued, and whether the catheter was intact when removed
- Completion of patient teaching and demonstration of understanding through patient's repetition of action or information

Labeling IV Containers

In addition to documentation in the patient record, specific information needs to be placed on labels attached to the IV container. All IV containers should be labeled with the patient's name and identification number, the name of the IV solution, a list of additives (including dosage), the date and time hung, initials of the person hanging the infusion, and the expiration dat e or time of the infusion.

Nursing Diagnoses

- Infection, potential for, related to invasive procedure
- Injury, potential for, related to obstruction of catheter
- Skin integrity, impaired: actual
- Fluid volume excess: actual or potential
- Fluid volume deficit: actual or potential

Patient/Family Teaching for Self-Management

Patients need to know the purpose of their therapy, the approximate duration of the treatment, and any movement restrictions to observe during the course of the infusion. In addition, patients should be taught to recognize and report the early signs and symptoms of infiltration or phlebitis. With electronic infusion devices, the patient should be instructed to call the nurse when an alarm sounds. Teaching activities to encourage patient cooperation and participation in care include the following measures:

- Discuss the signs and symptoms of possible infiltration or phlebitis, such as swelling, pain, burning, soreness, redness, or a cool feeling at the insertion site.
- Teach the importance of reporting symptoms to the nurse.
- Discuss the importance of not readjusting the flow rate or bending or lying on the tubing.
- Show the patient how to avoid placing pressure on the venipuncture site when attempting to sit up in bed, pushing the IV pole, and positioning the arm with the IV catheter.
- Demonstrate how to wash the arm and hand in the area of the IV to ensure that the IV remains clean and dry.

Home Care Considerations

Before initiating an electrolyte infusion in the home setting, ensure that the patient is in stable condition. Recent (past 24-hour) serum electrolyte values are recommended.

Patients and family or other caregivers who will manage infusions at home require extensive information related to management of all IV supplies and equipment. Storage requirements, infusion preparation, disposal of supplies, and management of all electronic equipment must be thoroughly understood before the patient or family attempts self-management. Return demonstrations and written instructions, including pump manuals and troubleshooting guides, are needed for all aspects of care that the patient or family will be managing. Emergency phone numbers are crucial. In addition, patients and families need information on unusual findings that they need to report, such as adverse effects, phlebitis, and infiltration.

 ## Geriatric Considerations

Many elderly people have compromised cardiovascular and renal systems. It is important to closely regulate and monitor infusions so a rapid infusion does not cause fluid overload and become a precipitating factor in congestive heart failure or pulmonary edema.

Chapter Resources
IV THERAPY PATIENT INFORMATION
What is IV Therapy?

This information has been compiled to answer patients' commonly asked questions about IV therapy. It explains the IV procedure, why IV therapy is used, what a patient feels while receiving IV therapy, and precautions patients should observe to make their IV therapy go smoothly.

IV stands for *intravenous,* meaning inside the vein. For IV therapy, a catheter (a soft plastic tube about the size of a needle) or needle is inserted into a vein, usually in your hand or arm. The catheter or needle is attached to tubing and a fluid container that provides a way to give you medications and fluids.

How Long Will the IV Stay in?

Your IV therapy may last only a few hours or up to several days. Your physician decides the duration of IV therapy.

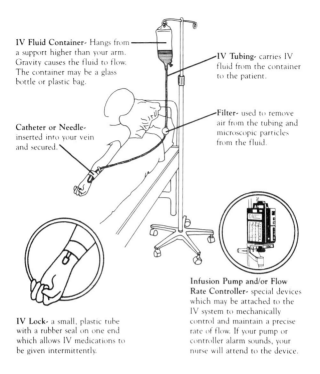

IV Fluid Container- Hangs from a support higher than your arm. Gravity causes the fluid to flow. The container may be a glass bottle or plastic bag.

IV Tubing- carries IV fluid from the container to the patient.

Catheter or Needle- inserted into your vein and secured.

Filter- used to remove air from the tubing and microscopic particles from the fluid.

IV Lock- a small, plastic tube with a rubber seal on one end which allows IV medications to be given intermittently.

Infusion Pump and/or Flow Rate Controller- special devices which may be attached to the IV system to mechanically control and maintain a precise rate of flow. If your pump or controller alarm sounds, your nurse will attend to the device.

Is IV Therapy Painful?

When the IV infusion is initiated, you will feel the insertion of the needle placing the catheter into your vein. As the IV solution enters your vein, it may sting for a few minutes, but the discomfort should stop in a short time.

If you feel any discomfort after the initial insertion, ask your nurse to check your IV site. Once the IV system is in place and secured, it should cause you minimal, if any, discomfort.

Is It Possible to Walk Around?

If you have permission to get out of bed, you may do so even while receiving IV therapy. If your IV is being regulated by a pump or controller, ask your nurse to unplug the instrument before you get up. It will be plugged in again when you return to bed.

While you are up and walking, push the pole slowly with your free arm while holding your arm with the catheter lower than the level of your heart. Keeping your IV arm lower than your heart prevents blood from backing up into the tubing and keeps the IV flowing at the correct rate. Never take the IV bag off the pole.

Is Bathing or Showering Allowed?

Depending on the type and location of your IV therapy, you may be allowed to shower or take a tub bath. Check with your nurse for permission or instructions regarding bathing or showering.

What Is Intermittent IV Therapy?

When continuous IV fluids are not needed, your IV catheter is disconnected from the IV tubing, and an IV lock is attached to it. The IV lock is a device that allows IV medications to be given as needed.

What Could the Patient Do to Help?

Observing the following precautions will help your IV procedure go smoothly:

- Promptly report to your nurse problems such as unusual swelling, redness, tenderness, or burning at the catheter site.
- Do not touch any of the clamps or controls on the IV tubing. Ask the nurse to make all adjustments.
- Do not remove the fluid container from the IV pole.
- Be careful not to pull on the IV tubing.
- Minimize your arm movements, particularly at the joints closest to the catheter site.
- Do not raise your arm too high; the catheter site must be below the IV fluid container for it to flow properly.
- Do not lie on your arm or any part of your body receiving the IV.
- Avoid lying on the tubing or letting it get tangled in the bed.
- Ask for help. Many tasks can be difficult with an IV. Your nurse will be glad to assist you.

What Happens After the IV Is Removed?

Immediately after your IV catheter is removed, pressure will be applied to the spot to seal the vein. After that, you may use your arm as you normally would.

If you have further questions about your IV therapy, ask your nurse or physician.

Infusion Therapy Audit

	Yes	No	N/A
The collection of data about the health status of a patient will be recorded and retrievable.			

Record Review

1. All IV solutions are sequentially recorded on the Infusion Record.
2. IV rates including rate changes are documented on the Infusion Record.
3. IV controller or pump use is documented at least every 24 hours according to agency policy.
4. Each shift documents a venipuncture site assessment on the Infusion Record.
5. Flushes are documented in conjunction with IV medication administration.
6. IV tubing changes are documented at least every 48 hours on the Infusion Record.

Patient Observation

1. IV solution hanging corresponds to the physician's order, information on Infusion Record, and patient care plan.
2. IV has a time strip marked in hourly increments (includes IVs regulated by controllers or pumps).
3. Time strip is initialed by the nurse hanging the bag.
4. The solution is being infused on time, within 30 minutes of schedule.
5. IV tubing is labeled with time of last tubing change.

Infusion Therapy Audit

	Yes	No	N/A
The patient's educational needs will be addressed.			
1. Patient has been instructed not to adjust flow rate of IV. "Did the nurses tell you not to make any adjustments to your IV?"			
2. Getting out of bed: "What have you been told about getting out of bed with your IV?"			
3. Controller/pump: "What have you been told to do if the alarm sounds?"			
4. Patient has been informed to report complications of IV therapy to the nurse. "What have you been told to report to your nurse?"			

SKILL CHECKLIST

Basic Procedures
1. Discontinues IV.
2. Labels bags and tubings according to policy.
3. Hangs new bags of solution after verifying order.
4. Correctly regulates hanging IV solution.
5. Changes IV tubing according to procedure.
6. Documents IV therapy on designated form: solution, rate, IV site status, tubing change, pump.
7. Flushes IV lock according to procedure.
8. Sets up IV pump: uses correct solution, primes tubing, adjusts rate, applies sensor.
9. Verifies correct IV pump setting when applicable.
10. Troubleshoots IV pump alarms.

 Study Questions

1. Select the intervention that may assist in improving the flow rate of an IV that is infused by gravity.

a. Position the IV bag so it is at least 36 inches above the patient's heart.
b. Restart the IV with a larger gauge IV catheter.
c. Retape the venipuncture site using sterile technique.
d. All of the above.

2. Which of the following statements best describes an infiltrated IV?
   a. The area around the IV catheter is inflamed and warm to touch.
   b. The IV is flowing sluggishly.
   c. There is tissue swelling and the surrounding tissue is cool to touch.
   d. There is a palpable cord along the vein.

3. When a nurse finds an IV is not flowing, the following is not suggested:
   a. Flush with normal saline in a tuberculin syringe.
   b. Remove the IV catheter, and relocate the IV site.
   c. Raise the height of the solution.
   d. Place the IV on a pump.

4. True or false: After an infiltration, the IV should be restarted below the area of infiltration.
   a. True
   b. False

5. True or false: Blood left in IV tubing can predispose the patient to an infection.
   a. True
   b. False

ANSWERS: 1. d   2. c   3. a   4. b   5. a

Venipuncture

2

Objectives

1. Discuss important aspects of patient preparation for insertion of an IV cannula.

2. Compare characteristics of veins and arteries.

3. Identify advantages and disadvantages of selecting each hand and arm vein for IV therapy.

4. Contrast characteristics of various venipuncture devices.

Venipuncture is a skill that is basic to IV therapy and can be learned and developed through frequent practice. Thorough understanding of both vein location and the venipuncture procedure increases confidence. Important elements of the procedure include patient preparation, vein selection, device selection, accurate insertion technique, knowledge of troubleshooting, and patient instruction.

Patient Preparation

Checking the patient's record for allergies and reviewing the physician's order and available laboratory results should be completed before approaching the patient. Supplies should be selected according to the purpose and duration of therapy and the patient's age and physical condition.

Patients who are unfamiliar with IV therapy may be frightened. When the patient is tense, the veins can constrict and make the venipuncture more painful and more difficult. Extreme anxiety can

be lessened by instructing the patient to inhale and exha
to avoid looking at the IV site, and to focus on a pleasan
These steps encourage patient cooperation:

1. Assume a confident attitude.
2. Greet the patient by name.
3. Introduce yourself.
4. Validate the patient's identification.
5. Explain the procedure in a way easily understood by the patient.
6. Ask for the patient's cooperation in holding his or her hand as still as possible.

Vein Selection

As a general rule, distal veins of the hands and arms should be used initially, and subsequent venipunctures should be proximal to previous sites. Arm veins are preferred for patients who do not have compromised vasculature. Veins commonly used for IV therapy include the basilic, cephalic, and metacarpal (Fig. 2-1). The extremity should be observed and palpated before a vein is chosen. Resiliency and location should be checked. An ideal vein is unused and relatively straight. The vessel should be verified as a vein and not an artery. The differences between veins and arteries include the following qualities:

Veins	Arteries
Dark-red blood	Bright-red blood
Slow blood return	Rapid, pulsating blood return
Valves at point of branching	No valves
Flow toward heart	Flow away from heart
Superficial location	Deep location surrounded by muscle
Multiple veins supply an area	Single artery supplies an area

Careful vein selection and assessment are crucial to a successful procedure. Observe the following guidelines for vein selection:

1. Use distal veins first.
2. Use the patient's nondominant arm if possible.
3. Choose a vein above areas of flexion.
4. Select a vein that is large enough to allow adequate blood flow around the catheter.

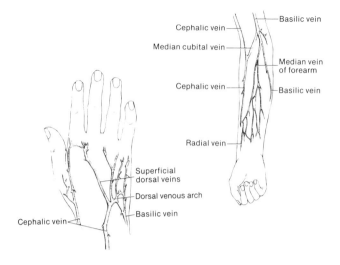

Fig. 2-1
Venous anatomy.
From Perry AG, Potter, PA: *Clinical nursing skills and techniques,* ed 3, St. Louis, 1994, Mosby.

5. Palpate the vein to determine its condition. Always choose soft, full, unobstructed veins when available.
6. Ensure that the site selected will not interfere with the patient's activities of daily living.
7. Select a site that will not interfere with planned surgery or procedures.

The following types of veins should be avoided if possible:

1. Previously used veins
2. Veins injured by infiltration or phlebitis
3. Sclerotic, hard veins
4. Veins of a surgically compromised limb, such as veins compromised by a mastectomy or placement of a dialysis access
5. Areas of flexion, including the antecubital fossa
6. Leg veins, because circulation is sluggish and complications are more frequent
7. Small, thin-walled branches of main arm veins
8. Affected extremity following a cerebral vascular accident

9. Bruised, red, swollen veins
10. Veins near infected area
11. Veins used for laboratory blood sampling

Advantages and Disadvantages of Hand and Arm Veins

Digital veins flow along the lateral aspect of the fingers and are joined to the dorsal veins by communicating branches.

Advantages: These may be the only veins available; they are easily secured with a padded tongue blade.

Disadvantages: They require small-gauge catheters, infiltrate easily, and are unsuitable for long-term therapy or infusion of irritating fluids and medications.

Superficial dorsal (metacarpal or hand) veins arise from the union of the digital veins.

Advantages: They permit arm movement and are easy to see and palpate; bones of hand splint catheter.

Disadvantages: Active patients may dislodge catheter; dressing becomes wet easily with handwashing; site will occlude if wrist restraint is applied.

Cephalic veins are located in the lower arm on the radial (thumb) side of the arm. They ascend along the outer region of the forearm into the antecubital region. Cephalic veins are smaller and usually curve more than basilic veins.

Advantages: The clinician may use a large-gauge catheter for rapid infusions; they are splinted by arm bones and are a good choice for infusion of irritating solutions.

Disadvantage: They curve more on the ascent up the arm than do the basilic veins; this is usually a disadvantage only when inserting long-line catheters.

Basilic veins are found on the ulnar side of the forearm, run up the posterior—or back—of the arm, and then curve toward the anterior surface, or antecubital region. They then ascend straight up the arm and enter the deep tissues.

Advantages: The advantages are the same as those of cephalic veins; usually basilic veins are straighter than cephalic veins.

Disadvantages: They may be prone to rolling; the patient may require awkward positioning of limb during venipuncture.

Median/antecubital veins arise from the veins of the forearm and commonly divide into two vessels: one that joins the basilic, and one that joins the cephalic. They are commonly used for blood sampling.

Advantages: They are easily accessed, large, and usually stable.
Disadvantages: They may limit patient arm movement and are
    often required for blood sampling.

Venipuncture Device Selection

Choosing the correct catheter is important to the outcome of
therapy. Steel butterfly needles are used in limited, short-term
situations. They are easy to insert but infiltrate easily. Improved
product design has resulted in many choices in short, peripheral
over-the-needle catheters (Fig. 2-2). Differences among the various
catheters include the following:

- Thickness of the catheter wall
  Effect: Rate of flow
- Sharpness of the insertion needle
  Effect: Slight alteration in insertion technique
- Softening properties of the catheter (Teflon does not soften;
  Vialon softens by a factor of 4; Aquavene softens by a factor
  of 50.)
  Effect: Catheter dwell time

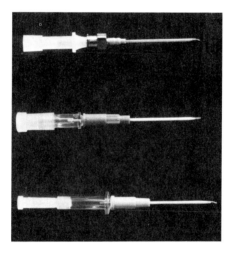

Fig. 2-2
Over-the-needle cannulas.
Courtesy Alton Ochsner Medical Foundation, New Orleans, LA.

- Safety design for prevention of needlestick injuries and blood contact
  Effect: Occupational safety (Fig. 2-3)
- Number of lumina available for simultaneous infusion of fluids
  Effect: Potentially incompatible fluids can be administered at the same time through the same peripheral line when a dual-lumen catheter is selected (Fig. 2-4)

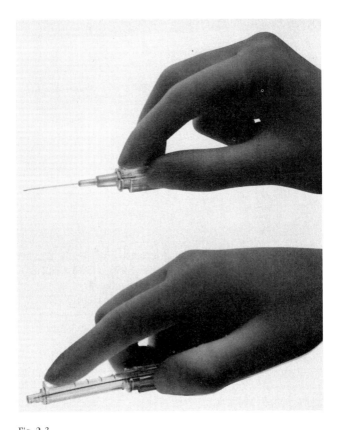

Fig. 2-3
Catheter safety system.
Courtesy Johnson & Johnson Medical Inc., Fort Worth, TX.

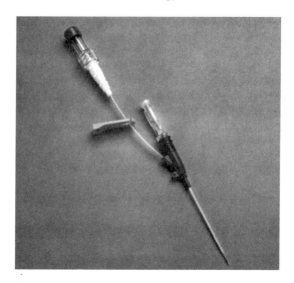

Fig. 2-4
Arrow dual-lumen catheter.
Courtesy Arrow International, Inc., Reading, PA.

Considerations when choosing a catheter include the size and condition of the vein selected, the viscosity of the fluid to be infused, the patient's age, and the expected length of therapy.

Consult the following list when selecting a catheter gauge:

1. 16 gauge—major surgery or trauma
2. 18 gauge—blood and blood products, administration of viscous medications
3. 20 gauge—most patient applications
4. 22 gauge—most patient applications, especially children and the elderly
5. 24 gauge—pediatric patients, neonates, and the elderly

CLINICAL ALERT: Choose the shortest catheter with the largest gauge (smallest bore) appropriate for the type and duration of the infusion. The larger the gauge number, the smaller the bore of the catheter.

Insertion Technique

Vein Location

To locate a suitable vein, find a comfortable position in a well-lighted area and apply a tourniquet 4 to 6 inches above the proposed site. The tourniquet should be tight enough to stop venous blood flow but not arterial flow. To encourage vein distention, ask the patient to clench and unclench the fist several times. When venous fill is difficult to achieve, placing the arm in a dependent position or applying warm packs may help alleviate the problem. The vein should then be stabilized by holding the skin taut, because stabilization of the vein before sticking is a key to atraumatic catheter insertion.

If the patient has a great amount of hair on the arm, clip the hair before venipuncture rather than shaving it, because shaving may nick the skin and create a potential site for infection. Check the refill capacity of the vein by running a finger along the vein. If the refill is sluggish, the vein will be prone to collapse. If a bifurcation exists below a desired site, enter the skin 2 to 3 cm below the bifurcation and proceed up into the main branch.

Catheter Insertion

1. Select the best available vein.
2. Clean the skin from the center outward with an approved solution (povidone-iodine, tincture of iodine, or 70% alcohol), and allow it to dry (Fig. 2-5).
3. Apply a flat, soft tourniquet 4 to 6 inches above the site.
4. Put on gloves.

Some people are extremely anxious about the pain of an IV insertion. For children, patients with a history of difficult IV starts, or those in whom some probing for vein location may be necessary, chances for a successful first needlestick can be improved if lidocaine cream ointment or an intradermal lidocaine wheal is used to numb the IV insertion site. Neither lidocaine ointment nor the lidocaine wheal can be used in patients who are allergic to lidocaine.

Use the following technique to create an intradermal lidocaine wheal through which the IV catheter may be inserted:

1. Hold a tuberculin syringe filled with 0.1 ml of 1% lidocaine bevel up at a 5 degree angle to the skin.
2. Insert only the bevel into the subcutaneous tissue.

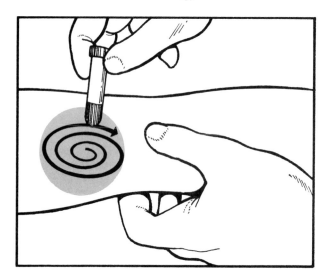

Fig. 2-5

Cleansing the venipuncture site. Wear gloves during this procedure.

3. Aspirate to be sure the needle is not in a vein.
4. Slowly inject the lidocaine solution.
5. Wait a few seconds for the lidocaine to take effect and insert the IV catheter through the wheal.
6. Anchor the vein; place your thumb over the vein to prevent movement and to stretch the skin taut against the direction of insertion.
7. Puncture the vein; hold the flash chamber of the catheter, not the hub. For a *direct approach,* place the needle bevel up at a 30- to 45-degree angle from the patient's skin (Fig. 2-6). Insert it in the direction of venous flow; and enter the vein. You may feel a "pop" and see a blood flashback. For an *indirect method,* enter the skin beside the vein and then direct the catheter to enter the side of the vein until you see a blood flashback.
8. Lower the needle until it is almost flush with the skin.
9. Advance the catheter into the vein an additional ¼ to ½ inch before removing the stylet; release skin tension, hold the stylet, and advance the catheter (Fig. 2-7).

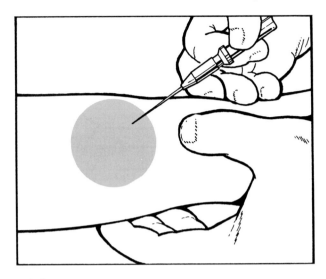

Fig. 2-6
Catheter insertion. Insert catheter bevel side up at 30 - to
45-degree angle in direction of blood flow. Wear gloves during
this procedure.

10. Release the tourniquet and remove the stylet.
11. Apply primed tubing or an intermittent injection cap.
12. Tape the IV catheter and tubing into place (Fig. 2-8).
13. Apply a sterile dressing.
14. Label the site (Fig. 2-9).

CLINICAL ALERT: When a stick is unsuccessful, use a new
catheter for a second attempt. Insert most catheters with one
continuous forward motion until the hub of the catheter is flush with
the patient's skin. If the catheter is not advanced to the hub,
dislodgment and infection occur more easily.

Securing and Taping Peripheral IV Sites

Procedures for securing a peripheral IV cannula vary among
agencies and institutions as well as among nurses. The basic
standards to be observed include the following:

   ▪ Secure the site so early signs of phlebitis or infiltration can be
     observed.

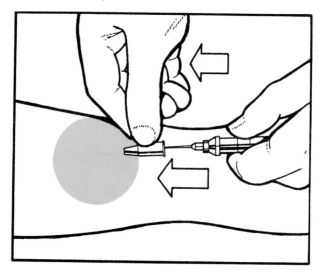

Fig. 2-7
Advance catheter until blood flashback is visible. Wear gloves during this procedure.

- Place tape above the catheter, neither directly over the catheter insertion site nor around the entire extremity; otherwise, blood flow may be impeded.
- Use a minimum amount of tape.
- Anchor the cannula hub to the skin to prevent movement of the catheter within the vein. Movement can cause mechanical phlebitis.
- Loop IV tubing close to the cannula to prevent kinking or pulling.
- Frequently check devices used to immobilize a hand or arm, such as splints and armboards, to ensure that the vein has not been constricted.
- Label the site completely (Fig. 2-9).

Patency

Patency of the IV site is indicated by blood return. One factor that may influence the rapidity of the blood return is the catheter gauge. In sites that have been in place, patency can be evaluated by observing for blood return in IV tubing when the solution is lowered

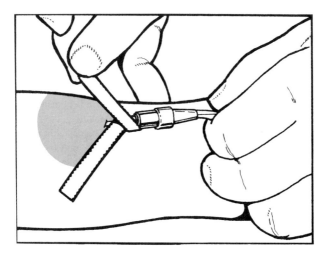

Fig. 2-8
Anchoring the catheter. Wear gloves during this procedure.

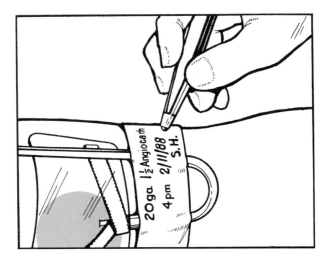

Fig. 2-9
Label insertion site with catheter gauge, date and time of insertion, and initials of person performing the procedure. Wear gloves during this procedure.

below the level of the IV site. Infiltration is indicated by coolness, pallor, and swelling at the site. Phlebitis is indicated by warmth and redness at the site.

Site Care

A sterile dressing is required at the peripheral IV cannula entrance site. The dressing should be changed whenever it becomes soiled, wet, or loose. Several types of dressings, including transparent dressings, sterile bandages, gauze, and tape, are acceptable as long as sterility is maintained. Povidone-iodine ointment may be applied to the IV site at the time of catheter insertion. Povidone-iodine and antibiotic ointments have not been shown to decrease infection, and they obscure site visualization.

Site Rotation

Venipuncture sites need to be changed on a planned basis to reduce the potential of phlebitis and infiltration. The frequency of site rotation depends on the catheter material. Catheters of Teflon or Vialon need to be changed every 48 to 72 hours. Aquavene catheters can remain in place for extended periods. A new site is always required if redness, tenderness, or infiltration occurs. If the device remains in place longer than 72 hours because of limited vein selection, the reason should be documented in the patient's record. A new site is chosen by moving up the patient's arm, or in a proximal direction.

Peripherally Inserted Central Venous Catheters

Peripherally inserted central venous catheters are available for insertion by nurses with advanced IV therapy skills as an alternative to physician-placed central venous catheters. These Silastic catheters may vary in length, gauge, and number of lumina. (See Chapter 4.)

Catheter maintenance

Refer to Chapter 3 for catheter procedures.

Venipuncture for Laboratory Sampling

Blood samples are most commonly drawn from an antecubital vein using vacuum collection devices. The antecubital is selected because the veins are large and have thicker walls than the veins that are lower in the arm and hand. When antecubital veins are not available, samples are drawn using a butterfly needle attached to a syringe, because the vacuum containers collapse the smaller veins.

CLINICAL ALERT: Draw blood samples from the arm without an IV whenever possible, since laboratory values may be altered by the IV fluids. If laboratory samples are drawn from the arm with an IV, stop the infusion for 1 to 2 minutes before drawing the blood sample.

Tips for Difficult Veins

With difficult veins, remember that systematic preparation is the key to a successful stick. The patient should be in a comfortable position with the arm lowered. Assume a confident attitude while reassuring the patient and urging him or her to relax.

Several techniques may increase the visibility of difficult-to-find veins:

- Wipe the skin with alcohol and tap it with fingers to make the vein more prominent.
- Place warm packs over the arm for several minutes.
- Transilluminate the vein with a fiberoptic light source.

Interventions to increase successful sticks in difficult situations follow.

Nursing Assessment	Nursing Intervention
Obese patient; unable to palpate or see veins	Create a visual image of the venous anatomy; select a longer catheter.
Fragile skin and veins; infiltration occurs after stick	Use minimal tourniquet pressure; if bounding pulse, do not use tourniquet.
Vein rolls with attempted stick	Anchor vein with thumb while sticking.
Patient in shock or has minimal venous return	Leave tourniquet on to promote venous distention; use 16- or 18-gauge catheter.

Infection Control Concerns
Patient Considerations

Infection at the venipuncture site is usually caused by a break in aseptic technique during the procedure. The following measures reduce patient risk:

1. Wash hands before starting an IV or working with the IV equipment.
2. Use an approved antiseptic to clean the patient's skin.
3. Clip hairs at the venipuncture site.
4. Do not reuse a catheter or needle.
5. Apply a sterile dressing to the site.

If an infection occurs at a venipuncture site, such as purulent drainage or cellulitis, the following care is required:

1. Culture the drainage before removing the catheter.
2. Remove the catheter by holding the hub to avoid touching the portion of the catheter under the skin.
3. Hold the catheter over a sterile container and use sterile scissors to cut the distal portion of the catheter so that it falls into a sterile container (Fig. 2-10).

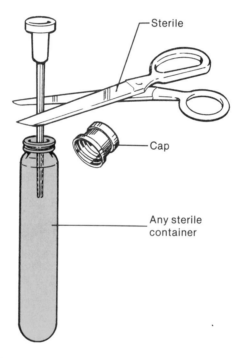

Fig. 2-10
Culturing the IV catheter.

4. Label the container and send it to the laboratory.
5. Restart the IV using all new supplies, including the tubing and solution.

Nurse Considerations

Both HIV and hepatitis virus are blood borne. When performing the venipuncture procedure, it is important for the nurse to adhere to the Centers for Disease Control (CDC) guidelines for invasive procedures. Recommended practices for nurses involved with IV therapy include the following:

1. Consider IV needles potentially infective. Do not recap needles after use. Have a puncture-resistant container at the bedside for disposal of used needles.
2. Wear gloves when inserting IV needles or handling tubings.
3. Wash hands thoroughly and immediately if they are accidentally contaminated with blood.

If a needlestick or a blood splash occurs, the nurse needs to be evaluated as soon as possible after exposure and periodically thereafter. Each professional needs to be acquainted with new information related to epidemiology, modes of transmission, and prevention of HIV and other blood-borne diseases. Further, the nurse should incorporate into daily practice universal precautions concerning blood, body fluid, and secretions.

Documentation Recommendations

Record the following information on the patient's dressing:

- Nurse's initials
- Date and time of procedure
- Catheter or needle gauge

Document the following information in the patient's record according to agency policy:

- Date and time of venipuncture
- Number of attempts required
- Site location
- Catheter gauge and length
- All IV supplies used
- IV fluids and flow rate, if infusion initiated
- Presence of any complications and actions taken to correct the problem
- Patient teaching and a reflection of understanding

Nursing Diagnoses

1. Skin integrity, impaired: potential related to catheter insertion
2. Infection, potential for, related to break in skin, contamination of supplies, or break in sterile technique at time of venipuncture
3. Anxiety related to invasive procedure
4. Altered comfort: pain associated with procedure or complications at insertion site

 ## Patient/Family Teaching for Self-Management

Patients who are receiving IV therapy need information that will enable them to protect their IV site and alert them to report complications to the nurse. Information should include the following:

1. Movement restrictions
2. Information to be reported
   a. Redness, swelling, or discomfort at site
   b. Blood in tubing
   c. Moisture on the dressing
   d. IV not infusing or infusion device alarms
3. Changing of the IV site (every 48 to 72 hours or immediately if complications occur)
4. How to bathe with the IV site

 ## Home Care Considerations

- Demonstrate catheter removal to the patient and caregiver in case it becomes accidentally dislodged.
- Instruct the patient in the frequency and technique of flushing the intermittent injection lock.
- Teach the patient to recognize signs of phlebitis and infiltration: presence of redness, induration, swelling, or pain. Inform the patient of the planned frequency of IV site rotation.

 ## Geriatric Considerations

- Arm muscles become less firm with aging. There is a loss of dermal skin thickness, which leads to paper-thin skin. Anchor catheters carefully to avoid tears and infiltration.
- Loss of subcutaneous fat makes tendons and veins prominent. Insert the catheter without a tourniquet if the skin is fragile and veins are visible and palpable.
- Vascular disease and dehydration may limit venous access.

Chapter Resources

Quality Assurance Monitoring—Universal Blood and Body Fluid Precautions to Minimize AIDS Transmission

	Yes	No	N/A
1. Gloves are worn for touching blood and body fluids, mucous membrane, or nonintact skin of all patients.			
2. Gloves are worn for handling items or surfaces soiled with blood or body fluids.			
3. Gloves are worn when staff member has a break in his or her skin.			
4. Gloves are *not worn* when item 1, 2, or 3 is not present or likely, such as when transporting patients.			
5. Gloves are worn for performing venipuncture and other vascular access procedures.			
6. Hands are washed immediately after gloves are removed.			
7. Hands or other skin surfaces are washed immediately and thoroughly if contaminated with blood or other body fluids.			
8. Used sharps, such as needles or scalpels, are placed in biohazard needle box.			
9. Needles are *not* purposely bent, broken, or recapped.			
10. Needle container is not overfilled.			
11. Disposable wastes and articles contaminated with blood or large amounts of body fluids are placed in impervious containers for a trash pickup.			
12. Spills of blood or body fluids are cleaned up with a 1 : 10 solution (prepared daily) of Clorox and water.			

Quality Assurance Monitoring—Universal Blood and Body Fluid
Precautions to Minimize AIDS Transmission–cont'd

	Yes	No	N/A
When the nurse is exposed to procedures that are likely to generate splashes or droplets, the following precautions should be implemented.			
1. Masks and protective eye wear are worn during procedures that are likely to generate droplets of blood or body fluid—for example, nasotracheal suctioning—to prevent exposure of mucous membrane.			
2. Gowns are worn during procedures that are likely to generate splashes of blood or other body fluids—for example, wound irrigation, patient bowel or bladder incontinence.			
3. Reusable items—for example, suction bottles and oxygen setups—are emptied with care to avoid splashing.			
4. All soiled linen is placed in laundry bag. Bag is *not* overfilled.			
5. Patients with diarrhea are treated the same regardless of presence or absence of AIDS.			
6. Patients who are coughing are treated the same regardless of presence or absence of AIDS.			

Venipuncture Audit

	Yes	No	N/A
1. Verify physician order.			
2. Check appropriate laboratory data.			
3. Check allergy data.			
4. Calculate flow rate.			
5. Choose and set up appropriate equipment: solution, set, venipuncture device.			
6. Wash hands.			
7. Correctly label IV with patient name, IV additives, rate of administration.			
8. Introduce self to patient.			
9. Assess patient identification.			
10. Explain procedure to patient and answer patient questions appropriately.			
11. Choose appropriate vein: location, size, condition.			
12. Apply tourniquet without occluding arterial flow.			
13. Cleanse area according to agency policy.			
14. Perform venipuncture according to accepted procedure using no more than two attempts.			
15. Attach tubing to IV cannula and establish flow of solution.			
16. Anchor needle and apply dressing to venipuncture site according to accepted procedure.			
17. Label venipuncture site with date, catheter gauge, catheter length, and nurse's initials.			
18. Set flow rate according to prescribed rate.			
19. Check for infiltration.			
20. Place IV pole on same side of bed as IV site.			
21. Record procedure in patient record according to agency policy.			

? Study Questions

1. When selecting a vein for an IV start, all the following are true except:
   a. Use proximal veins first.
   b. Avoid areas of flexion.
   c. Catheter size should be based upon size of vein.
   d. Blood flow around a catheter is an important consideration.

2. Which of the following is characteristic of veins:
   a. Blood flows away from the heart.
   b. A single vein supplies a given area.
   c. Blood return is rapid.
   d. Valves are present at points of branching.

3. All the following information should be documented on the IV site dressing except:
   a. Date and time of the procedure.
   b. Catheter gauge.
   c. Initials of nurse who started the IV.
   d. None of the above: The dressing is sterile.

4. True or false: Basilic veins are found on the ulnar side of the forearm and are the vein of choice in most adult IV applications.
   a. True
   b. False

5. True or false: Dorsal veins of the hand are the vein of choice in most adult IV applications.
   a. True
   b. False

ANSWERS: 1. a   2. d   3. d   4. a   5. b

Central Venous Catheters

3

Objectives

1. List the types and features for central venous access devices.

2. Describe the drug or solution administration procedures for central venous access devices.

3. Discuss the procedure for blood sampling from venous access devices.

4. Identify the major complications associated with central venous access devices.

5. List the patient and family education needs associated with daily, weekly, and monthly maintenance of central venous access devices.

Long-term venous access without repeated venipuncture is required for persons with certain medical conditions. Catheters, implantable ports, or both may be placed for continuous or intermittent infusions, simultaneous infusion of incompatible drugs, administration of viscous or high-volume fluids, blood products, blood sampling, short-or-long hyperalimentation, hemodialysis, central venous pressure monitoring, or high-flow administration in trauma or urgent situations. Central venous catheters are commonly used to administer fluids for hydration, chemotherapy, antimicrobials, analgesics, and parenteral nutrition in many varied settings such as acute care, ambulatory care, extended care, and home care.

In any such setting the nurse is a key member of the team responsible for drug or fluid administration and therapeutic monitoring of the catheter, port, and infusate, and of the patient. Nurses involved with the care of these catheters must be able to recognize complications and initiate appropriate interventions. Procedures for care and maintenance for the catheter and port may vary from agency to agency, and numerous central venous access devices are now available, posing additional challenges. Therefore, safe and prudent nursing care is necessary to ensure successful catheter use and longevity. (See Table 3-1 for types and characteristics of central venous catheters.)

Catheter and Implantable Port Composition

Catheters and implantable ports have become more versatile in their composition and design. The material selected to compose a catheter or port is often dependent on the type of the device and

Text continued on p. 49.

Table 3-1   Central venous catheters

Types of Catheters	Characteristics
Subclavian catheter: single and multilumen (dual-, triple-, or quadruple-lumen available)	Short-term use (less than 60 days)
	Polyurethane and Silastic material
	Added mechanical barrier available
	Vitacuff or Surecuff with antimicrobial activity, placed at or near insertion site
	Catheters with new antiseptic surface; for example, antimicrobial agents silver-sulfadiazine and chlorhexidine, both antimicrobial agents, reduce incidence of catheter-related infection
	Sutured in place
	Volume 0.5 to 0.6 ml/lumen
	Sterile dressing required for duration of catheter placement
	Allows simultaneous administration of potentially incompatible medication and fluids (applies to the multilumen catheter *only*)
	Requires heparinization of each lumen every 12 hours
	Can be repaired if damaged

Table 3-1   Central venous catheters—cont'd

Types of Catheters	Characteristics

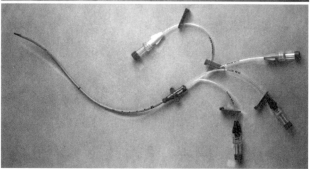

Multilumen subclavian catheters.
Courtesy Arrow International, Reading, PA

Types of Catheters	Characteristics
Tunneled catheters: single-, dual-, or triple-lumen, such as Hickman-Broviac catheters	Long-term use (1 to 2 years) Silastic material Subcutaneously tunneled in place Dacron cuff Volume 1.8 ml/lumen uncut adult catheter Sterile environment until exit site healed (usually 14–21 days); dressing optional Requires scheduled flushings with heparinized saline when not in use Repair kits available

Continued.

Table 3-1   Central venous catheters—cont'd

Types of Catheters	Characteristics

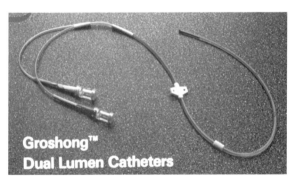

Hickman and Broviac catheters.
Courtesy Bard Access Systems Inc., Salt Lake City, UT

Central venous catheter with three-position valve and closed distal tip, such as Groshong catheter	Same as tunneled catheter except it requires scheduled flushings with normal saline when not in use NOTE: Always *vigorously* flush the Groshong catheter. Do *not* clamp catheter following flushing. Repair kits available

Groshong dual lumen catheter.
Courtesy Bard Access Systems Inc., Salt Lake City, UT

Table 3-1   Central venous catheters—cont'd

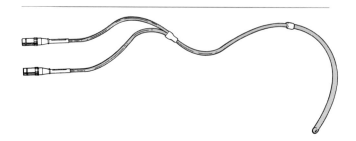

Implantable ports: venous placement single- and dual-lumen	Long term use (1 to 2 years) Metal (stainless steel or titanium) or plastic portal chamber with silicone septum connected to Silastic/Silicone catheter Self-sealing dense silicone septum allows up to 2000 punctures Portal chamber sutured and catheter tunneled in place Requires Huber needle in place for port access Volume 2 ml port and lumen (adult) Maintain sterile environment when port accessed; change Huber needle and extension at least every 5 to 7 days when port is accessed for continuous infusion therapy Port requires at least monthly heparinization

Continued.

insertion procedure for that catheter or port. Polyurethane is commonly used for short-term percutaneously placed catheters. It is a material stiff enough to allow for percutaneous insertion that then softens after insertion in response to body temperature. The softening makes the catheter more biocompatible once placed within the vein. Additionally, polyurethane has a tensile strength that permits the catheter to be constructed with thinner walls and smaller external diameters. This decreases the volume of foreign

Table 3-1   Central venous catheters—cont'd

Types of Catheters	Characteristics
Implantable ports: venous placement single- and dual-lumen—cont'd	Minimal self-care requirements Nurse and patient instructional material available from manufacturers Does not require a dressing when not in use

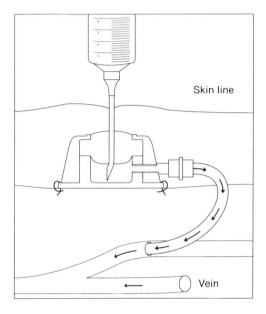

Cross-section of implantable port with needle access.
Courtesy SIMS Deltec, Inc., St. Paul, MN

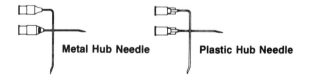

Huber needles.
Courtesy SIMS Deltec, Inc., St. Paul, MN

Table 3-1   Central venous catheters—cont'd

Types of Catheters	Characteristics

CLINICAL ALERT: The implantable port is also available for epidural, intraarterial, and intraperitoneal placement. Administer IV fluids only through the *venous* port. Use other sites only for infusions of medications or fluids specific to that placement site. Be sure to check the product information accompanying each port for instructions and use (Fig. 3-1).

Types of Catheters	Characteristics
Peripheral venous assess system: PAS Port (Fig. 3-2)	Long-term use (1 to 2 years) Titanium portal chamber with silicone system connects to Silastic catheter Self-sealing silicone septum allows up to 2000 punctures

Continued.

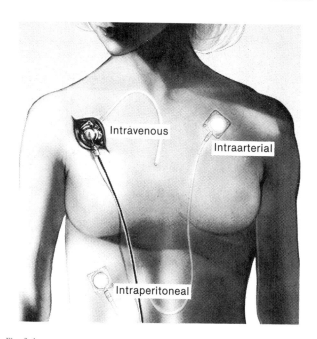

Fig. 3-1
Placement of IV, intra-arterial, and intraperitoneal ports.
Courtesy SIMS Deltec, Inc., St. Paul, MN

Table 3-1   Central venous catheters—cont'd

Types of Catheters	Characteristics
CathLink 20 (Fig. 3-3)	May be implanted in the chest or forearm
	System portal is usually implanted under the skin in the patient's forearm or in the chest. The catheter is inserted into the major arm veins until the tip is positioned in the superior vena cava. The catheter is then connected to the portal providing venous access.
	Use only 20- to 22-gauge ½ inch Huber needle to access PAS Port. CathLink may be accessed via over-the-needle IV catheter (minimum 20 gauge; 1¾ inch length) into the funnel-shaped entrance until resistance is felt; advance the catheter into CathLink 20 port while simultaneously withdrawing the needle.
	Volume 1-2 ml port and lumen (adult)
	Maintain sterile environment when port accessed
	Port requires at least monthly heparinization
	Minimal self-care requirements
	Nurse and patient instructional material available from manufacturer
	Does not require a dressing when not in use

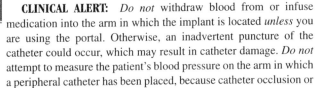

CLINICAL ALERT: *Do not* withdraw blood from or infuse medication into the arm in which the implant is located *unless* you are using the portal. Otherwise, an inadvertent puncture of the catheter could occur, which may result in catheter damage. *Do not* attempt to measure the patient's blood pressure on the arm in which a peripheral catheter has been placed, because catheter occlusion or other damage to the catheter could occur.

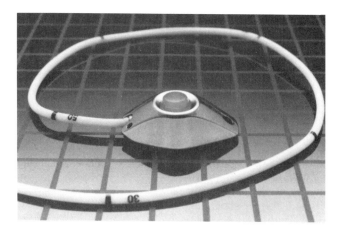

Fig. 3-2
Peripheral implantable venous access system port.
Courtesy SIMS Deltec, Inc., St. Paul, MN

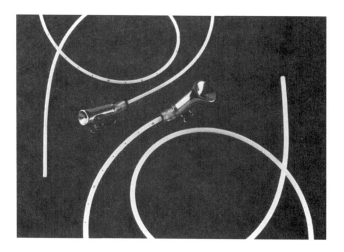

Fig. 3-3
Courtesy Bard Access Systems Inc., Salt Lake City, UT

material within the vein. A polyurethane catheter is now available (Arrowguard, Arrow International, Reading, PA) that has been bonded with colonization-resistant surface-treated antiseptic agents, silver sulfadiazine, and chlorhexidine along the entire indwelling length of the catheter. A recent randomized, comparative trial of 405 central venous catheters showed that antiseptic surface catheters were two-times less likely to be colonized and four times less likely to produce catheter-related bloodstream infection than were those in a control group of noncoated catheters.

The majority of tunneled central venous catheters and implantable port catheter lumens are constructed of Silastic or other silicone material. Other possible features are bonding of the anticoagulant agent heparin on the catheter lumen surface; a patented, three-position, pressure-sensitive Groshong valve located at the catheter tip; and a Dacron Cuff/SureCuff/VitaCuff/Vita Guard attached to a specific portion of the catheter and designed to provide protection against infections related to central venous catheters.

Implantable ports contain a reservoir that leads to the catheter and self-sealing silicone septum for access to the reservoir. The reservoirs may be composed of titanium, plastic, stainless steel, or a combination of these materials. The various ports differ in size and profile, single- or dual-lumen structure, place of implantation, and port access (Fig. 3-4). Most implantable ports have septums that lie perpendicular to the skin so that they may be accessed from the top with a Huber needle. The new CathLink implanted port has a patented funnel-shaped entrance for port access and uses a standard over-the-needle IV catheter (minimum length 1¾ inch).

Although the peripherally inserted and placed implanted ports have the advantage of a less traumatic implantation procedure than conventional chest-placed devices, they have limitations on blood sampling and blood product infusions.

Insertion

Catheter insertion is usually performed by a physician with the patient under local anesthesia. Sterile technique is maintained during the procedure. The catheter is inserted via percutaneous placement or a venous cutdown procedure. It is then threaded into the subclavian or jugular vein or the superior vena cava at or above the junction of the right atrium. A subcutaneous tunneling procedure or suturing of the catheter is used to secure catheter placement. Before administration of IV fluids or drugs, a catheter-

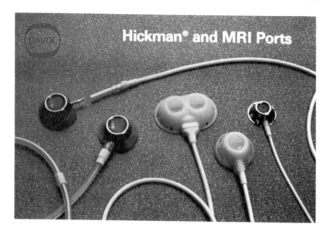

Fig. 3-4
Hickman and MRI ports.
Courtesy Bard Access Systems Inc., Salt Lake City, UT

imaging radiograph is recommended to confirm catheter placement.

For the CathLink, the system portal is usually implanted under the skin in the patient's forearm or chest. The catheter is inserted into the major arm veins or subclavian vein until the tip is positioned in the superior vena cava. The catheter is then connected to the portal providing venous access.

WARNING: System flushing recommendations are 10 ml normal saline after infusion of medication and 20 ml normal saline after infusion of blood, total parenteral nutrition (TPN), or known incompatible medications.

Hemodialysis and Apheresis Catheters

These catheters are specifically designed for prolonged vascular access for hemodialysis, hemoperfusion, or apheresis therapy via the jugular or subclavian vein. Occasionally these catheters are placed in the femoral vein. The catheters are composed of polyurethane, Silastic material, or a combination of both; may have a Dacron Cuff to facilitate tissue growth, and are inserted similar to the way venous access tunneled catheters are inserted. Hemodialysis/apheresis catheters are divided into two separate lumens by a septum allowing a blood exchange process (Fig. 3-5). The lumen gauges are usually 12 gauge to 14 gauge to allow for exceptional

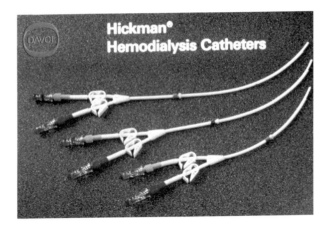

Fig. 3-5
Hickman hemodialysis catheters.
Courtesy Bard Access Systems Inc., Salt Lake City, UT

pressurized flow rates (300 to 400 ml/min) or high-volume viscous infusion/apheresis. Care and maintenance includes the following:

1. A directive that the catheter is *not* to be used for any purpose other than the prescribed therapy
2. Sterile technique for access and site care
3. Daily monitoring of the catheter integrity and exit site
4. Maintenance of catheter patency between therapies by the creation of a heparin lock in each lumen of the catheter.
   a. Inject 5000 units of heparin/ml into each lumen, *equal* to the priming volume of each lumen (e.g., arterial volume is 1.3 ml; venous volume is 1.4 ml).
   b. Ensure that each lumen is totally filled, then vigorously inject the flush solution and clamp the extension tubing while under positive pressure (e.g., maintain thumb on syringe plunger as you withdraw syringe/needle from the extension tubing).
   c. Attach a sterile injection cap to each clamping extension.

WARNING: The heparin solution must be aspirated out of both lumens *immediately* before use of the catheter to prevent systemic heparinization of the patient.

Critical Elements of Nursing Management of Central Venous Catheters

Aseptic Technique

Strict aseptic technique is required to maintain venous integrity and to prevent serious infection. A rubber-topped Luer-Lok cap is used to provide a sterile closed system when the catheter is not directly connected to IV tubing. This cap must fit securely to prevent any contamination or loss of blood. All tubing, needle junctions, or injection caps must be prepared with povidone-iodine before needle insertion to prevent introduction of microorganisms into the catheter.

Infection Control

Recommendations for nurse's protection against infection include disposing of needles or blood-contaminated caps and tubings into puncture-resistant containers; wearing gloves during catheter management procedures such as blood sampling; and washing hands thoroughly and immediately after accidental contamination with blood.

Catheter Maintenance Procedures

Catheter maintenance procedures may vary from one setting to another and according to each manufacturer's recommendations. Heparinization of central venous catheters varies in frequency, volume of solution, concentration of heparin dilution, type of device, and age and weight of the patient. Confirm with the physician managing the patient's care and the agency/institution for the nursing management protocol regarding heparinization of central venous catheters/implantable ports. Consider the patient with an alteration in coagulation factors or heparin allergy/intolerance with the frequency of the intermittent device use. Potentially these patients may require low concentration (e.g., 10 units heparin/ml) or alternative flushing solution (e.g., sodium citrate 1.4% solution). The specific protocol for each device should be consulted before use. Tables 3-2 and 3-3 summarize the recommended nursing management for central venous catheters for adults and children, respectively. The suggestions outlined thereafter are within the guidelines of each product's requirements.

Table 3-2 Adult central venous catheters: Recommended nursing management

Type	Heparinization	Dressing	Blood Sampling
Central Venous Catheters			
Short-term use			
Subclavian			
-Single lumen -Dual lumen -Triple lumen	After each use, flush *each* lumen with 5 ml normal saline (N/S), then heparinized saline 2 ml (100 u/ml). For catheter *NOT* in use, flush *each* lumen with heparinized saline 2 ml (100 u/ml) *every 12 hours.*	Daily sterile dressing change at the site for duration of catheter placement. Change Luer-Lok injection caps *every 72 hours.*	Shut off all IVs for *1 full minute.* Withdraw 5 ml blood. Discard. Withdraw blood sample. Flush lumen with 5 ml N/S, then heparinize or resume IV. *For TPN: Shut off IV for 10 minutes.*
Long-term use			
Tunneled catheters			
Single, dual, and triple lumens -Hickman -Quinton -Raaf	After each use, flush *each* lumen with 5 ml N/S, then heparinized saline 2 ml (100 u/ml) For catheter *NOT* in use, flush *each* lumen with heparinized saline 2 ml (100 u/ml) daily/ biweekly	Daily sterile dressing change at the exit site for initial 14–21 days. Thereafter, cleanse exit site daily (Betadine/alcohol). Apply clean dressing. Change Luer-Lok injection caps *weekly.*	Shut off IVs for *1 full minute.* Withdraw 5 ml blood. Discard. Withdraw blood sample. Flush lumen with 5 ml N/S, then heparinize or resume IV. *For TPN: Shut off IV for 10 minutes.*

Grosbong
-Single lumen
-Dual lumen
-Triple lumen

Does not require heparin to maintain* catheter patency. *Use force when flushing.* Flush *each* lumen with 5 ml N/S after each use—except for TPN, then flush with 30 ml N/S. For catheter *NOT* in use, flush with 5 ml N/S weekly.

Daily sterile dressing change at the exit site for initial 14–21 days. Thereafter, cleanse exit site daily (Betadine/alcohol). Apply clean dressing. Change Luer-Lok injection caps *weekly*.

Shut off all IVs for *1 full minute.* Withdraw 5 ml blood. Discard. Withdraw blood sample. Flush lumen with 30 ml N/S *vigorously*, then resume IV or apply injection cap. *For TPN: Shut off IV for 10 minutes.*

Implantable Vascular Access Devices

-Davol Port
-Infuse-A-Port
-Life Port
-Omega Port
-Port-A-Cath

After each use, flush *each* port with Huber needle— 10 ml N/S, followed by 3–10 ml heparinized saline (100 u/ml).*† For port *NOT* in use, flush *each* port within 3–10 ml heparinized saline (100 u/ml)* *every 30 days* (venous placement).‡

Sterile biooclusive dressing when port accessed. Sterile strips at new incision site for 3 days. When incision site healed and port not accessed, no dressing required. Change Huber needle access tubing every 5–7 days for continuous access of port.

Shut off all IVs for *1 full minute.* Withdraw 5 ml blood. Discard. Withdraw blood sample. Flush with 20 ml N/S, followed by 3–10 ml heparinized saline (100 u/ml)* or resume IV. *For TPN: Shut off IV for 10 minutes.*

Continued.

Table 3-2   Adult central venous catheters: Recommended nursing management—cont'd

Type	Heparinization	Dressing	Blood Sampling
Peripheral Inserted Catheter			
-Longline PICC§	After each use, flush lumen with 2 ml N/S, then heparinized saline 1 ml (100 u/ml). For catheter *NOT* in use, flush lumen with heparinized saline 1 ml (100 u/ml) every 12 hours.	Sterile dressing change after first 24 hours, then every 72 hours. Change Luer-Lok injection caps every 72 hours.	Shut off all IVs for *1 full minute*. Withdraw 2–3 ml blood. Discard. Withdraw blood sample. Flush lumen with 2–5 ml N/S; then heparinize or resume IV. *For TPN: Shut off IV for 10 minutes.*

*Selected oncologists use 2 ml to 5 ml heparinized saline (100 u/ml).

†Check manufacturer's specific recommendations regarding volume. Oncologists use heparin 10 ml (100 u/ml).

‡Assess patient, disease, platelet count with frequency/volume/concentration of heparinization schedule.

§Use 5 ml or larger syringes when flushing and/or blood sampling from PIC catheter.

Table 3-3   Pediatric central venous catheters: recommended nursing management

Type	Heparinization	Dressing	Blood Sampling
Central Venous Catheters			
Short-term use			
Subclavian			
-Single lumen -Multilumen	After each use, flush *each* lumen with 2 ml normal saline (N/S), followed by 1 ml heparinized saline solution, 10 u/ml, after each use or at least BID.	Daily sterile dressing change at site for duration of catheter placement. Gauze dressing change every 24 hours. Change Luer-Lok injection caps every 24 hours.	Shut off all IVs for *1 full minute.* Withdraw 3 ml blood and discard. Withdraw blood sample. Flush lumen with 2 ml N/S, then heparinize or resume IV. *For TPN: Shut off IV for 10 minutes.*
Long-term use			
Tunneled catheters			
-Broviac	After each use, flush the lumen with 2 ml N/S, then 1 ml heparinized saline (10 u/ml). For catheter *NOT* in use, flush the lumen with 1 ml heparinized saline (10 u/ml) daily.	Daily sterile dressing change at the exit site for initial 14 days. Gauze dressing change every 24 hours. Thereafter, cleanse exit site daily with Betadine. Apply sterile 2 × 2. Change Luer-Lok injection caps *weekly.*	Shut off all IVs for *1 full minute.* Withdraw 3 ml blood and discard. Withdraw blood sample. Flush lumen with 2 ml N/S, then heparinize or resume IV. *For TPN: Shut off IV for 10 minutes.*

Continued.

Table 3-3   Pediatric central venous catheters: recommended nursing management—cont'd

Type	Heparinization	Dressing	Blood Sampling
Implantable Vascular Access Devices			
-Port-a-Cath	After each use, flush the port with Huber needle—5 ml N/S followed by 2 cc heparinized saline (100 u/ml). For port *NOT* in use, flush port with 2 ml heparinized saline (100 u/ml) *every 30 days* (venous placement).	Sterile bioocclusive dressing when port accessed. Sterile strips at new incision site for 3 days. When incision site healed and port not accessed, no dressing is required. When port is accessed for continuous infusion, change needle and extension tubing every 5–7 days.	Shut off all IVs for *1 full minute.* Withdraw 3–5 ml blood (depending on size of child) and discard. Withdraw blood sample. Flush with 5 ml N/S, then heparinize or resume IV. *For TPN: Shut off IV for 10 minutes.*

Peripheral Inserted Catheter

-Longline PICC -Single lumen -Dual lumen (Use gentle pressure on syringe plunger for PIC catheters)	Use 3 to 5 ml or larger syringe. After each use, flush lumen: *Pediatrics*: 2 ml of normal saline in a 5 ml syringe or larger, followed by 1 ml heparinized saline (10 u/ml) after each use or at least BID. *Special Care Nursery (neonates)*: 0.5 ml normal saline/preservative free, in a 5 ml syringe or larger, followed by 0.5 ml heparinized saline (4 u/ml). Intermittent flush schedule every 4–8 hours—consult with physician orders.	Sterile dressing change after first 24 hours, then every 72 hours. Change Luer-Lok injection caps every 72 hours.	Shut off all IVs for *1 full minute*. Withdraw 1–2 ml blood and discard. Withdraw blood sample. Flush lumen with 2.5 ml N/S, then heparinize or resume IV. *For TPN: Shut off IV for 10 minutes.*

I. Site Care
   A. Site cleansing: All preparation solutions should be applied with friction, working outward from the insertion site. Typical products used: povidone-iodine with 3 swabs, 70% isopropyl alcohol with 3 swabs, hydrogen peroxide to remove crusting. Alternate products: chlorhexidine in place of povidone-iodine, application of ointment to site at discretion of physician.
   B. Change gauze dressing every 24 hours.
   C. Change biooclusive dressing every 3 to 5 days or more frequently to maintain an occlusive seal. Consider moisture permeability of dressing. Consider patient status (e.g., diaphoresis, secretions, immunocompromised).
   D. With all types of dressings, the dressing should be changed in conjunction with any extension set change. Dressings should be adapted to catheter location (e.g., jugular catheter site). Consideration should be given to the use of sterile gloves and mask when performing dressing changes, especially if the patient is immunocompromised.
   E. Coil tunneled catheter and tape securely to skin when catheter is not in use.
II. Cap change (depends on the frequency of catheter access)
   A. Change subclavian catheter every 3 to 5 days.
   B. Change tunneled catheter every 7 days.
   C. Change cap when rubber coring occurs.
   D. Change cap at dressing change or catheter flushing.
III. Needle and tubing change for implantable port
   A. Change sterile needle and tubing for each bolus access.
   B. Change sterile needle and tubing for continuous infusion every 5 to 7 days.
IV. Blood sampling
   A. To ensure a pure blood sample from multilumen catheters, turn off *all* IV fluids 1 full minute (TPN solutions, 10 minutes) before blood or fluid discard.
   B. Recommended discard for laboratory samples should equal 3 times the volume of each catheter lumen (range: 2 to 6 ml) for all the adult central venous catheters.
   C. Obtain laboratory sample via vacutainer or syringe.
   D. Flush catheter immediately with normal saline or heparin solution.
   E. Resume previous catheter function or heparin lock the

device. Note specifics on blood sampling for peripheral PAS port and CathLink.

V. Heparinization—The volume and concentration of the heparin solution and frequency of flushing remain a controversial issue in catheter patency management

A. Volume

1. It is accepted that the volume of the heparinized saline flush be equal to 2 times the volume capacity of the catheter lumen/implantable port.

2. Use between 1 and 2 ml per catheter/lumen (child) for tunneled catheter and implantable port.

3. Use approximately 2 ml per catheter/lumen (adult) for tunneled, subclavian catheters, and PICC lines.

4. Use approximately 5 ml for implantable port (adult).

5. The amount of heparin and the frequency of flush should be such that the patient's clotting factors are not altered. It is helpful to standardize the volume and concentrations used to flush the various central venous access devices to decrease confusion in trying to remember the flushing protocol for each device. See Appendix A for sample physician's orders for adult standard flush protocol orders.

B. Concentration of heparin (10–1000 units/ml)

1. Per physician discretion, normal saline or low-dose heparin (e.g., 10 u/ml) is indicated for a flush when intermittent medications are administered more than qid and a continuous infusion is not maintaining line patency. 1.4% sodium citrate solution is an alternative to heparin for heparin allergy or intolerance, heparin-induced thrombocytopenia, or patients with low platelet counts (e.g., 20,000/mm^3 or less).

2. Individualized adjustments in heparinization are indicated for pediatric patients who approach adult sizes (e.g., 50 kg).

C. Frequency

1. Subclavian catheters and PICC lines: every 12 to 24 hours

2. Tunneled catheters: daily to weekly

3. Implantable ports: monthly

D. To ensure a heparin lock, maintain a positive pressure (keep a forward motion on the syringe plunger as needle is removed from cap or port) while injecting the heparin solution into the catheter to prevent a backflow of blood into the catheter tip.

VI. Catheter repair—Most subclavian and tunneled catheters have specific repair kits that may be obtained from the manufacturer

A. Obtain the recommended repair kit specific to the lumen gauge of the catheter (Fig. 3-6).

B. Maintain a sterile environment during the catheter repair procedure.

C. Clamp the desired catheter lumen to be repaired before cutting or splicing the lumen.

D. Follow the manufacturer's guidelines for inserting the new lumen link or connector and repairing the catheter step by step.

1. Use of adhesive product
2. Cutting of the damaged catheter
3. Use of a splicing device
4. Use of suture material
5. Use of protective splice material
6. Splinting and stabilization of the catheter repair section
7. Limitations on catheter use after repair

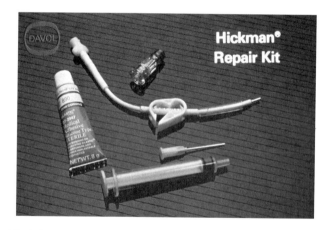

Fig. 3-6
Hickman repair kit.
Courtesy Bard Access Systems Inc., Salt Lake City, UT

   E. Use caution when cementing the new catheter lumen
      connector; for example, avoid getting the cement inside the
      catheter lumen.
   F. Flush the repaired catheter lumen with heparinized saline
      solution per physician request.
   G. Some tunneled catheter repair kits have restrictions limiting
      use of repaired catheter lumen for 4 to 8 hours after catheter
      repair.
   H. Document the catheter repair procedure results in the
      patient's medical record.

Accessing an Implantable Port

Because the port is located beneath the skin surface, the boundaries
specific to each device and the resilience of the silicone septum
need to be known before needle access. This procedure requires
aseptic technique using sterile supplies.

   1. Wash hands and apply gloves.
   2. Cleanse portal site with povidone-iodine swabs, starting over
      the portal and moving outward in a spiral motion to cover an
      area 5 inches in diameter.
   3. Attach tubing with a Huber needle to a syringe filled with
      saline.
   4. Locate the portal septum by palpation (Fig. 3-7).

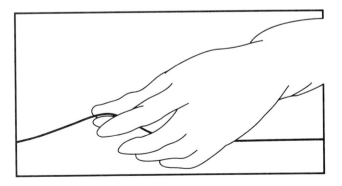

Fig. 3-7
Palpating the implantable port.
Courtesy SIMS Deltec, Inc., St. Paul, MN

5. Insert the needle perpendicular to the septum and push it slowly but firmly through the skin and portal septum until it comes to rest at the bottom of the portal chamber.

6. Aspirate for a blood return; flush the system with normal saline to confirm that fluid flows through the system.

   a. Note any unusual resistance to flow or any swelling around the injection site. Either may be a sign of insufficient needle penetration, incorrect needle placement, catheter blockage, or a leaking portal system, catheter, or connection.

   b. For bolus injection of medication, remove the empty saline syringe, replace it with the drug-filled syringe, and administer the injection. At the completion of the injection, flush the catheter with normal saline and then heparin lock the device while withdrawing the needle from the portal septum (Fig. 3-8).

   c. For a continuous infusion, remove the empty saline syringe, replace it with IV infusion tubing, and secure the tubing. Because the Huber needle remains in the portal chamber during the infusion, secure the needle to prevent inadvertent dislodgment by placing a 2×2 gauze dressing underneath the needle and applying antibacterial ointment around the needle site. Finally, apply a semipermeable occlusive dressing over the entire area. Secure extension tubing to minimize needle dislodgment (Fig. 3-9).

 CLINICAL ALERT: Use the Huber needle at a 90-degree bend for continuous infusion. Use only a 20 - to 22-gauge ½-inch 90-degree bend needle to access the PAS Port system peripherally inserted ports.

 ## Documentation Recommendations

- Daily assessment of port or exit site, skin or catheter integrity, and catheter placement
- Procedure access for each catheter or device
- Heparinization or normal saline flush—drug, concentration, dose, volume, date, and time
- Injection cap or extension tubing changes
- Site care management
- Patency of catheter, blood sampling, and infusion of medications or fluids

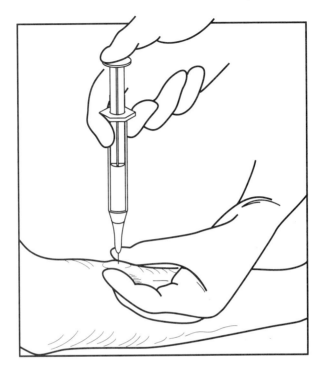

Fig. 3-8
Bolus injection into implantable port.
Courtesy SIMS Deltec, Inc., St. Paul, MN

- Patient symptoms related to catheter malfunction or potential complications associated with central venous catheter
- Patient and family education regarding understanding (verbalized or return demonstration) of catheter self-care management

Nursing Diagnoses

- Skin integrity, impaired: potential related to erosion of skin at exit site or frequent implantable port access
- Injury, potential for, related to venous obstruction, catheter dislodgment, catheter migration, or catheter occlusion

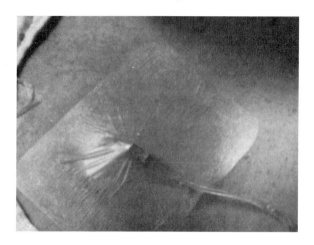

Fig. 3-9
Continuous infusion with implantable port.
From Perry AG, Potter PA: *Clinical nursing skills and techniques*, ed 3,
St. Louis, 1994, Mosby.

- Infection, potential for, related to contamination of supplies, break in sterile technique when managing catheter, performing site care, accessing catheter, or changing dressings
- Knowledge deficit regarding ongoing self-management of catheter
- Self-concept, disturbance: body image, related to placement of venous access device

 ## Patient/Family Teaching for Self-Management

- Assess the patient's ability and willingness to learn, availability of caregiver, home environment, and previous experience or expectations.
- Describe purpose and function of the catheter or device. (See Chapter Resources for patient information on caring for the venous access device.)
- Instruct the patient regarding preoperative and postoperative procedures.
- Explain self-care management issues: Completing site care, changing injection cap, and flushing catheter with heparin

Table 3-4   Troubleshooting tips—central venous catheters

Nursing Assessment	Nursing Interventions
Deeply Implanted Port Unable to palpate port	Note portal chamber scar Use deep palpation technique or seek assistance of second person to locate port
Do not feel needle stop against portal chamber	Use 1½- or 2-inch Huber needle
Unable to Obtain Blood Return	Try to change catheter alignment by raising the patient's arm on same side as catheter Roll the patient to opposite side Ask the patient to cough, sit up, take a deep breath Try infusing 10 ml of normal saline into catheter Reaccess catheter or implantable port with new sterile needle
Unable to Inject Fluid or Medication	Follow steps to obtain blood return If unable to inject fluid or obtain blood return, notify the physician Catheter placement should be determined by radiographic examination

solution or normal saline require demonstration with return demonstration to facilitate learning and integration of necessary skills.

- Review symptoms related to each potential complication with emergency self-management techniques and reporting of that information immediately to the physician.
- Reinforce the troubleshooting tips related to potential catheter malfunctions with appropriate intervention strategies.
- Provide information on obtaining, storing, and disposing of supplies and availability of 24-hour hotline for problems.

Table 3-5   Potential complications—central venous catheters

Nursing Assessments	Nursing Interventions
Air Embolus	Clamp central line
May occur during connections or disconnections of syringes and IV tubing	Instruct the patient to lie on left side with head down; Trendelenburg position
	Notify the physician
Sudden onset of symptoms	Monitor vital signs
Chest pain	Remain with the patient
Cyanosis, anxiety	Administer O_2
Increased pulse and respirations	Initiate peripheral IV
Decreased blood pressure	
Catheter Dislodgment	Note presence or absence of suture in securing subclavian catheter or Dacron cuff protruding from exit site of tunneled catheter
Medication or fluid leaking from catheter or exit site	
	Report finding to physician
	Secure catheter and extension tubing with tape
Catheter Migration	Notify physician to determine catheter placement
Unable to inject fluid or medication	
Catheter Occlusion	Gently flush catheter with appropriate normal saline flush
Unble to inject fluid or medication	*Do not use force* (catheter may rupture)
	Notify the physician; there is a potential need for injection of fibrinolytic agent
	Inject urokinase 1 ml (5000 units/ml) into catheter port using a 5-ml syringe

Table 3-5   Potential complications—central venous
catheters—cont'd

Nursing Assessments	Nursing Interventions
	After 10 minutes, try to aspirate the clot
	If necessary, repeat aspiration at 5-minute intervals for 30 minutes
	Declotting procedure may be repeated using two doses of the fibrinolytic agent; wait 1 hour between procedures
	Hydrochloric acid (HCl) has been used to restore catheter patency of catheters obstructed by drug precipitate including etoposide, calcium salts plus sodium bicarbonate, parenteral nutrition solution, or heparin plus an incompatible antibiotic (amikacin or vancomycin). Instill 0.2 to 1 ml of solution (0.1 molar HCl) into obstructed catheter. One to several hours may be required to restore total patency. HCl is proposed to work by lowering pH, which increases the solubility of these agents
	Upon establishing catheter patency, withdraw 5 ml of fluid and discard before flushing catheter lumen with normal saline; resume previous catheter function or heparin lock the device

Continued.

Table 3-5   Potential complications—central venous catheters—cont'd

Nursing Assessments	Nursing Interventions
	For TPN and lipid solutions, if urokinase does not clear the blockage, an ethanol 70% solution may be instilled and left in place for 1 hour. Follow procedure for urokinase instillation. This may help to clear the catheter of lipid material deposition.
Catheter Sepsis	Culture catheter exit site, port site, and tension tubing, and obtain a blood sample from peripheral site
Inflamed, reddened, painful catheter exit or port site	
Purulent exudate	Notify physician
Elevated temperature, chills	Administer appropriate prescribed antibiotics
May or may not be able to aspirate or infuse	*Do not access* an inflamed port site
Catheter/Port Drug Extravasation	
Possible causes:	
Catheter misplaced out of vessel into soft tissue	
Catheter has rupture secondary to vigorous flushing	
Implantable port—Huber needle dislodged from port septum because of anatomical location, excess adipose tissue, or movement or activity of patient	
"Pinch-off sign"—compression of catheter between clavicle and first rib	
Thrombus or fibrin sheath formed at the distal end of the catheter	

Table 3-5   Potential complications—central venous
catheters—cont'd

Nursing Assessments	Nursing Interventions

Symptoms:
  Stinging/burning pain and swelling along catheter site infusion
  Redness
  Warmth
  Leaking of fluid at catheter exit site or at Huber needle insertion site
	Stop the infusion
	Do not use the catheter/implantable port
	Notify the physician
	Determine the cause of extravasation
	May need a chest x-ray or venogram to determine catheter placement
	Remove a ruptured catheter

Fibrin Sheath
  Partial or total occlusion at the tip of the catheter form platelet aggregation and fibrin deposition; results in a one-way valve effect and diminishes withdrawal of blood from the catheter
  Symptoms:
    Retrograde flow of infusate back up the length of the catheter
    Ability to infuse fluids but not aspirate (partial occlusion)
    Reverse ball effect: fibrin or precipitate deposits accumulate within the port reservoir around the port/catheter outlet—aspiration is possible but on attempt to flush the catheter, the obstruction lodges against the port/catheter outlet, totally occluding the flow
	Notify physician—potential for administration of lytic agent (urokinase) or prophylactic oral anticoagulant; radiograph of catheter for position, tip location, catheter integrity, and thrombosis formation; change in catheter flushing solution or frequency

Continued.

Table 3-5   Potential complications—central venous catheters—cont'd

Nursing Assessments	Nursing Interventions
Superior Vena Cava Syndrome Potential causes: mediastinal tumor growth (lung, breast, esophageal, head and neck, and lymphoma) or growth secondary to central venous access placement Symptoms: progressive upper extremity, neck, and facial edema with dilation of the superficial veins of the chest, neck, and arms	*Stop* the infusion *Do not* use the catheter/ implantable port Notify the physician Monitor the patient Initiate oxygen per nasal cannula Administer treatment as ordered for fibrinolytics, anticoagulants May require immediate treatment for tumor (chemotherapy/radiation therapy)

Vessel Thrombosis
May be related to diameter of catheter in relation to patient's vessel size
Symptoms:
    Edema and tenderness of neck, shoulder, and arm on the same side of the catheter
    Shortness of breath, cough, cyanosis of face and upper extremities
	Notify the physician to determine catheter placement via radiograph

Home Care Considerations

- Keep supplies and equipment used for catheter management in a secure place.
- Schedule daily or intermittent catheter flushings at the same time every day to coincide with the patient's activities of daily living.
- Reinforce to the patient or caregiver to report abnormal findings immediately to the physician, such as elevated temperature, inflamed port or exit site, catheter malfunction, and unusual discomfort related to catheter.

- Discard all supplies used for catheter care into a puncture-resistant container such as an empty coffee can in preparation for garbage pickup.

Geriatric Considerations

Consider neuromuscular and sensory deficits that may be present, such as visual and hearing losses and arthritic joints. Plan individualized self-care teaching of catheter maintenance. Printed materials may require large print for reading ease. Return demonstration techniques may require more simplistic steps to facilitate ease in use of the supplies. Assess ability of patient and caregiver and determine if additional resources, such as a home-care agency, are needed to provide self-care catheter maintenance.

Chapter Resources
CARING FOR YOUR VENOUS ACCESS DEVICE
What Is a Venous Access Device?

Your physician has recommended a *venous access device* because your treatment requires frequent administration of intravenous fluids, drugs, and blood products or blood samples need to be taken frequently.

These medications or fluids can be delivered directly into the bloodstream by inserting one end of a *catheter* (thin tube) or accessing a *port* into a large vein or artery. The other end of the catheter or port extends from a small incision in the skin. Drugs or fluids can then be injected, via a needle or tubing, through the external end of the catheter/port.

Where is the Venous Access Device Placed?

Your physician will insert the device while you are under a local or general anesthetic. The following illustration shows some of the most common locations for catheter and port placement.

What Does a Venous Access Device Look Like?

Following are pictures of some common venous access devices. Your physician has selected the device that is most appropriate for you.

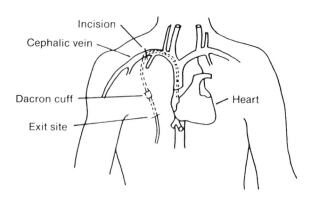

MULTILUMEN SUBCLAVIAN CATHETER
Patient Information
This catheter is composed of pliable polyurethane material and allows easy access to your vascular system (bloodstream). Because of its unique design (three separate ports), more than one medication or IV fluid can be given at one time. The catheter is used for short-term situations (usually 2 to 8 weeks) to give medication or to take blood samples. It is inserted by a physician using sterile technique while you are under a local anesthetic. Catheter placement is usually checked by getting a radiograph at the end of the procedure. The catheter is held in place by sutures securing the small wing-tip device next to the skin. It is important to keep this area free of germs.

GROSHONG CATHETER
Patient Information
This catheter is composed of a transparent silicone rubber material and allows easy access to your vascular system (bloodstream). Because of its unique design (a patented two-way slit valve next to a rounded, closed tip), it requires minimal catheter care. The catheter may have a single, double, or triple lumen and is usually in place months to 2 years. It is inserted by a physician using sterile technique and a local anesthetic. Catheter placement is usually checked by getting a radiograph at the end of the procedure. A Dacron fiber cuff is placed below the skin to hold the catheter in place and to prevent infection.

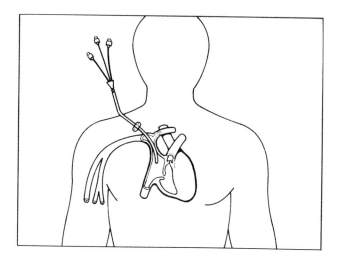

Multilumen subclavian catheter.

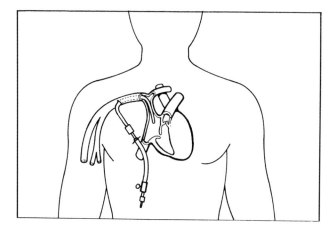

Groshong catheter.

TUNNELED CATHETER
Patient Information
The tunneled catheter, or Hickman catheter, is a flexible silicone tube that gives easy access to your vascular system (bloodstream). The catheter can be used to draw blood for laboratory samples or to give chemotherapeutic drugs and other medications, IV fluids, blood or blood components, and nutritional support. The catheter is inserted using a local anesthetic—you cannot feel it inside your body. With the aid of a radiograph fluoroscope, the catheter is placed into your upper chest and directed to the upper right chamber (right atrium) of your heart. After insertion, the catheter is sutured into place. A Dacron fiber cuff is placed below the skin to hold

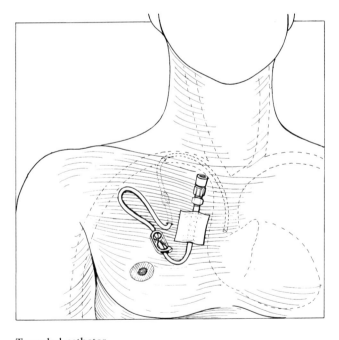

Tunneled catheter.
Pharmacia Deltec, St. Paul, MN

the catheter in place and to prevent infection. When you no longer need the catheter, it can be removed by your physician or nurse.

IMPLANTABLE VENOUS ACCESS DEVICES (PORTS)
Patient Information

An implantable venous access device (port) has two major parts: a catheter and a small chamber, called a portal. In the center of the portal is a self-sealing silicone septum. Some implantable venous access devices have more than one portal, making it possible for more than one medication or fluid to be given through the system at the same time.

An implantable venous access device is placed by a doctor, usually in a hospital or outpatient operating room. An anesthetic is used at the insertion site to make the area numb during the placement procedure.

The catheter is put through the skin and into a vein in the chest. The tip of the catheter is threaded through the vein to a point just above the heart. The other end of the catheter is tunneled under the skin for a short distance. An incision is made and the portal is placed

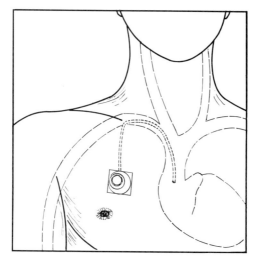

Placement of an implantable venous access device.

under the skin. The catheter is then attached to the portal. After the incision is closed, the entire device is under the skin.

PERIPHERALLY PLACED IMPLANTABLE VENOUS ACCESS DEVICES (PERIPHERAL PORTS)
Patient Information

A peripherally placed implantable venous access device has two major parts: a catheter and a very small chamber, called a portal. In the center of the portal is a self-sealing silicone septum.

A peripherally placed implantable venous access device is placed by a doctor, usually in an outpatient operating room. An anesthetic is used at the insertion site to make the area numb during the placement procedure.

The catheter is put into a vein in the lower arm. The tip of the catheter is threaded through the vein to a point just above the heart. The other end of the catheter is tunneled under the skin for a short distance. An incision is made and the portal is placed under the skin. The catheter is then attached to the portal. After the incision is closed, the entire device is under the skin.

PERIPHERALLY INSERTED CENTRAL VENOUS CATHETERS (PICC LINES)
Patient Information

A peripherally inserted central venous catheter is a very small, flexible, hollow tube with an injection cap on one end.

This catheter can be placed by a doctor or a specially trained nurse at the bedside, in the office, or in the home. An anesthetic is used at the insertion site to make the area numb during the placement procedure.

The catheter is put through the skin into a vein in the lower arm. The tip of the catheter is threaded up through the vein. The other end of the catheter comes out through a small opening on the lower arm.

CARE OF THE VENOUS ACCESS DEVICE
Flushing the Catheter or Port

Flushing the catheter helps keep the catheter clean and prevents it from becoming blocked.

Your catheter should be flushed every _____ hours/days with _____ solution.

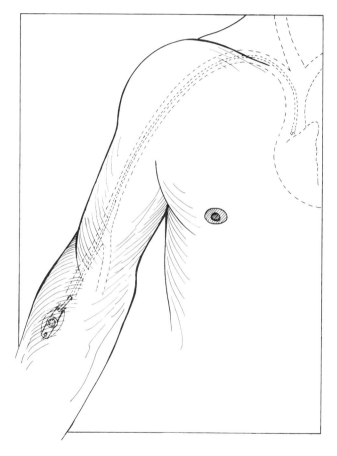

Placement of a peripherally inserted implantable venous access device.
Pharmacia Deltec, St. Paul, MN

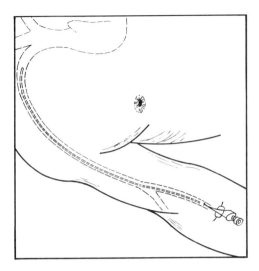

Placement of a peripherally inserted central venous catheter.

What You Need

- 0.9% normal saline
- Heparin tubex, 2 ml (100 u/ml)
- Heparin syringe holder
- Alcohol swabs
- Povidone-iodine wipes
- 20-gauge × 1-inch sterile needles
- 5- or 10-cc sterile syringes
- Tape
- Puncture-proof container (for disposal of used needles and syringes)

What To Do

1. Wash your hands for 10 seconds using warm, soapy water, then rinse.
2. Dry your hands on a clean towel.
3. Prepare heparin and/or normal saline syringe.
4. Cleanse the catheter cap with povidone-iodine, then alcohol.
5. Inject heparin or normal saline into catheter cap.

6. Withdraw the needle, continuing to press down on the plunger with your thumb.
7. Discard the syringe and needle in the puncture-proof container.
8. Wash your hands for 10 seconds using warm, soapy water, then rinse.
9. Dry your hands on a clean towel.

CARE OF THE "EXIT SITE"
Dressing Change

The dressing at the exit site needs to be changed regularly to avoid infection and allow you to inspect the catheter exit site. Your dressing change should be done according to the schedule ordered by your physician or nurse.

Your dressing should be changed _____ times a day/week.

What You Need

- Bag for disposal of used items
- Alcohol swabs
- Povidone-iodine swabs
- Povidone-iodine ointment
- Hydrogen peroxide
- Sterile cotton-tipped swabs
- Sterile gauze dressing
- Sterile transparent dressing
- Sterile tape
- Sterile disposable gloves

Changing the Dressing

1. Wash your hands for 10 seconds using warm, soapy water, and rinse.
2. Dry your hands on a clean towel.
3. Carefully remove and discard the old dressing (if you have a dressing).
4. Wash your hands for 10 seconds using warm, soapy water and rinse.
5. Dry your hands on a clean towel.
6. Examine the site for redness, swelling, tenderness, or drainage. If you note any, finish changing the dressing and take your temperature. Notify your physician, nurse, or home-care agency.

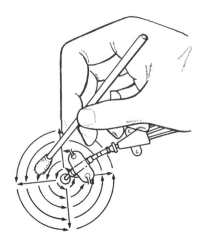

Cleansing of the exit site.

7. Carefully clean the catheter exit site with povidone-iodine swabs or alcohol swabs. Starting at the exit site, work in a circular motion around and away from the catheter exit site.
8. Allow the area to dry for 10 seconds. Pat the site with a sterile, dry gauze sponge.
9. Clean the catheter/port:
    - Using a sterile alcohol swab, grasp the catheter near the exit site.
    - Use a second alcohol swab to gently wipe the catheter, beginning at the exit site and ending at the catheter tip.
10. Prepare catheter for flushing. If you are flushing the catheter at this time, follow the instructions for flushing the catheter.
11. Coil the catheter, and *tape it in place.*
12. Wash your hands for 10 seconds using warm, soapy water, then rinse.
13. Dry your hands on a clean towel.

CHANGING THE CATHETER CAP

The catheter cap is used for needle access and needs to be changed regularly.

Your catheter cap should be changed every _____ days.

What You Need

- New sterile cap
- Alcohol swabs
- Catheter clamp (attached to catheter)

What To Do

1. Wash your hands for 10 seconds using warm, soapy water, then rinse.
2. Dry your hands on a clean towel.
3. Be sure the catheter is securely clamped over the reinforced sleeve. (*Do not* clamp the Groshong catheter—this catheter does not need a clamp.)
4. Wipe with an alcohol swab around the area where the cap is connected to the catheter.
5. Unscrew the old cap and discard.
6. Pick up the new cap by the top and remove the protective covering over its base.
7. Attach the new cap by firmly screwing it onto the catheter.
8. Release the catheter clamp.
9. Follow the directions your doctor or nurse has given you regarding whether to leave the clamp in place.
10. If the catheter requires flushing, follow the procedures listed under "Flushing the Catheter."
11. Wash your hands for 10 seconds using warm, soapy water, then rinse.
12. Dry your hands on a clean towel.

POTENTIAL COMPLICATIONS

For years catheters have been used safely by many patients. The risk of complications can be minimized with proper care.

The following potential complications should be reported immediately to your physician or nurse.

- Pain
- Shortness of breath
- Bleeding from catheter site
- Redness, swelling, or tenderness at or near the catheter site
- Drainage at or near the catheter site
- Temperature greater than 100° F

TROUBLESHOOTING TIPS

Don't expect problems, but be prepared if they should occur. Below is a list of potential problems with information about what to do if they occur.

Catheter Flushing

If your catheter resists the flushing solution, don't force the solution into the catheter. First, change your body position; take a deep breath, exhale, or cough. If your catheter still resists the flushing solution, stop and call your physician or nurse.

Catheter Damage

Keep sharp objects away from your catheter. If the catheter is accidentally cut or punctured, clamp the catheter or tubing by folding the catheter back onto itself. Secure it with a rubber band. Report catheter damage to your physician or nurse immediately.

Blood in Catheter/Tubing

Follow catheter flushing steps.

Pump Malfunction

Check and if necessary replace the battery or electrical plug; check the start and stop function; check for clamped tubing.

Bleeding or Irritation at Exit Site

If you note pain, redness, swelling, or oozing at the exit site, you should call your physician immediately. These signs may indicate an infection. Avoid possible infections by following your physician's instructions regarding activity.

Infection

Call your physician if you experience fever or chills. Infection may also cause you to note a foul odor, feel pain or heat, or observe swelling or oozing at the exit site. To prevent infection, wash your hands before beginning any procedure, wear a mask if you have a cold, avoid persons who are ill, and do your procedure in a well-ventilated but draft-free place.

Loose or Disconnected Filter

If the filter is loose or completely detached, clean the catheter adapter and replace the filter with a new filter. Do not use the same filter again. Use tape to secure the filter to the catheter adapter.

Pain on Injection

If you feel discomfort during injection, try injecting more slowly (about ½ ml every 30 seconds). If pain continues, call your physician.

Inadequate Pain Relief

Call your physician immediately if you have pain between injections or no pain relief at all. Your physician may want to change your medication or check catheter placement.

OTHER QUESTIONS
How Will I Know if Something Is Wrong?

If you are unable to inject your medication, the filter may be clogged or you may have a catheter obstruction. Try changing the filter. If this does not help, call your physician.

If you notice redness and swelling at the catheter exit site or have a low-grade temperature (98.6° to 100° F), or if you have a feeling of general discomfort that lasts more than 24 hours, this may indicate the beginning of an infection.

If your temperature spikes (goes higher than 100° F), this may also indicate an infection.

Contact your physician as soon as you suspect that something is wrong.

May I Bathe or Swim?

You should ask your physician this question. The answer will depend on your health and risk for infection. It will also depend on how long you have had the catheter in place. If your physician approves swimming, the catheter and exit site must be covered with an appropriate waterproof dressing. When finished, you will need to cleanse and dress the exit site.

Does the Exit Site Always Need a Bandage?

This depends on how long the catheter or port has been in place. Check with your physician or nurse to see if you should keep your incision or exit site covered with a dressing or bandage.

What if I Get a Cold?

If you have a cold, your physician may instruct you to wear a mask when you are caring for the catheter, especially during the filter and cap change procedure.

What Happens if the Catheter Is Damaged?

If the damage is far enough away from the exit site, it can be repaired. If there is too little catheter to work with, you may need to have the catheter replaced. Clamp the catheter above the damaged area, then contact your physician or nurse immediately.

What if I Break a Needle in the Cap?

Replace the filter and injection cap, following the directions described earlier.

What Do I Do if I Run Out of Supplies?

Call the company, pharmacy, physician, or nurse that is providing your supplies. You should always have extra supplies on hand so that you will not run out.

What Happens if the Catheter Gets Pulled Out?

The catheter is anchored with sutures underneath your skin. Therefore, it is unlikely to get pulled out. The catheter may stretch a bit and may seem like it has slipped out. If you think your catheter is slipping out, do not try to test it by pulling on it. Call your physician.

What if I Become Allergic to the Povidone-Iodine or Tape?

There are many choices for antiseptic solutions and tape. Check with your physician or nurse if you think you are having an allergic reaction. He or she can determine which tapes and antiseptics are best for you.

Should Someone Else Learn the Procedure?

Having another person available who has been trained in all of the necessary procedures is important. If you become too ill to perform a procedure, the other person could perform it for you.

ST FRANCIS REGIONAL MEDICAL CENTER

PHYSICIAN'S ORDERS
UNLESS OTHERWISE DIRECTED BY THE PRESCRIBING PHYSICIAN
BY UNDERLINING, THE PHARMACY SHALL DISPENSE GENERICALLY.
BEAR DOWN - YOU ARE MARKING TWO COPIES

DOES NOT APPLY TO HEMODIALYSIS CATHETERS

Date	Time	ADULT STANDARD FLUSH PROTOCOL ORDERS	Nurse
		Per physician discretion, Normal Saline or low dose heparin (eg. 10u/ml) is indicated for a flush when intermittent medications are	
		administered more than qid and a continuous infusion is not maintaining line patency. 1.4% Sodium Citrate solution is an	
		alternative to heparin in the following situations: Heparin Allergy or Intolerance; Heparin Induced Thrombocytopenia;	
		Leukemic Patients with low platelet counts, eg. 20,000 or less.	
		(Check the box indicating the appropriate Protocol.)	
		1) **Peripheral IV Lock:**	
		☐ 2ml Normal Saline after each use or at least q-12 hours. 8am-8pm.	
		2) **Peripheral Inserted Long Line Catheter:** *(circle type)* Single lumen Dual lumen	
		(circle lumen gauge) 23 ga 22ga 20ga 18ga 16 ga other___	
		☐ 2ml Normal Saline (5ml syringe or larger) followed by 1 ml heparin 100u/ml in <u>each</u> lumen after	
		each use or at least q 12 hours. 8am-8pm.	
		(See Standard Flush Protocol Orders For Sodium Citrate if Indicated.)	
		3) **Central Venous Catheter:** *(circle type)* Single lumen Dual lumen Triple lumen Quad lumen	
		(circle type) Hickman Quinton-Raff Subclavian Other:	
		(circle hub color) white red blue brown grey other_____	
		☐ 5ml Normal Saline followed by 2ml heparin 100u/ml in <u>each</u> lumen after each use or at least daily	
		for catheter not in use. 8am. (<u>Arrow Subclavian Catheter</u> - Flush each lumen q 12 hours. 8am-8pm)	
		(See Standard Flush Protocol Orders For Sodium Citrate if Indicated.)	
		4) **Groshong Catheters:** *(Circle Type)* Single lumen Dual lumen Triple lumen	
		(circle hub color) white red blue brown grey other_____	
		☐ 5ml Normal Saline in each lumen after each use or weekly, if not in use. (Use force when flushing.)	
		☐ Use 30 ml Normal Saline flush after TPN	
		(See Standard Flush Protocol Orders For Sodium Citrate if Indicated.)	
		5) **Implanted Vascular Access:** *(circle type)* Single port Dual port - (left/right)	
		(circle type) Port-a-cath Infuse-a-port Life port Davol Port Other:	
		☐ 10ml Normal Saline in each port after each use.	
		☐ 10ml heparin 100u/ml in each port at least once per month if not in use. *(When port is accessed	
		for intermittent therapy, flush port daily.)	
		(See Standard Flush Protocol Orders For Sodium Citrate if Indicated.)	
		6) **Other:** (write in)	
		ALLERGIES:	

Can Some Chemicals Hurt the Catheter?

Some chemicals can damage the catheter, so it is important not to use anything on or near the catheter unless you check with your physician or nurse.

Acetone, which is found in nail polish remover and tape removers, is especially harmful and should not be used on or around the catheter.

How Long Can the Catheter or Port Stay in Place?

The catheter or port is designed to stay in place for long periods of time, but each patient's situation is unique. The better you take care of your catheter or port, the longer it will last.

What Support Services Can I Access?

Your physician and other members of your health care team are available to answer your questions about your venous access device while you are in the medical center. They can also help you make arrangements for supplies and home care nursing after you go home.

You will be in charge of caring for your venous access device when you are at home. If you have questions at any time, call and ask for the nursing staff on the unit you were on during your hospital stay or your home care agency staff.

? Study Questions

Match the word in column I with the correct definition in column II

Column I		Column II
1. Groshong valve	_____	a. Acts as a barrier, reducing the risk of organism migration causing an infection
2. Tunneled central venous catheter	_____	b. A device that is accessed through the skin via a noncoring needle
3. Multilumen catheter	_____	c. Surgically placed beneath the subcutaneous tissue to an exit site on the chest wall

4. Implantable port   _____   d. A slit that keeps the catheter lumen closed when not in use

5. Catheter cuff   _____   e. Contains separate channels, or lumens, each running the entire length of the catheter

6. Fill in the blanks: When obtaining a blood specimen from a tunneled venous access device in an adult, withdraw _____ ml for blood discard; obtain the requested blood specimen; flush the tunneled catheter with _____ ml normal saline; then _____ if the venous access device is not in use.

7. Usual maintenance frequency for a normal saline or heparin flush (daily/weekly/monthly):
    a. _____ subclavian catheter
    b. _____ tunneled venous access device (catheter)
    c. _____ Groshong catheter
    d. _____ implantable port

    Select one best answer.

8. Patient or family education for home management of central venous access devices includes which topics:
    a. Exit site care, blood sampling procedure, and heparinization
    b. Heparinization, and/or normal saline flushing, signs and symptoms of complications, catheter exit site care
    c. Blood sampling procedure, heparinization, signs and symptoms of complications
    d. Venous access device patient education materials only

9. Air embolus related to a disconnected central venous access device may result in which symptoms:
    a. Headache, dyspnea, engorged neck veins, fever
    b. Tachycardia, hypertension, dyspnea, chest pain
    c. Hypotension, bradycardia, chest pain, cyanosis
    d. Cyanosis, chest pain, tachycardia, hypotension

10. Nursing practice guidelines to ensure implantable port access and infusion therapy include which steps:
    a. Wash hands, palpate port, access port, infuse solutions

    b. Palpate port, wash hands, access port, infuse solutions

    c. Wash hands, access port, obtain blood return, infuse solutions

    d. Wash hands, palpate port, access port, obtain blood return, infuse solutions

ANSWERS: 1. d   2. c   3. e   4. b   5. a
6. 5 ml; 5 to 10 ml; flush with heparin   7a. q 12 hours
7b. daily or weekly   7c. weekly   7d. monthly   8. b
9. d   10. d

Peripherally Inserted Central Catheters

4

Objectives

1. List the types and features of the peripherally inserted central catheters (also called PIC catheters, or PICCs).

2. Describe the drug or solution administration procedures for PICCs.

3. Discuss the procedure for blood sampling from PICCs.

4. Identify the major complications associated with PICCs.

5. List the patient and family education needs associated with daily, weekly, and monthly maintenance of PICCs.

The use of PICCs is on the rise in all health care settings. Recent advances in catheter technology and in the theoretical and clinical expertise of the professionals in the practice of intravenous therapy have had a significant impact on patient care and improved outcomes. PIC catheters can remain in place from weeks to months to provide multiple infusion therapies such as chemotherapy, hydration therapy, blood products, analgesia, antimicrobials, and parenteral nutrition. Additionally, the catheter's uses are increasing because they fill a void between the simple peripheral venous access catheters and surgically placed long-term indwelling catheters and ports.

Catheter Placement Guidelines

The PIC catheter can be inserted at the patient's bedside or in the home setting by nurses with advanced IV therapy skills as an alternative to physician-placed central venous catheters. The placement of these catheters by nurses requires special training and demonstrated competency. The initial education course and the ongoing education and competency program should include topics such as anatomy and physiology of the vascular system, device selection criteria, patient assessment, aseptic technique, procedural technique, suturing technique, product evaluation, potential complications (emphasizing prevention, recognition, and nursing interventions), care management, quality improvement issues; expected and unexpected patient outcomes, and program planning. Observation of clinical competence should be performed in the appropriate patient care setting under preceptorship of a clinical expert. Protocols for meticulous care and management of the PICC should be in place to facilitate prudent nursing practice guidelines. Some states have specific nurse practice regulations regarding PIC catheter insertion. It is the responsibility of the institution or agency to establish qualifications within that organization and the responsibility of each nurse to be knowledgeable of both the state nurse practice regulations and agency policies.

Indications and Contraindications

Currently the PICC is considered appropriate for IV therapy greater than 7 to 14 days and can remain in place weeks to months. The type and size of PICC depends on such considerations as the duration and type of therapy, expected catheter uses, desired flow rates, tip placement, and patient preferences. There are no limitations for use related to age, gender, or diagnosis. These catheters are particularly advantageous for high-risk groups such as neonate, pediatric, geriatric, malnourished, and immunocompromised populations. Patients with medical conditions such as inability to undergo surgical procedure for vascular access, neurologic conditions contraindicating changes in head positions, and physical disability for positioning, such as kyphosis, may benefit from PIC catheter placement.

Contraindications for use include dermatitis, cellulitis, burns at or about the insertion site, and previous ipsilateral venous thrombosis. The PICC is *not* suitable for high-fluid-volume infusions, rapid bolus injection, hemophoresis, or hemodialysis. Conditions requiring careful assessment are contractures, mastectomy, existing thrombophlebitis, radiation therapy, pacemaker wires, crutch walking, and potential future use of the extremity for dialysis arteriovenous fistula.

Catheter Products Description

These catheters are made of a soft, biocompatible silicone elastomer, Silastic, or flexible polyurethane radiopaque material (Fig. 4-1). Like tunneled catheters, PICCs are available in single lumen or multilumen designs and have an open-ended tip or a valve that closes the catheter tip when it is not in use (Fig. 4-2). They may vary in length (33 to 60 cm) and should be longer than the length measured for the patient to ensure adequate tip placement. The gauge size (23 gauge = 2 French to 14 gauge = 6 French) should be large enough to facilitate the infusion of the prescribed infusates and blood sampling but small enough for the selected vein.

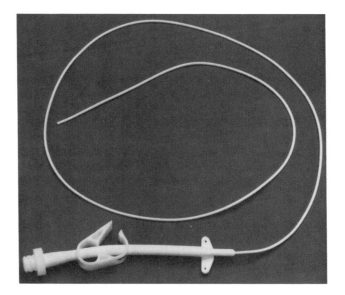

Fig. 4-1
Peripherally inserted central venous catheter.
Courtesy Cook Incorporated, Bloomington, IN

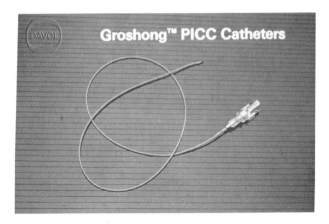

Fig. 4-2
Groshong PICC catheter.
Courtesy Bard Access Systems Inc, Salt Lake City, UT

   Product designs are differentiated mainly by the type of device used for venipuncture, the internal guidewire or stylet, and the catheter material. Venipuncture device designs (Fig. 4-3) include over-the-needle sheaths that strip away or slide off after insertion of the catheter; a scored butterfly needle that breaks and strips away from the catheter; and a small-gauge needle for over-the-wire technique. A flexible, blunt-tipped stylet or guidewire positioned within the catheter is important for ease of insertion and to reduce the risk of coiling or reversing direction while advancing the catheter. When using the breakable needle design, the risk of catheter shearing is reduced when internal guidewires or stylets are used, because the stylet or guidewire would be cut before transecting the catheter.

Principles of Catheter Insertion

- Verify the physician's order and obtain patient's informed consent.
- Identify the appropriate vein for insertion. In most adult patients the basilic vein is more suitable for cannulation than the cephalic vein because of the basilic's larger size and straighter, less tortuous shape. The cephalic, medial-cephalic, and medial-

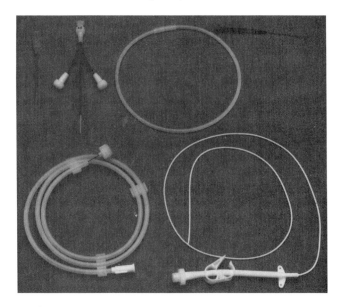

Fig. 4-3
Peripherally inserted central venous insertion set.
Courtesy Cook Incorporated, Bloomington, IN

basilic veins may also be successfully used for venipuncture.
Figure 4-4 provides vasculature identification and upper extremity vein anthropometric measurements. In infants and neonates,
other veins such as the temporal, external jugular, or saphenous
can be used for placement.

- Ensure accurate placement by measuring the distance from the
  insertion site to the catheter tip termination point. Add a
  predetermined length (5-8 cm) to allow sufficient length for
  securing the catheter.
- Catheter placement should be performed with strict aseptic
  technique, including nurse surgical hand scrub; use of hair cover,
  mask, sterile gown, gloves, and drapes; and appropriate patient
  skin antiseptic preparation.
- Silastic catheters must remain free of external particular matter
  before and during insertion. Rinsing the gloved hand with sterile
  water or saline before handling the catheter will prevent glove
  powder contact with the catheter.

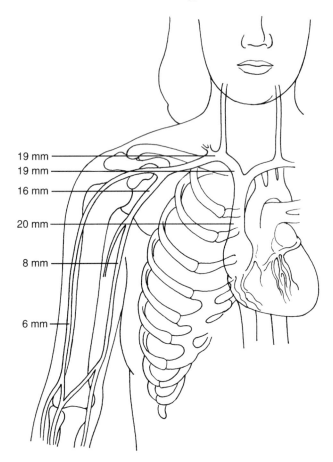

Fig. 4-4
Vasculature identification: upper extremity vein and anthropometric measurements.
Courtesy Gesco International, Inc, San Antonio, TX

- Place the patient in a comfortable, convenient position. For central venous tip placement, the patient should be lying flat with arm extended at a 90-degree angle to the body. To help prevent catheter malposition into the jugular vein, the patient should turn

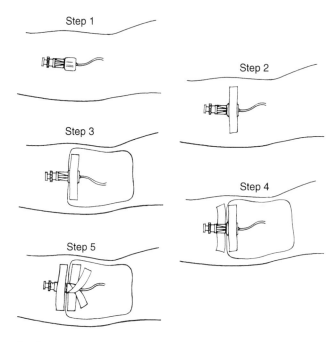

Fig. 4-5
Securing the PER-Q-Cath.
Courtesy Gesco International Inc, San Antonio, TX

his or her head toward the accessed side and place the chin on
chest.

- After the skin prep and application of the sterile drape, the
  venipuncture is performed.
  - Advance the catheter to the predetermined length.
  - Validate blood return.
  - Flush with heparinized saline solution.
  - Attach the injection cap or extension tubing.
  - Secure the catheter with sutures or sterile strips.
- Refer to the PIC catheter product recommendations or contrain-
  dications for catheter suturing. Figure 4-5 illustrates securing the
  PIC catheter with tape and transparent bioocclusive dressing.

- Stabilization of the catheter directly at the site reduces introduction of microorganisms with the in-and-out motion of the catheter through the skin.
- Standards of practice recommend that any catheter tip located within the central venous system be verified through radiographic examination to ensure proper location before any infusion.

The technique for placement of the PIC catheter will vary according to the product selected.

I. Breakaway Needle Technique: Use a specifically designated introducer for venipuncture; advance the catheter to the desired endpoint; then remove the introducer from the venipuncture site, break it in half, and peel it away from the catheter.
   A. *Advantages:* The catheter hub is attached by the manufacturer; minimizes blood exposure; most popular technique for manufacturers; many products available.
   B. *Disadvantages:* The procedure may be awkward for clinician; potential exists for catheter damage during insertion procedure.

II. Through-the-Cannula Technique: Use a large-gauge angiocatheter for venipuncture; remove the stylet; thread the desired endpoint through the angiocatheter; remove the angiocatheter over the PIC catheter; attach the hub to the distal end of the PIC.
   A. *Advantages:* Eliminates potential for catheter damage insertion; variety of products available; removeable catheter hub allows for easier repair.
   B. *Disadvantages:* Slightly more complex insertion procedure; requires larger introducer unit; catheter hub must be attached by clinician.

III. Guidewire Technique: Use a solid introducer needle to make a venipuncture, and thread a guidewire through the needle and into the vein. Remove the needle, and thread the catheter over the guidewire and into the vein. Advance the catheter into the vein slowly, using a gentle touch to avoid trauma. After threading the catheter to the desired length, remove the guidewire.
   A. *Advantages:* Reduced potential for catheter damage during insertion procedure; multiple products available.
   B. *Disadvantages:* More complex insertion procedure; potential for vein wall perforation and increased trauma to vein wall intima.

Catheter Maintenance Procedure

I. Dressing change: Provide a sterile environment for the duration of the catheter placement; the dressing should be changed at scheduled intervals and coincide with tubing and injection cap changes. Remove the dressing carefully, stabilize the hub, then gently pull the dressing away from the hub toward the venipuncture site parallel to the skin, to avoid pulling the catheter out from the insertion site. Inspect the insertion site and surrounding area for any signs of infection (e.g., drainage, edema, erythema, pain). If purulent drainage is present, obtain a culture using a sterile swab and send it to the laboratory for evaluation; report the incident to the physician promptly. During all dressing changes, verify that the catheter length remaining outside the patient corresponds with the initial placement measurement to determine if catheter migration has occurred.

CLINICAL ALERT: The initial dressing (first 24 hours) requires a sterile gauze and tape dressing over the insertion site to absorb any bloody drainage. Change this dressing within 24 hours, and follow agency protocol for the sterile dressing procedure. Monitor the insertion site for hematoma, edema, discoloration, and mechanical phlebitis.

II. Heparin flush: The amount of heparinized saline necessary to flush the catheter should be equal to the catheter/extension set volume plus approximately 0.2 ml. The priming volume of catheters varies with catheter gauge and length. Usually, *1* ml/lumen is adequate to maintain patency. Guidelines recommended by the manufacturer may include the following.

   A. Adult, intermittent use: Flush with 100 u/ml heparin every 12 hours and after each use.

   B. Child or neonate, intermittent use: Flush with 10 u/ml heparin every 8 hours and after each use.

   C. Home care maintenance: Flush every 24 hours.

III. Blood sampling: Blood sampling may be obtained from the infant or adult PIC catheter with proper technique. For consistently good blood sampling, use a larger catheter, greater than 3 French. The pliable soft walls of the catheter may collapse if a strong vacuum is applied; instead, use a 5-ml syringe with a push/pull technique rather than a vacutainer to obtain the blood sample specimen. Normal saline—10 to

20 ml—should be used for catheter flushing after blood sampling. Refer to the product manufacturer's guidelines regarding contraindications related to small size of catheter for blood administration and blood sampling. See Chapter 3, Tables 3–2 and 3–3, pages 54 and 57.

IV. Catheter declotting: The PIC catheter may be cleared by using urokinase according to the product manufacturer's recommendation with a physician's order. The small volume of the PICC must be taken into consideration as well as the potential for catheter rupture. Figure 4-6 illustrates a recommended declotting procedure.

 CLINICAL ALERT: *Never apply excessive force* or pressure when flushing the PIC catheter or when encountering severe resistance because of the danger of dislodging a clot or rupturing the catheter.

V. Catheter removal:

A. Place the patient in a supine position and remove the dressing: position the patient's arm at a 45- to 90-degree angle to the body.

B. Apply gloves.

C. Slowly pull the PIC catheter out, using a gentle, hand-over-hand technique. This process should take about 60 seconds.

D. Examine the site, note any abnormalities, and apply a small sterile pressure dressing to insertion site.

E. Measure and examine the PIC catheter to make sure the entire catheter has been removed.

F. Compare its length with the length documented in the insertion procedure.

VI. Catheter repair or exchange: Refer to the PIC catheter manufacturer's guidelines for catheter repair options and kits. PIC catheter exchange should be done only by personnel skilled in the procedure.

VII. Precautions for syringes and infusion pumps.

A. Syringes: All PIC product manufacturers recommend a minimum syringe size of 5-ml for any PIC catheter maintenance procedure. Small-diameter syringes, such tuberculin syringes, can create very *high pressure* (120 to 150 PSI). If the catheter becomes occluded, the small syringe could rupture or force that which is causing the occlusion downstream into the patient.

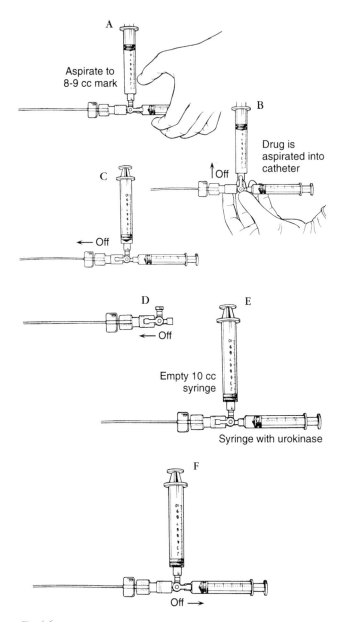

A — Aspirate to 8-9 cc mark

B — Drug is aspirated into catheter — ↑ Off

C — ← Off

D — ← Off

E — Empty 10 cc syringe — Syringe with urokinase

F — Off →

Fig. 4-6
Declotting peripherally inserted central catheters.
Courtesy Gesco International Inc, San Antonio, TX

B. Infusion pumps: Large-volume, small-volume, volumetric, linear, and rotary peristaltic pumps have all been used successfully with PIC catheters. When using infusion pumps to administer infusates, be sure the mechanism's alarm feature *does not exceed 15 PSI.*

Refer to Table 4-1 for PIC catheter troubleshooting tips and Table 4-2 for PIC catheter potential complications.

Documentation Recommendations

- Catheter insertion: catheter brand, gauge/size, lot number, and insertion site; location of tip placement; length of PICC inserted and length of external segment; date, time, and any problems encountered during insertion; radiograph confirmation of PIC catheter tip placement; the type of dressing; patient and caregiver education regarding understanding of catheter self-care management; and heparin or normal saline flush—drug, concentration, dose, volume, date, and time.
- Duration of PICC placement: assessment of insertion site; length of external segment of PICC; dates and description of sterile dressing and cap changes; presence and quality of blood return or blood sampling; heparin or normal saline flush—drug, concentration, dose, volume, date, and time; any infusion problems and interventions.

Nursing Diagnoses

- Injury, potential for, related to venous obstruction, catheter dislodgment, catheter migration, or catheter occlusion
- Infection, potential for, related to contamination of supplies, break in sterile technique when managing the catheter, performing site care, accessing catheter, or changing dressings
- Knowledge deficit regarding ongoing self-management of catheter

Patient/Family Teaching for Self-Management

- Assess the patient's or caregiver's ability and willingness to learn, the availability of the caregiver, the home environment, and previous experience or expectations.
- Describe the purpose, function, and potential duration of placement for the catheter. (See patient information on page 78.)
- Instruct the patient on the insertion procedure.

Table 4-1   Troubleshooting tips for peripherally inserted central catheters

Nursing Assessment	Nursing Intervention
Accidental catheter removal	Apply pressure dressing at the insertion site for at least 5 minutes, and notify physician. Assess the source of catheter removal, and measure the catheter length to determine if measurements coincide with catheter insertion measurements.
Fluid leak at insertion site	May be related to a hole or tear in the catheter or a loose connection between catheter and connection tubing. Follow agency guidelines for catheter repair or exchange. Use sterile technique and apply new connection/extension tubing. *Never use scissors to remove tape or dressing.*
Inability to aspirate blood	May be due to catheter occlusion or a PICC too small for blood sampling. Follow flushing protocol; reposition the patient's arm; and use push/pull technique with a 5-ml syringe. Venipuncture may be required to obtain blood sample.
Mechanical phlebitis	Related to sensitivity of PICC insertion. Elevate extremity; apply warm compresses qid for 72 hours. Consult with physician for catheter removal.
Pain, redness, drainage at insertion site	May be related to movement of the PIC catheter, skin or suture irritation, or infection. Reposition the catheter hub; remove sutures if skin is healed; apply sterile dressing; monitor skin irritation or infection; and obtain cultures. Consult with physician for catheter removal.

Table 4-1   Troubleshooting tips for peripherally inserted central catheters–cont'd

Nursing Assessment	Nursing Intervention
Pain in arm, ear, shoulder	May be due to thrombosis of the superior vena cava, misplacement of the PICC in the internal jugular vein, or internal PICC leak. *Notify* the physician: need radiograph, venogram, or ultrasound to determine PICC placement. Consider catheter removal.
Pump occlusion alarm	Assess for kink in IV tubing or in PICC at dressing site and for occlusion in catheter. Palpate the IV tubing and catheter with hand to detect kinks and reposition tubing and catheter; for suspected occlusion use the catheter-flushing protocol. If unable to obtain catheter patency, notify the physician. Potential exists for declotting PICC.
"Stuck catheter"	Catheter will appear to be firmly held within the vessel—potential causes are vasospasm, vasoconstriction, and thrombophlebitis. Remove the PICC dressing, apply moderate tension on the catheter with tape below the insertion site, and apply a sterile dressing. Apply warm compresses, and attempt catheter removal in 8, 12, and 24 hours.

- Explain self-care management issues: site care, dressing and injection cap changes, flushing of the catheter with heparin or the normal saline.
- Review the symptoms related to each potential complication; teach emergency self-management techniques, and emphasize the need for prompt reporting of that information to the physician or nurse.
- Reinforce the troubleshooting tips related to potential catheter malfunctions with appropriate intervention strategies.

Table 4-2   Potential complications for peripherally inserted central catheters

Nursing Assessment	Nursing Interventions
Air Embolus Symptoms: Chest pain, dyspnea, air hunger, tachycardia, hypotension, confusion, restlessness	Immediately place patient into a left-lateral, steep Trendelenburg position. Notify physician, initiate O_2, and remain with the patient.
Arterial Puncture Symptoms: Bright red color blood flashback, *pulsatile blood flow*	Withdraw cannulation immediately, apply pressure at venipuncture site for at least 5 minutes, and observe for hematoma. *Know venous anatomy* before inserting the device; observe dark red blood flashback/nonpulsatile flow on venipuncture for *venous access*.
Bleeding	Excessive bleeding more than 24 hours after PIC catheter insertion. Requires further evaluation for coagulation status. Obtain physician orders for prothrombin time/partial thromboplastin time; apply moderate pressure dressing; and change sterile dressing when applicable.
Cardiac Arrhythmia Symptom: Irregular heart rate	Potential need to reposition PICC tip to middle to lower third of superior vena cava to allow normal arm movements. Securing/suturing catheter at the insertion site prevents internal and external catheter migration.
Catheter Embolism Symptoms: Catheter shear, "pinch off" syndrome Related to catheter product or catheter insertion technique	Apply a tourniquet proximal to the site to prevent catheter fragment migration into central veins. Notify the physician; obtain a radiograph; and prepare for catheter fragment removal.

Table 4-2   Potential complications for peripherally inserted central catheters—cont'd

Nursing Assessment	Nursing Interventions
Catheter Malposition or Migration: Referred pain in jaw, ear, teeth, or shoulder	During catheter placement, the risk of entry into the internal jugular vein can be reduced by turning the patient's head toward the same side, while advancing the catheter. Spontaneous migration may occur during coughing, sneezing, or vomiting; Periodic PICC tip verification by radiograph may be required on long-term PICC placement.
Catheter Occlusion Symptoms: Resistance to flush or fluid infusion, inability to perform blood sampling	Follow agency guidelines for flushing, blood sampling, and declotting catheter.
Cellulitis Symptoms: Pain, tenderness, erythema at insertion site and/or surrounding subcutaneous tissue	Notify the physician. Remove the catheter; administer prescribed antimicrobials; and observe insertion site.
Nerve Damage Symptoms: Numbness, tingling, or weakness in area of insertion site	Notify the physician. Remove the catheter; reposition the extremity; and use sterile technique to apply a new dressing.
Thrombosis/ Thrombophlebitis: Symptoms: Pain, erythema, and tenderness at the insertion site; slowing of the infusion rate	Observe and note osmolarity of infusate. Notify the physician; initiate prescribed therapies.

Table 4-2   Potential complications for peripherally inserted central catheters—cont'd

Nursing Assessment	Nursing Interventions
Sepsis Symptoms: Elevated temperature, pain, tenderness, chills	Notify the physician. Administer prescribed therapies; potential for catheter removal. *Use sterile technique* for catheter insertion, care, and maintenance.

- Provide information on obtaining, storing, and disposing of supplies and on the availability of professional care.
- Suggest that the patient carry a medical-alert card identifying the PICC type, tip location, insertion and external catheter length, and date of insertion.

Home Care Considerations

- Ensure radiograph verification of PICC tip location for PIC catheter central venous placement.
- Remind patient to keep supplies and equipment used for catheter management in a secure place.
- Have the patient immediately report to the physician or nurse such abnormal findings as elevated temperature, catheter malfunction, or unusual discomfort related to the catheter.
- The patient or caregiver should discard all supplies used for catheter care into a puncture-resistant container.
- If the catheter was placed at a tertiary care center, communicate to the home care agency expectations for duration, type, and complexity of therapy.

Geriatric Considerations

Consider age-related physiological changes such as loss of subcutaneous tissue, fragile skin, neuromuscular and sensorydefects, visual and hearing losses, and arthritic joints. Assess the patient's and caregiver's ability to provide catheter site care, dressing changes, and catheter heparinization. Plan individualized self-care teaching of catheter maintenance using demonstration and return demonstration techniques. Consider large print for educational materials.

? Study Questions

Select one best answer.

1. Which of the following statements about PICCs is correct?
   a. PICCs are inserted into the subclavian vein.
   b. PICCs are commonly inserted into the basilic or cephalic vein.
   c. PICC tip placement is in the jugular vein.
   d. PICC tip placement is in the right atrium.

2. PIC catheter placement confirmation is determined by which event?
   a. Aspiration of venous blood
   b. Observation of catheter pulsation
   c. Measurement of the catheter external length
   d. Radiograph confirming tip placement in superior vena cava

3. Contraindications for PIC catheter placement include which factors:
   a. Neonate, geriatric, immunocompromised, malnourished patients
   b. Hemophoresis, hemodialysis, high-volume, or rapid infusions
   c. Long-term parenteral nutrition therapy
   d. Intermittent therapy for antimicrobials

4. Care and maintenance of PIC catheter and insertion site include which of the following?
   a. Sterile dressing at the insertion site for duration of catheter placement
   b. Sterile dressing at the insertion site during initial 30 days only
   c. Sterile dressing at the insertion site for initial 30 days, then clean dressing technique
   d. Sterile 4 × 4 gauze dressing covered with an Ace bandage for the duration of catheter placement

5. Select the correct blood-sampling guidelines for PICCs:
   a. Blood sampling can be obtained from all PICCs at any time.
   b. Use a small syringe (<3 ml) to obtain better vacuum in the syringe.
   c. Assess size and PICC placement, use a 5-ml or larger

syringe, use push/pull technique, flush with 10 ml normal saline after the blood sample; flush catheter with heparin.
   d. Assess size and PICC placement, use a 10-ml syringe, use push/pull technique, and vigorously flush the catheter after the blood sample.

6. A patient accidentally pulls out his PIC catheter. What should you do?
   a. Notify the physician, and apply gauze dressing.
   b. Immediately apply pressure dressing at the site for at least 5 minutes, notify the physician, and measure catheter length.
   c. Restrain the patient, notify the physician, and apply gauze dressing.
   d. Prepare to resuscitate the patient.

7. Documentation for PIC catheter management includes which steps?
   a. Assess insertion site, PIC catheter, dressing, infusate.
   b. Auscultate the PIC catheter for bruits; assess dressing and infusate.
   c. Ask the patient to describe how the PIC catheter and infusate are functioning.
   d. Assess insertion site and dressing; measure the length of the external catheter; palpate external catheter for kinks; observe quality of blood return or blood sampling.

8. A fluid leak at the insertion site may be corrected by which actions:
   a. Slow the infusion rate because the vein is irritated.
   b. Notify the physician to obtain orders for new PICC insertion.
   c. Stop the infusion, use sterile technique to apply new dressing, palpate the PIC catheter tubing for kinks, assess catheter tubing connections, and then initiate the fluid infusion.
   d. Remove the PIC catheter.

9. If you encounter resistance in removing a PIC catheter, follow these guidelines:
   a. Remove the dressing, apply tension on the catheter, and vigorously flush the catheter.
   b. Remove the dressing, apply warm compresses, wait 30 minutes, then withdraw the catheter.

    c. Remove the dressing, apply tension to the catheter by taping it to arm, and then withdraw the catheter.

    d. Remove dressing, apply moderate tension on the catheter with tape below the insertion site, apply sterile dressing, apply warm compresses, then wait 8, 12, or 24 hours before attempting to remove the catheter.

10. Sudden or *new* pain in the jaw, ear, arm, or shoulder may be related to which causes:

    a. Sepsis, mechanical phlebitis, catheter occlusion

    b. Bleeding, cellulitis, thrombophlebitis

    c. Catheter malposition or migration

    d. Accidental catheter removal

ANSWERS: 1. b   2. d   3. b   4. a   5. c
6. b   7. d   8. c   9. d   10. c

IV Fluids

5

Objectives

1. Discuss the processes by which fluid balance is maintained.

2. Identify important measures of electrolyte balance.

3. Name the two major fluid compartments in the body.

4. Define the terms *isotonic, hypotonic,* and *hypertonic.*

5. Name isotonic, hypotonic, and hypertonic IV fluids.

The body's fluid and electrolyte needs are altered by a variety of diseases and conditions. When an individual is ill, these needs are constantly changing. IV therapy is prescribed to correct deficiencies and achieve balance by supplying maintenance requirements of water and electrolytes and replacing any ongoing losses.

Fluid Balance
Fluid Compartments
Although a small amount of body fluid is transcellular, it is primarily intracellular or extracellular. Intracellular fluid (ICF)—fluid within the cells—accounts for approximately 25 liters of fluid in an average-size adult. Extracellular fluid (ECF) is in the spaces between cells (interstitial space) and in the intravascular fluid or plasma. Approximately 15 liters of fluid are contained in the ECF—12 liters in the interstitial space and 3 liters in the plasma or intravascular space. ECF values are similar to chemistry laboratory values (Table 5-1).

Table 5-1   Comparison of electrolyte values for ICF, ECF, and serum values on laboratory reports

Electrolytes	ICF	ECF	Normal Laboratory
Sodium	2–10 mEq/L	138–142 mEq/L	135–145 mEq/L
Potassium	135–155 mEq/L	3.8–5 mEq/L	3.5–5 mEq/L
Chloride	4–10 mEq/L	92–105 mEq/L	100–110 mEq/L
Calcium	< mg/dl	<5 mg/dl	8.5–10.5 mg/dl
Magnesium	80 mg/dl	1–2 mg/dl	1.7–3.4 mg/dl

Approximately two-thirds of the total body fluid is in the ICF space, and one-third is in the ECF space. Fluids shift from one compartment to the other as the concentration of electrolytes (solutes) is altered in the body. Fluids always move from the compartment with the lowest concentration of solutes to that with the greatest concentration. *Dehydration,* or body fluid loss, leads to *greater* concentration of electrolytes in the *extracellular* compartment. This is treated with the administration of IV fluids. Fluid retention in the ECF compartment is treated with sodium restriction and restriction of fluid amounts.

Losses of ECF may be difficult to assess if the patient has pooling of fluids in the bowel, peritoneum, or intestinal spaces, such as in intestinal obstruction, peritonitis, hepatic failure, and burns. These areas are sometimes referred to as a "third space." Surgical patients usually manifest reabsorption after pooling in the third space by an increased urine output 48 to 72 hours after the operation. This can often be anticipated, and fluids are adjusted accordingly. As fluid from the third space is reabsorbed into the circulation, the patient is monitored for fluid overload.

CLINICAL ALERT: Headache and confusion may indicate ICF volume changes. Thirst and nausea may indicate ECF volume changes. Noninvasive assessments of plasma volume include examining jugular veins, checking pulse rate, and measuring blood pressure.

Water Balance

Water is essential for life; people can live several weeks without food but only a few days without water. Water maintains blood volume, regulates temperature, transports electrolytes and nutrients to and from cells, and is a part of many biological reactions.

Table 5-2   Normal fluid intake and loss in an adult eating 2500 calories per day (approximate figures)

Intake		Output	
Route	Amount of Gain (ml)	Route	Amount of Loss (ml)
Water in food	1000	Skin	500
Water from oxidation	300	Lungs	350
Water as liquid	1200	Feces	150
		Kidney	1500
TOTAL	2500	TOTAL	2500

From Phipps WJ, Long BC, Woods NF, Cassmeyer VL: *Medical-surgical nursing: concepts and clinical practice,* ed 4, St Louis, 1991, Mosby.

Chemically, water and electrolytes work in concert to maintain water balance. Water intake is regulated through the sensation of thirst; water and electrolytes are continuously lost and replaced. Water balance is maintained primarily by the kidneys' response to the concentration of solutes present in the filtered body water.

Actual body water content depends on such variables as age, sex, body composition, and disease processes. Adults are composed of approximately 60 percent water, and infants of approximately 77 percent. Women have a slightly lower water content than men because of a larger amount of body fat. There is an inverse relationship between body water and adipose tissue (fat): the more adipose tissue, the less body water. Many disease processes alter body water; Examples are renal failure, congestive heart failure, and gastrointestinal dysfunction. These abnormal conditions alter the concentration of electrolytes present in the ICF and ECF and cause a shift in fluid between compartments.

Water balance is monitored through body weight. An otherwise unexplained weight change of 1 kg (2.2 pounds) represents a gain or loss of 1 liter of body water. An individual's average daily water intake and water output is approximately 2500 ml (Table 5-2).

Electrolyte Balance

Attaining and maintaining electrolyte balance are critical components of IV therapy, since imbalances can be fatal. Electrolytes are related to at least four fundamental physiological processes: water distribution in the ICF and ECF, neuromuscular irritability, acid–base balance, and maintenance of osmotic pressure.* IV therapy is directed at restoring lost electrolytes; once the electrolytes are replaced, the metabolic acid–base balance corrects itself. There are respiratory acid–base disturbances that cannot be corrected with IV therapy alone, such as hyperventilation causing an increased pH secondary to blowing off CO_2 or hypoventilation with CO_2 retention resulting in decreased pH or acidosis. The primary regulation of fluid and electrolyte status is determined by renal function. Proximal tubules of the kidney are responsible for reabsorption, filtration, and secretion of electrolytes.

CLINICAL ALERT: Elderly patients are at particular risk for compromised fluid and electrolyte status. Arteriosclerosis, heart failure, cardiomyopathy, diabetes, hypertension, and many other chronic conditions place patients at risk for diminished renal function and renal failure. Monitor renal function by closely monitoring intake and output records and changes in the blood urea nitrogen (BUN) level.

The electrolytes of greatest importance in fluid therapy are discussed in the following sections.

Sodium

More than any other electrolyte, sodium influences the distribution of body water. Because sodium attracts water, it is the primary factor determining the volume of extracellular space. Sodium is administered intravenously as sodium chloride. Sodium disorders are considered extracellular volume disorders. High sodium concentrations in the plasma (hypernatremia) result from conditions such as an impaired sense of thirst, hyperventilation, fever, head injuries, decreased secretion of antidiuretic hormone (ADH), diabetes insipidus, and the inability of the kidneys to respond to ADH.

Low sodium concentrations in the plasma (hyponatremia) involve an increase in the proportion of water to salt in the blood.

---

*Osmotic pressure refers to the pull or force created by random movements in a compartment or area. Fluids always flow from areas of lesser concentration of solute to areas of greater concentration. Concentration in the blood plasma is largely determined by serum proteins, such as albumin. The osmotic influence (osmolality) of an IV fluid is a key consideration when determining which type of IV fluid to administer in a particular situation.

Hyponatremia results from a disturbance in the ADH secretory mechanism, such as head injury and severe physiological and psychological stress (this disturbance is called SIADH—syndrome of inappropriate ADH secretion). Hyponatremia may also occur when hypotonic fluids are given to such patients at a time when ADH secretion is excessive.

Hypernatremia	Hyponatremia
Serum sodium >145 mEq/L	Serum sodium <135 mEq/L
Hypotension	Hypertension, increased intra-cranial pressure
Hypervolemia	Hypovolemia
Dry mucous membranes	Increased salivation
Urine volume <30 ml/hour	Low urine specific gravity
Altered mental status	Altered mental status
Coma and death	Coma and death

CLINICAL ALERT: Hypernatremia is corrected slowly—over 48 hours or more—because rapid treatment can produce serious consequences, including loss of consciousness and death. Use normal saline to correct hypernatremia, because normal saline is less concentrated than the serum of a patient with severe hypernatremia. Administer hypertonic sodium chloride solutions 3% to 5%, to correct severe hyponatremia and follow with diuretics that will result in the loss of more water than sodium. Instill these solutions cautiously while monitoring closely both neurological and cardiovascular status.

Potassium

Potassium—the major electrolyte of the ICF—is required to maintain osmotic balance and cell membrane electrical potential and to the move glucose into the cell. Plasma potassium, or the potassium found in the ECF and measured by laboratory testing, is influenced by dehydration, blood pH, dietary intake, and diuretic therapy. When potassium balance between the ICF and ECF is altered, cellular metabolism is affected along with the cardiovascular, renal, respiratory, and neuromuscular systems.

Elevated serum potassium levels are referred to as hyperkalemia; reduced serum potassium levels are called hypokalemia. Acidosis drives potassium out of cells, resulting in hyperkalemia; alkalosis drives potassium into cells, resulting in hypokalemia.

Hyperkalemia	Hypokalemia
Serum K^+ >5 mEq/L	Serum K^+ <3.5 mEq/L
Conduction disorders of heart	Ectopic cardiac activity
ECG: peaked T-wave, widened QRS, lengthened P-R	ECG: flattened T-wave, depressed ST segment
Diarrhea, abdominal pain	Decreased bowel sounds, ileus
Neuromuscular irritability	Muscle weakness, paresthesias
Oliguria or anuria	Polyuria
Cardiac failure	Digitalis toxicity

Potassium is administered intravenously as potassium chloride. Hypokalemia is treated with oral or IV administration of potassium chloride (KCI). A potassium deficit is slowly corrected to avoid development of transient hyperkalemia. Treatment of hyperkalemia depends on the rate at which the potassium level increased. Immediate treatment measures may include IV administration of calcium gluconate, sodium bicarbonate, glucose, or insulin. In mild states of hyperkalemia, oral and IV intake of potassium is restricted.

CLINICAL ALERT:

1. Urine output of at least 30 ml/hr should be verified before beginning IV potassium administration.
2. If the administration rate exceeds 20 mEq/hr, cardiac monitoring is suggested.
3. Potassium chloride should never be administered directly in a concentrated form by IV push because of the danger of cardiac arrest.
4. KCI should be thoroughly mixed when adding to an IV bag to prevent layering of potassium at the bottom of the bag.
5. A low dose of lidocaine may be added to the KCI solution to diminish the burning sensation patients frequently complain of when IV infusions contain potassium greater than 40 mEq/L.

Chloride

Chloride is the major electrolyte in the ECF. Chloride levels in blood are passively related to those of sodium, so that when serum sodium increases, chloride also increases. Factors causing losses or gains of chloride frequently affect sodium levels. Increased chloride levels are caused by dehydration, renal failure, or acidosis. Decreased chloride levels result from fluid losses in the gastrointestinal tract (nausea, vomiting, diarrhea, and gastric suction).

Chloride Excess	Chloride Deficit
Serum Cl^- >110 mEq/L	Serum Cl^- <100 mEq/L
Dehydration	Fever
Hyperventilation	Nausea and vomiting
Urine output less than 30 ml/hr	Tissue wasting (burns)

Chloride is always administered intravenously in conjunction with sodium and potassium.

Calcium

Calcium, the most abundant electrolyte in the human body, is stored primarily in the skeleton. Greater than 99 percent of skeletal calcium is unavailable for day-to-day electrolyte regulation. Calcium is present in the blood in two forms: free, ionized calcium that is circulating, and calcium that is bound to protein. The bound form attaches to the plasma protein (albumin) and other complex substances such as phosphates. For this reason it is important to correlate serum calcium concentration with the serum albumin level.

Calcium levels have an effect on neuromuscular function, cardiac status, and bone formation. Disturbances in calcium balance result from alterations in bone metabolism, secretion of parathyroid hormone, renal dysfunction, and altered dietary intake.

Hypercalcemia	Hypocalcemia
Serum Ca^{++} >10.5 mEq/L	Serum Ca^{++} <8.5 mEq/L
Decreased mental alertness	Neuromuscular irritability, such as numbness and tingling, hyperactive reflexes, and seizures
Abdominal pain, muscle weakness, nausea and vomiting, and hypertension	Bone pain

Acute symptoms of hypocalcemia are treated with IV administration of calcium gluconate or calcium chloride. Oral calcium supplements are used for chronic hypocalcemic states.

Hypercalcemia treatment includes supportive measures to lower the serum calcium level and to correct the underlying cause. Sodium chloride infusion and the administration of thiazide diuretics, usually furosemide (Lasix), are given to enhance the body's excretion of calcium. IV administration of calcitonin and pamidronate (aredia) may be given to inhibit bone resorption in bone-destructive conditions.

Magnesium

Magnesium is normally obtained from dietary intake. Excretion of magnesium is through the kidneys. Hypomagnesemia is far more common than hypermagnesemia. Conditions associated with magnesium deficits include prolonged malnutrition or starvation, alcoholism, and long-term IV therapy without magnesium supplementation. Symptoms are potentiated by hypocalcemia. Hypermagnesemia occurs most often in patients with renal failure, those with diabetic ketoacidosis, and those who use excessive amounts of antacids or laxatives.

Magnesium Excess	Magnesium Deficit
Serum Mg^{++} >3.4 mEq/L	Serum Mg^{++} <1.7 mEq/l
Lethargy	Disorientation
Absent deep tendon reflexes	Hyperactive reflexes
Hypotension	Tremors, tetany
Depressed respirations	

Magnesium sulfate solutions can be administered intravenously to correct deficits, although monitoring is required to avoid cardiac effects. Magnesium excess may be treated with the IV administration of calcium gluconate, which reverses the action of magnesium. Glucose or insulin may be given to enhance the renal excretion of magnesium.

Fluid and Electrolyte Loss

The major components of body fluids are water and electrolytes. Water losses occur when water leaves the body through the kidneys, lungs, skin, and gastrointestinal tract. Kidneys are the organs principally responsible for regulating the volume and concentration of all body fluids. When given optimal amounts of water and electrolytes, a normally functioning kidney can maintain water and electrolyte balance. However, during serious illness the kidneys are sometimes unable to make the final adjustments for fluid and electrolyte balance.

Water loss from the lungs and skin increases with elevated temperatures in the environment, fever, rapid respiratory rate, and a loss of skin covering. Examples of situations resulting in skin-covering loss are surgical procedures, burns, and wounds. Gastrointestinal losses increase when vomiting and diarrhea are present. Fluid and electrolyte losses are replaced through the intake of food and water.

Assessments and Findings of Fluid and Electrolyte Balance

Assessments	Findings
Compare total fluid intake and total fluid output	Intake should be approximately the same as output
Compare daily weight obtained at approximately the same time on the same scale	A gain of 1 kg of body weight corresponds to 1 liter of fluid
Review serum electrolyte laboratory values	*Fluid excess:* Electrolyte level is diluted; thus, laboratory values are decreased *Fluid deficit:* Electrolyte levels are concentrated, resulting in increased laboratory values
Observe clinical status	Condition of mucous membranes, skin, heart rate, presence of thirst, and mental alertness

IV Fluids

IV fluids are classified as isotonic, hypotonic, or hypertonic solutions depending on the effect a fluid has on the ICF and ECF compartments (Table 5-3).

Table 5-3   IV fluids

Fluid and Tonicity	Comments
Saline Solutions	
0.33% Sodium chloride Hypotonic	Extremely hypotonic; used only with close observation
0.45% Sodium chloride Hypotonic	Does not supply calories
	Does not supply calories
0.9% Sodium chloride Isotonic	Used to expand plasma volume; provides sodium and chloride in excess of plasma levels; given primarily with blood transfusions and to replace large sodium losses, as in burns, gastrointestinal fluid loss; *contraindicated* in congestive heart failure, pulmonary edema, renal impairment, sodium retention
	Does not supply calories
3% Sodium chloride Hypertonic	Correction of severe sodium depletion
	Does not supply calories
5% Sodium chloride Hypertonic	Maximum daily amount not to exceed 400 ml; can result in fluid volume excess and pulmonary edema
	Does not supply calories
Dextrose in Water Solutions	
5% Dextrose in water Isotonic	Used to maintain fluid intake or to reestablish plasma volume; does not replace electrolyte deficits; aids in renal excretion of solutes; *contraindicated* in head injuries; may increase intracranial pressure
	Supplies 170 calories/L
10% Dextrose in water Hypertonic	Used for peripheral nutrition
	Supplies 340 calories/L

Table 5-3   IV fluids—cont'd

Fluid and Tonicity	Comments
20% Dextrose in water Hypertonic	Irritating to veins; acts as a diuretic; may increase fluid loss; central line required Supplies 680 calories/L
50% Dextrose in water Hypertonic	Must be given through a central line Supplies 1700 calories/L
70% Dextrose in water Hypertonic	Used to provide calories to persons with compromised renal and cardiac status; central line required Supplies 2400 calories/ LDextrose in Water and Saline Solutions
5% Dextrose and 0.2% NaCl Isotonic	Supplies 170 calories/L
5% Dextrose and 0.3% NaCl Isotonic	Supplies 170 calories/L
5% Dextrose and 0.45% NaCl Hypertonic	Used to treat hypovolemia and to promote diuresis in dehydration; used to maintain fluid intake; maintenance fluid of choice if no electrolyte abnormalities Supplies 170 calories/L
5% Dextrose and 0.9% NaCl Hypertonic	Supplies 170 calories/L
10% Dextrose and 0.9% NaCl Hypertonic	Supplies 340 calories/L
Multiple Electrolyte Solutions	
Ringer's solution Isotonic	Electrolyte concentrations of sodium, potassium, calcium, and chloride are similar to normal plasma levels Supplies calories only when mixed with dextrose

Continued.

Table 5-3   IV fluids—cont'd

Fluid and Tonicity	Comments
Lactated Ringer's solution Isotonic	Electrolyte concentrations similar to plasma levels: lactate for correction of metabolic acidosis; used to replace fluid losses due to bile drainage, diarrhea, and burns; fluid of choice for acute blood loss replacement; *contraindicated* in congestive heart failure, renal impairment, head injury, liver disease, respiratory alkalosis Does not supply calories
5% Dextrose and lactated Ringer's solution Hypertonic	Used to replace gastric fluid losses; not to be given with blood products; *contraindicated* in congestive heart failure, renal impairment Supplies 170 calories
5% Dextrose and electrolyte #2 Hypertonic	Electrolyte maintenance solution Supplies 170 calories

Isotonic Solutions

Isotonic solutions are used to expand ECF volume. Fluid initially stays in the intravascular compartment. These solutions contain the same concentration of solute to fluid as that in body fluid and exert the same osmotic pressure as ECF in a normal, steady state. Isotonic fluids are indicated for intravascular dehydration.

Normal saline, or 0.9% NS, lactated Ringer's solution, and 5% dextrose and water all function as isotonic solutions. If an isotonic solution is infused into the intravascular system, fluid volume increases. One liter of isotonic solution expands the ECF by 1 liter. Three liters of isotonic fluid is required to replace 1 liter of blood loss.

Hypotonic Solutions

Hypotonic solutions exert less osmotic pressure than the ECF. Infusion of excessive hypotonic fluids can lead to intravascular fluid depletion, hypotension, cellular edema, and cell damage. Because these solutions can cause serious complications, the patient and the infusion should be monitored closely. The hypotonic solutions of 0.45% sodium chloride and 0.3% sodium chloride provide free water, sodium, and chloride to aid the kidneys in the excretion of solutes. Hypotonic solutions are administered for cellular dehydration.

CLINICAL ALERT: Never administer sterile distilled water intravenously except when using it as a drug diluent, because plain distilled water has an extremely hypotonic effect on red blood cells and can lead to lysis of the red blood cells.

Hypertonic Solutions

Hypertonic solutions exert greater osmotic pressure than ECF. These solutions are used to shift ECF into the blood plasma by diffusing fluid from the tissues to equalize the solutes in the plasma. Rapid administration of a hypertonic solution can cause circulatory overload and dehydration. Hypertonic IV fluids include 5% dextrose in 0.9% saline, 5% dextrose in lactated Ringer's solution, and dextrose and water solutions of 10% dextrose and greater.

Documentation Recommendation

1. Volume and composition of all administered fluids
2. Fluid intake and output
3. Fluid deficit
   a. Eyes: dry conjunctiva, reduced tearing, sunken appearance
   b. Mouth: dry, sticky mucous membranes; dry, cracked lips
   c. Skin: diminished turgor
   d. Neurological: reduced central nervous system (CNS) activity
   e. Cardiac: Narrowed pulse pressure, lowered blood pressure
   f. Weight; loss
   g. Other: fever, source, and amount of any body fluid loss
4. Fluid excess
   a. Eyes: orbital edema
   b. Skin: warm, moist; edema in dependent areas

   c. Cardiac: bounding pulse, vein distention
   d. Respiratory: dyspnea, crackles, wheezes, increased rate, pulmonary edema
5. Electrolyte imbalance
   a. Sodium excess: urine volume and patient temperature
   b. Sodium deficit: increased viscosity of saliva, increased urine volume, all mental status changes, and signs and symptoms of increased intracranial pressure, such as headache and increased blood pressure
   c. Potassium excess: irregular heart rate, diminished urine volume, ECG changes
   d. Potassium deficit: muscle weakness, dysrhythmias

 ## Nursing Diagnoses

- Fluid volume deficit, related to excessive fluid loss from abnormal routes (vomiting, diarrhea, indwelling tubes), diuretic therapy, burns, trauma, and surgical procedures
- Fluid volume deficit, related to inability to receive or absorb fluids, such as in hypermetabolic states (fever), head injury, coma, and electrolyte imbalance
- Fluid volume excess related to excess fluid or sodium intake

 ## Patient/Family Teaching for Self-Management

- Stress that IV fluids do not provide sufficient calories to meet basic energy needs, and when indicated, encourage small, frequent meals.
- Teach signs and symptoms of fluid excess and deficit, such as significance of weight gain, edema, shortness of breath, dyspnea on exertion, and recognition of gastrointestinal losses.
- Teach measurement of fluid intake and output so patients and family members can participate in record keeping.

 ## Home Care Considerations

Successful home infusion therapy depends on patient motivation, disease stability, and the availability of venous access. A capable person must be present in the home during the infusion to monitor patient changes.

- Instruct patients and caregivers to monitor weight gains and losses and to report significant findings.
- Reinforce the need to report all abnormal findings to the physician, such as shortness of breath, dyspnea on exertion,

edema, elevated temperature; discuss an emergency plan with the patient and caregiver.

- Monitor electrolyte status on a planned basis; ideally, electrolytes should be obtained within 24 hours of initiating infusion therapy; obtain results of recent BUN, creatinine, blood glucose values, and any other tests relevant to the patient's condition.
- Plan oral fluid and electrolyte supplements with the physician.
- Clearly document all education provided.

Geriatric Considerations

Many older individuals experience diminished homeostasis due to the reduced capacity of various body systems. Nurses caring for elderly patients should carefully monitor the patients' clinical status, laboratory results, vital signs, and intake and output.

- Common alterations in fluid and electrolytes affecting the cardiovascular patient include hypovolemia, hypervolemia, potassium and calcium imbalance, heart failure, and dysrhythmias. Correction of imbalances and prevention of serious complications caused by the imbalances lead to increased survival rates.
- Obstructions of the urinary tract are likely to result in fluid and electrolyte imbalances. Removal of the obstruction results in diuresis, which can significantly alter fluid and electrolyte status.
- In acute or chronic renal failure, patients have a tendency to develop hypervolemia, hyperkalemia, hypocalcemia, and metabolic acidosis. Sodium is generally retained.
- Elderly postoperative patients, especially following intestinal surgery, are at high risk for fluid and electrolyte imbalances, particularly fluid overload and sodium and potassium imbalances.

Chapter Resources

EVALUATION FOR FLUID IMBALANCE

Assessments	Findings
Blood pressure	*Fluid deficit:* Fall in systolic blood pressure (BP), decreased pulse pressure, and postural hypotension
	Fluid excess: Increased BP, no postural changes

Assessments	Findings
Pulse	*Fluid deficit:* Weak, thready pulse
	Fluid excess: Bounding pulse; increased pulse rate; tachycardia may be present with *either* fluid *excess* or *deficit*
Jugular vein	*Fluid deficit:* Flat neck veins
	Fluid excess: Vein distention visible; pulsation higher than 2 cm above sternal angle when head of bed raised 45 degrees
Respirations	*Fluid deficit:* Rare crackles and wheezes; dry, thick secretions
	Fluid excess: Crackles and wheezes; moist secretions
Edema	*Fluid deficit:* Infrequent edema
	Fluid excess: First found in dependent parts, such as sacral edema in persons on bed rest; pedal edema in ambulatory persons
Skin turgor	*Fluid deficit:* Loose, toneless skin; skin tense when lifted with two fingers; inaccurate assessment in elderly
	Fluid excess: Good skin turgor
Intake and output	*Fluid deficit:* Output greater than intake; slow urine output; high specific gravity
	Fluid excess: Intake greater than output; rapid urine output; low specific gravity
Weight	*Fluid deficit:* Weight loss
	Fluid excess: Weight gain

CLINICAL ALERT: Major alterations in fluid balance can occur before clinical signs and symptoms are present. Approximately 3 days following major abdominal surgery, fluid can move rapidly from the abdominal cavity and interstitial space to the intravascular compartment, creating fluid overload. Expect significant change in the patient's output at this time.

Study Questions

1. Approximately two-thirds of the total body fluid is in which space?
   a. Intracellular
   b. Extracellular
   c. Transcellular
   d. None of the above

2. Dehydration leads to increased electrolyte concentration in which space?
   a. Intracellular
   b. Extracellular
   c. Transcellular
   d. None of the above

3. An otherwise unexplained weight change of 1 kg (2.2 pounds) represents:
   a. 0.25 liter body water
   b. 0.50 liter body water
   c. 1 liter body water
   d. 1.5 liter body water

4. Before administering IV potassium to an adult, verify that urine output is at least:
   a. 20cc/hour
   b. 30cc/hour
   c. 40cc/hour
   d. Not a consideration

5. Electrolyte values in a patient experiencing fluid volume deficit are expected to be:
   a. Increased
   b. Unchanged
   c. Decreased
   d. Not reflected in electrolyte values

6. A postoperative patient is experiencing a fluid volume deficit. Which types of fluid do you expect will be ordered to expand the ECF volume?
   a. Isotonic solution
   b. Hypotonic solution
   c. Hypertonic solution
   d. Packed red blood cells

ANSWERS: 1. a   2. b   3. c   4. b   5. a   6. a

IV Medication Administration

6

Objectives

1. Identify goals of therapeutic drug monitoring.

2. List immediate actions to be taken in the event of an adverse drug reaction.

3. Describe advantages and disadvantages of various methods of IV drug administration.

4. Discuss features that differ among IV pumps.

5. Review steps the nurse can take to avoid medication errors.

More medications are being administered intravenously than before, and nurses are assuming greater responsibilities related to IV medication administration. With increased usage has come a greater understanding of the benefits and risks of this treatment modality. Many technical improvements have been made in equipment, and innovative and time-saving measures have been developed to increase the efficacy of this practice. This chapter addresses principles of IV medication administration, methods of delivering drugs intravenously, and information on select drugs.

General Principles
Indications for IV Drug Administration

IV drug administration is beneficial for several reasons:

1. Assurance that effective concentrations of the drug are achieved rapidly

2. Control over onset of peak serum drug concentrations

3. Production of a biological effect when a drug cannot be absorbed by the oral route
4. Drug administration to patients who are unable to take oral medications

Drug Dose Calculations

Because drugs for IV medication administration are injected directly into the vascular system, IV doses are often lower than those administered through other routes. Although the doses of many drugs administered intravenously are calculated according to the patient's weight, doses are adjusted also according to drug distribution and the patient's absorption ability, metabolism, and excretion, and observed signs and symptoms.

Serum albumin levels are important to drug distribution, because drugs bind to receptor sites on plasma proteins (especially albumin) and tissues. Only a drug that is not bound to a plasma protein or to a tissue is able to exert a therapeutic effect, so patients with *low* serum albumin levels have *more* adverse effects. This occurs because more free (unbound) drug is available to exert a therapeutic effect. Drug binding influences both drug effectiveness and the duration of the effect.

Drug metabolism and excretion are the two components involved in drug elimination from the body. Metabolism refers to the transformation of the drug to a water-soluble form that allows excretion to occur. Metabolism occurs mainly in the liver, and most drugs are excreted by the kidneys. Patient age and underlying disease affect elimination. Elderly people usually have diminished liver and kidney function and less muscle mass than younger persons. Any disease process that alters hepatic or renal function also can cause a prolonged drug effect and increase the likelihood of adverse drug effects.

A drug's half-life is defined as the time required for plasma levels of the drug to fall to half of the original level. Drug half-life is influenced by both metabolism and excretion rates. In addition, the half-life determines the frequency of doses that must be administered to maintain a steady drug state. Some drugs, such as heparin, must be administered continuously to effectively maintain blood levels. However, antibiotics and various other drugs may be given intermittently. When a new drug is given, loading doses are frequently required to reach therapeutic plasma concentrations rapidly. Therapeutic blood plasma levels are altered by increasing or decreasing the drug dose or by changing the amount of time between doses.

CLINICAL ALERT: Because the kidney and the liver are the major organs involved in drug excretion, the half-life of a drug is extended in patients with renal or liver disease and in the elderly.

Therapeutic Drug Monitoring

Therapeutic drug monitoring (TDM) is an important tool that is used to adjust drug dosages when drugs that have a narrow therapeutic range are administered or when patients with complex conditions receive drugs that are known to cause toxic responses. TDM is expected when giving aminoglycosides.

Some goals of therapeutic drug monitoring include the following:

- reducing drug toxicity
- improving the effectiveness of therapy
- reducing the incidence of therapeutic failure
- documenting careful use of potentially toxic medications

To monitor drug dosages closely, periodic drug peak and trough levels are drawn. Accurate laboratory analysis of peak and trough drug levels depends on accurate communication of the time of drug administration and of the time of the blood sampling. Trough levels are measured before administration of a subsequent dose, and peak levels are drawn within 30 minutes of the completion of a dose. The intensity of monitoring depends on the clinical circumstances. In relatively low-risk situations, only the steady state concentration is measured. Medium monitoring includes analysis of two blood levels before steady state and the steady state level. Maximal monitoring, used with very unstable patients, involves measuring the drug level immediately after a loading dose is given, as well as at least two levels before steady state and the steady state levels. Trough levels greater than 2 µg are associated with increased toxicities (see Table 6-1 for a listing of some IV peak and trough levels).

Combination Drug Therapy

Combination therapy refers to intended drug interactions. Drugs are often administered in combination to potentiate a desired effect that is enhanced by the interaction of two or more drugs; for example, meperidine (Demerol) and promethazine (Phenergan) are often administered together to enhance sedation and postoperative pain control. Metabolism, excretion, and binding can all be affected when multiple drugs are administered.

Complications of IV Drug Administration

Every complication that may develop with IV therapy is present when drugs are administered intravenously, including infiltration, phlebitis, and the potential for embolism or infection. Some drugs may damage surrounding tissue if an infiltration or extravasation occurs. Adverse or unplanned effects such as diminished drug potency and toxicities can occur often when multiple drugs are administered. Mild adverse effects are called side effects; serious adverse effects are called toxicities.

Adverse Drug Reactions

Adverse drug reactions can range from expected side effects of a drug to hypersensitivity reactions and death. According to the Food and Drug Administration, an adverse reaction is any undesirable experience associated with the use of a medical product in a patient. Adverse drug reactions (ADRs) are more narrowly defined by agencies and institutions, so it is necessary to be aware of agency policy for reporting adverse drug reactions. Hypersensitivity reactions, drug incompatibilities, and unexpected reactions are common examples of reportable adverse drug reactions.

Almost any drug can produce hypersensitivity (allergic) reactions in susceptible patients. Unless a person has had a previous allergic episode, there is no way to predict who may experience this medical emergency. Hypersensitivity reactions occur more quickly when drugs are given intravenously than when given by other routes. High-risk patients are very young patients and elderly patients suffering altered renal and hepatic function, patients with a history of multiple allergies, patients receiving investigational drugs, and those receiving more than one drug at a time.

High-risk drugs known to cause adverse reactions include the following:

Amphotericin B
Antibiotics
Anticoagulants
Antineoplastic agents

Corticosteroids
Dextran
Digoxin
Dyes used for diagnostic testing
Lidocaine
Phenytoin

The onset of a reaction is usually sudden, although reactions may be delayed as much as 30 to 60 minutes. Usually a more rapid onset correlates with a more severe reaction. The extent of a reaction is related to the dose of drug administered and the patient's degree of hypersensitivity. Mild reactions include urticaria, pruritus, and erythema. Sudden onset of inflammation and itching is the most common hypersensitivity reaction. Stop the drug and treat the patient symptomatically with antihistamines such as diphenhydramine HCI (Benadryl).

More severe reactions may include laryngeal edema, bronchospasm, and hypotension. Signs and symptoms of anaphylaxis include angioedema (swelling of the mouth, tongue, extremities, and area around the eyes), respiratory distress (wheezing, cyanosis), skin reactions (itching, blotchy skin wheals), and symptoms of circulatory collapse (rapidly falling blood pressure, weakness, thready pulse, and vertigo). Patients feel fear, panic, and a sense of impending doom. Suffocation resulting from laryngeal edema is the most common cause of death following an anaphylactic reaction. Many people have a recurrence of anaphylaxis within 24 hours. Take the following steps when reactions are identified:

1. Stop the medication immediately.
2. Keep an IV line open.
3. Observe the patient's respiratory status; if the patient has respiratory difficulty, keep him or her in an upright position if possible while summoning help.
4. Notify the physician.
5. Prepare to administer emergency medications.
6. Monitor vital signs.
7. Begin resuscitation if a respiratory or cardiopulmonary arrest occurs.

CLINICAL ALERT: Epinephrine (Adrenalin) followed by diphenhydramine (Benadryl) is the combination of choice for treating anaphylaxis. Other drugs that may be given include hydrocortisone (Solu-Cortef) and aminophylline (Theophylline).

Drug incompatibility

Potential incompatibility of medications is a concern whenever patients receive multiple intravenous regimens. Information on drug stability and compatibility is complex and changes frequently as administration systems and solutions change. New research and additional experience result in changes in drug treatment recommendations. Because of conflicting literature and the complexities involved with compatibility information, absolute statements are difficult to make and consultation with a pharmacist is important.

Drug stability is affected by temperature. Refrigeration improves stability, and higher temperatures reduce stability. Always follow the manufacturer's recommendations for drug diluent to ensure drug stability.

Compatibility is most influenced by pH. Drugs with similar pH are compatible; those with significantly different pH are incompatible and should not be administered together. Although compatibility charts are helpful tools, they should be used judiciously, because conflicting information is often presented as a result of varied study conditions.

Incompatibility occurs when either two drugs or a drug and an IV solution are mixed to make a product that is unsuitable for safe administration. Physical, chemical, and therapeutic changes in the drug result from incompatibility. These changes result in loss of drug activity, unexpected adverse reactions, precipitate formation, and adverse clinical changes in the patient such as anaphylaxis, multiple pulmonary infarctions, and platelet aggregation.

Physical changes in the drug are the most common and the easiest to detect visually. These may be a change in color or precipitate formation. A precipitate formation is often determined by the concentration of the drug, the pH of the solutions, the sequence of additives, and the amount of standing time since admixture. Precipitation can occur immediately, hours later in the tubing or filter, or later in the IV catheter, thus causing occlusion. Visual inspection cannot detect very small precipitates.

Chemical changes result in irreversible drug degradation. The product resulting from chemical change is less active than expected, and therefore the therapeutic effect is altered. Chemical effects are often not detected with a visual inspection.

Therapeutic changes occur when two or more drugs combine to produce an effect that is pharmacologically antagonistic or synergistic, an effect usually considered adverse.

IV Drug Administration Rate

The IV drug administration rate is determined by the amount of drug that can be given over 1 minute. When the administration rate is not known, an IV medication should be administered at the rate of 1 mg/min.

CLINICAL ALERT: Always refer to the package insert or a reference text when administering an unfamiliar drug.

Methods of IV Medication Administration

IV drugs may be given using a variety of techniques. The method chosen depends on the desired effect and the available supplies and equipment. When selecting a method, the clinician should consider the following variables that can affect serum levels of drugs: flow rate, location of injection site, drug volume, and fluid volume of the tubing. Descriptions of various methods follow.

IV Push

High concentrations of medication are administered directly into an IV lock or through an injection port to achieve rapid and predictable serum levels. The IV injection is usually given over 5 minutes or less. This method of drug administration is designed to administer bolus doses.

1. Procedure
   a. Insert the syringe with medication into the IV lock or through an injection port as close to the IV cannula as possible after cleansing the port with an alcohol swab.
   b. Clamp off the primary IV line (if applicable).
   c. Administer the drug at prescribed rate.
   d. Use a second syringe to administer flush solution.
   e. If the medication bolus was given directly into an IV lock, flush the lock with 2 to 3 ml of normal saline or heparinized saline according to policy; continue exerting pressure on the syringe while withdrawing it to prevent a backflow of blood into the IV catheter.
2. Advantages
   a. The drug response is rapid and predictable; this method is frequently used in emergency situations.
   b. The nurse is able to observe the patient throughout the procedure.
3. Disadvantages

a. Adverse effects can be expected at the same time and rate as therapeutic effects.

b. The IV push method has the greatest risk of adverse effects and toxicity, because serum drug concentrations are sharply elevated.

CLINICAL ALERT: Flush IV tubing after administering a drug to ensure that the complete dose is delivered; otherwise a portion of the drug may remain in the port or may layer in the IV tubing. Administer the flush at the same rate as the medication bolus, because the flush pushes medication from the tubing into the patient's vein.

IV Piggyback

IV piggyback is a type of intermittent drug infusion. IV medication is diluted in a small bag or syringe of D5W or normal saline and administered as a drip over approximately 30 minutes. The administration time varies according to the volume of solution intended for infusion. When medication is attached to a primary IV line with a secondary set, the primary line requires a one-way or back-check valve.

1. Procedure
   a. Spike medication container with an IV administration set.
   b. Hang the medication container at or above the level of the primary IV (Fig. 6-1).
   c. The drug may be administered simultaneously with a compatible IV fluid; if the fluid entering the IV cannula is not compatible with the medication, flush the line with 2 to 3 ml of normal saline before beginning medication infusion and stop the flow of the main solutions; if the primary infusion cannot be interrupted, consider using a dual-lumen catheter or administering the medication through a second site as an intermittent infusion.
   d. Infuse the drug at prescribed rate.
   e. After drug administration, the secondary set may remain attached to the IV set or be removed until the next dose; if the line is removed, cap the end of the line with a new needle or cannula.
2. Advantages
   a. Incompatibilities are avoided.
   b. A larger drug dose can be given at a lower concentration

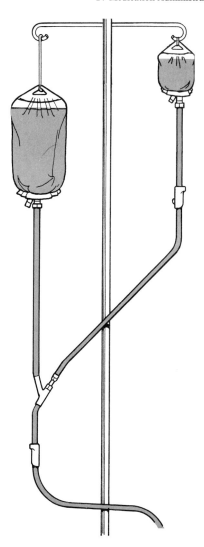

Fig. 6-1
Piggyback IV medication.

per milliliter than would be practical with the IV push method.

3. Disadvantages
   a. Administration rate is not controlled precisely unless the infusion is electronically monitored.
   b. IV set changes can result in the wasting of a drug assumed to have been given.
   c. Bags are available with only D5W and normal saline solutions.
   d. The added volume of 50 to 100 ml of IV fluid can cause fluid overload in some patients.

Intermittent Infusion

The drug is prepared in the same manner as an IV piggyback solution. Instead of a secondary IV line being attached to the existing infusion, an intermittent infusion is attached directly to an IV lock.

1. Procedure
   a. Flush IV lock with 2 to 3 ml of normal saline.
   b. Insert the infusion into the IV lock and secure the junction with tape.
   c. Infuse the drug at the prescribed rate.
   d. After drug administration, flush the lock with normal saline or heparinized saline solution; exert a positive pressure on the syringe when withdrawing from the IV lock to prevent a backflow of blood into the IV catheter.
2. Advantages and disadvantages are the same as for the piggyback method.

Volumetric Chamber

Medication is added to the volume control chamber and diluted with IV fluid. Infusion is generally over 15 minutes to 1 hour (Fig. 6-2).

1. Procedure
   a. Add medication to the chamber.
   b. Add the required amount of IV fluid.
   c. Infuse the drug at the prescribed rate.
   d. Following completion of the drug infusion, resume the IV infusion or flush the IV lock.

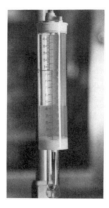

Fig. 6-2
Volumetric chamber.
From Perry AG, Potter PA: *Clinical nursing skills and techniques,*
ed 3, St Louis, 1994, Mosby.

2. Advantages
    a. Runaway infusions are avoided without the use of electronic equipment.
    b. May be used to transport patients without a pump.
    c. Volume of fluid in which the drug is diluted can be adjusted easily.
3. Disadvantages
    a. The drug must travel a long distance before it reaches the patient; there is a significant time delay during very slow infusion rates before the drug dose reaches the patient.
    b. When the chamber empties and the infusion is slowed, a large amount of the drug can remain in the IV tubing.
    c. Incompatibilities may develop when the chamber is used for multiple drugs.
    d. It is necessary to change the labeling on the chamber each time a new solution is added.

Continuous Infusion

Medication is added to a large volume of parenteral solution and administered continuously. These infusions are usually regulated

with an IV pump or controller to ensure an accurate flow rate
(Fig. 6-3).

1. Procedure
   a. Place time-tape on bag, even when a pump or controller
      is used, to verify administration rate.
   b. Spike the IV container with an IV administration set.
   c. Regulate flow rate.
   d. Observe the patient at least every hour during the
      infusion; many medications require more frequent patient
      monitoring.
2. Advantages
   a. Admixture and bag changes can be performed every 8 to
      24 hours.
   b. Constant serum levels of the drug are maintained.
3. Disadvantages
   a. When it is not monitored electronically, there is an
      imprecise control over the administration rate.
   b. Drug compatibility problems may develop if the line is
      used to administer piggyback or IV push medications.

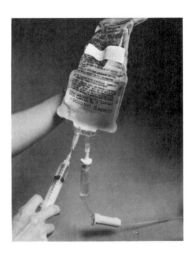

Fig. 6-3
Injecting medications into IV solutions.
From Perry AG, Potter, PA: *Clinical nursing skills and techniques,*
ed 3, St Louis, 1994, Mosby.

CLINICAL ALERT: Inadequate drug mixing can result in serious and undesired drug effects. To ensure adequate mixing of any drug added to an IV solution, do not add a medication to a hanging bag. Follow these guidelines:

1. Use a long needle—at least 1 inch in length—to inject drugs into the bag; otherwise a concentration of the drug may remain in the port.
2. To assist with mixing, use force when injecting a medication.
3. Agitate or rotate the bag several times to aid in mixing the drug with the IV solution.

If the added drug is not as dense as the IV solution, the medication floats to the top of the solution; if the drug is more dense than the IV solution, it remains at the bottom of the container. Incomplete mixing of any drug results in drug delivery that is not consistent. Aminophylline is a drug that is less dense than most IV solutions; potassium chloride is more dense than most IV solutions.

Special Drug Manufacturer Packaging

Many innovative premixed and partially mixed medications are available from drug manufacturers. These packages allow medication to be admixed in their original packaging at the time of administration. There is no one best system; however, patient needs may be best met with specialty packages. Use of the medications is convenient and reduces wastage and labor costs. The major disadvantage associated with special packaging is an increase in cost per dose. Consult the manufacturer's directions for procedures related to administration.

Use of Infusion Devices

The volume and complexity of IV drug administration have increased dramatically. This is due to the rapid improvements in the capabilities of electronic control devices. Device reliability has improved as well as capabilities. Changes will likely continue to occur rapidly as technology improves to meet the challenges of acute care and ambulatory care.

IV pumps and controllers are designed to regulate flow rates precisely and are used widely with medicated IVs. Fluids are delivered at a preselected rate, and most record the amount of fluid infused, automatically prime tubings, and offer prompts to assist with pinpointing infusion problems. Most machines are accurate within 2 percent of the selected rate. They vary according to ease

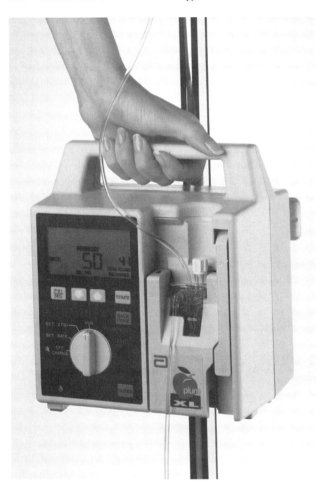

Fig. 6-4
Abbott Plum XL Infusion Pump.
Courtesy Abbott Laboratories, Abbott Park, IL.

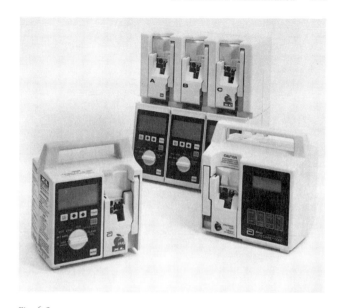

Fig. 6-5
Abbott Infusion Pumps: Plum XL3: Plum 1.6 w/dataport;
Plum XL.
Courtesy Abbott Laboratories, Abbott Park, IL.

of use, pressure-monitoring capabilities, size, programmability, microrate-infusion capability, need for special tubings, battery life, availability of printouts, and method of operating.

Devices may administer one to four or more channels simultaneously and include automatic piggybacking, direct syringe or vial delivery, back priming and automatic air elimination, dose calculation, and safeguards against free-flow. In the ambulatory setting, small nonelectronic elastomeric devices are widely used (Fig. 6-4). Always check the manufacturer's recommendations for specific device features. See Fig. 6-4, 6-5, and 6-6.

IV Controllers

Controllers deliver fluids with the aid of gravity. The IV fluid container must be placed approximately 36 inches above the IV site

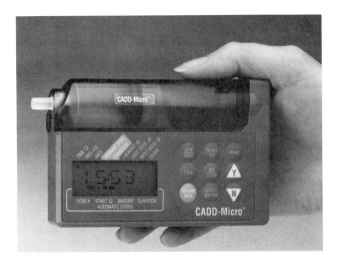

Fig. 6-6
CADD-Micro Ambulatory Infusion Pump Model 5900.
Courtesy SIMS Deltec Inc., St Paul, MN.

to overcome venous resistance and operate properly. A photoelectric eye monitors the flow rate. Controllers are designed to sound an alarm when resistance is detected and thus are useful for the detection of infiltrations.

IV Pumps

Pumps are used to deliver accurate flow rates. Infusion pumps allow concentrated medications and small volumes of fluid to be administered over prolonged time periods. Pumps also increase the accuracy of rapid infusions. Pumps provide pressure to fluid delivery when it is necessary to overcome filter resistance, viscous solutions, small-gauge catheters, and patient activity (Fig. 6-7). When the pump senses resistance, it attempts to maintain the IV flow rate by increasing the pressure of fluid delivery. Many pumps allow the user to set occlusion pressure limits. This is useful if an IV catheter is in an area where it partially occludes with movement (positional IV) or in other situations in which either higher-than-

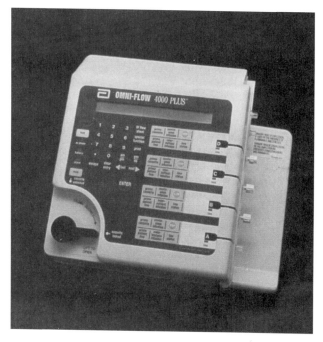

Fig. 6-7
Omni-Flow 4000 Plus infusion pump.
Courtesy Abbott Laboratories, Abbott Park, IL.

normal or lower-than-normal pressures are desired (such as in chemotherapy administration). Select features of IV pumps and related comments follow.

Features	Comments
Operating mechanism	Operate with a diaphragm, piston (syringe), or peristaltic mechanism
Pressure	The maximum pressure applied before an occlusion alarm sound varies; some pumps allow variable settings according to the desired applications (IV, arterial, epidural)

Features	Comments
Programmability	Allows portions of the total daily dose to be given at desired times, rates, and intervals; usually able to accommodate at least a 24-hour drug supply for ambulatory patients
Bolus doses	Pumps designed for patient-controlled analgesia administration have the capacity to deliver bolus doses of drug on demand
Flow rate	Can range from 0.1 to 2000 ml/hr according to machine selected
Variable pressure	Variable pressure settings allow solutions of different viscosity to be administered
Multiple infusions	One to four solutions may be regulated at different rates by one machine; some have piggyback options
Alarms	Alarm conditions can include occlusion, machine malfunction, empty container, air in line, door open, and low battery; the number of safety alarms varies according to model
Tamper-proof settings	Desirable especially for use with children and with narcotic infusions
Energy source	Pumps are designed to operate on electrical or battery power. Many use electrical power and have battery back-up. Most ambulatory pumps are battery powered, although some are spring operated or designed for onetime use
Size	Wide range of sizes available; ambulatory pumps are designed specifically to deliver small volumes of 50 to 100 ml; the pump and a bag are worn by the patient to allow mobility; may have a piston or peristaltic action
Cost	Wide range according to features; dedicated tubing costs also vary widely according to the manufacturer

Considerations When Working With Pumps and Controllers

If the pump monitors flow with a sensor, follow these guidelines:

1. Fill the administration set's drip chamber to the fill line or half full to allow the sensor to monitor the drip accurately; most drip sensors are placed at the top of the chamber. Splashes in the chamber may cause inaccurate rates.
2. Most tubing cassettes should be inverted for priming.
3. Verify accurate functioning at regular intervals.
4. Always follow manufacturer's directions.
5. Do not use tubing clamps with a pump or controller.

CLINICAL ALERT: Some pumps and tubings allow a free flow of IV solution when the pump door is opened or if the IV tubing is removed from the pump. This results in the patient receiving a bolus of a potent medication. *Always* close the manual clamp on an IV tubing set before opening the pump door.

Avoiding Medication Errors

As in the administration of all medications, the potential for error is a concern. This concern is particularly serious in IV administration because of rapid drug absorption. To minimize the risk of errors, always follow the five "rights" of medication administration: right drug, right dose, right patient, right time, right route. In addition, observe the following precautions:

1. Always read the label on all drugs and verify the medication(s) with the physician's order before administration.
2. Resolve questions about unfamiliar drugs before administration; know the expected dosage ranges, administration rates, incompatibilities, adverse effects and antidotes, and the intended usages of the drugs.
3. Clarify ambiguous medication orders; encourage the use of only approved abbreviations in physician orders.
4. Consider the possibility of drug interactions and take appropriate precautions.
5. If a patient has had an allergic reaction in the past, be cautious, especially when adding a new drug; when starting a new drug, particularly an antibiotic of the same type as one the patient has been allergic to in the past, question the possibility of another reaction.

6. Before administering a drug, check the patient's armband and record for the presence of allergies.

7. Verify dosage calculations with another person to avoid mathematical errors; when possible, refer to calculation tables for medications frequently administered.

8. Chart medications immediately after administration to avoid the possibility of administering a repeat dose.

9. To the extent possible, reconstitute drugs so that they can be administered at a rate of 1 mg/min.

10. Encourage the implementation of standardized IV drug dilutions to simplify administration rate calculations.

11. If handwriting is illegible or nonstandard abbreviations are used, confirm the medication order with the physician.

Select Drug Information

Antimicrobial Agents

Antibiotic, antifungal, and antiviral agents are frequently administered intravenously. These drugs may be administered prophylactically to decrease the incidence of infection after certain operations, empirically to initiate therapy directed against the most likely infecting organism before receipt of culture and sensitivity reports, or therapeutically. Therapeutic coverage is achieved based on culture and sensitivity reports. Antibiotics act either by inhibiting bacterial cell wall synthesis and producing a defective cell wall or by altering intracellular function of the bacteria, as in electron transport and target DNA binding. The categories of antimicrobial agents most widely used are discussed in the following sections.

Cephalosporins

Cephalosporins are widely used, relatively safe antibiotics. There is a wide dosage range between toxic drug levels and subtherapeutic drug levels. Adverse effects are similar to those of penicillins; approximately 3 percent to 5 percent of individuals who have adverse reactions to penicillin have adverse reactions to cephalosporins. Those who have had anaphylaxis are most susceptible to an allergic reaction with a cephalosporin. Adverse effects may include hypersensitivity, phlebitis, diarrhea, neutropenia, and altered liver function. Aminoglycosides are chemically inactivated by cephalosporins. The following target organisms are affected by cephalosporins:

1. First generation: Most gram-positive organisms and some gram-negative organisms.
2. Second generation: Increased gram-negative action, decreased gram-positive effectiveness.
3. Third generation: Expanded gram-negative coverage, decreased gram-positive coverage.

Aminoglycosides

Aminoglycosides are used most often to treat bacteremia, systemic infections, and urinary tract infections. IV administration is always used to achieve a systemic effect, because the drugs are not absorbed from the gastrointestinal tract. Target organisms include gram-negative aerobes, staphylococci, and mycobacteria. The mechanism of action is interference with bacterial protein synthesis and replication.

One of the major differences among the various aminoglycosides is toxicity incidence. Adverse effects are a concern when using aminoglycosides because of the narrow range between therapeutic and toxic effects. To monitor drug dosages closely, draw periodic drug peak and trough levels. Trough levels are measured before administration of a subsequent dose, and peak levels are drawn within 30 minutes of the completion of a dose. Trough levels greater than 2 μg are associated with increased toxicities (see Table 6-1 for a listing of some IV drug peak and trough levels). Adverse effects of aminoglycosides include the following:

1. Nephrotoxicity. Persons who already have diminished renal function are particularly at risk for developing this effect; when other nephrotoxic drugs are administered, this effect is potentiated.
2. Ototoxicity. Tinnitus, loss of high-frequency hearing, and altered balance may all result from ototoxicity.
3. Neuromuscular blockade. Respiratory depression or paralysis can occur in conjunction with anesthetics.

Penicillins

Penicillins act by inhibiting bacterial cell wall synthesis. Most gram-positive organisms and some gram-negative cocci are sensitive to penicillins. Adverse effects can include cutaneous reactions, gastrointestinal symptoms (especially diarrhea), hypersensitive reactions, and renal damage (see Table 6-2 for a listing of cephalosporins, aminoglycosides, and penicillins).

Table 6-1 Serum drug level monitoring

Drug	Trough	Peak
Aminoglycosides (gentamicin, tobramycin, amikacin)	Within one-half hour of next dose Serum level: <2 μg/ml	One-half hour after end of 30-minute infusion, or 15 minutes after end of 1 hour infusion Serum level: 5 to 10 μg/ml
Vancomycin	Within one-half hour of next dose Serum level: <10 μg/ml	1 hour after end of infusion Serum level: 20 to 40 μg/ml
Digoxin-IV	5 to 24 hours after last dose, just before next dose preferred Serum level: 0.8 to 2 μg/ml	Do not draw
Aminophylline	Just before dose Serum level: 10 to 20 μg/ml	1 hour after dose Serum level: 10 to 20 μg/ml
Dilantin-IV	Just before dose Serum level: 10 to 20 μg/ml	One-half hour after end of infusion

Table 6-2 Aminoglycosides, cephalosporins, and penicillins

	Generic Name	Trade Name
Aminoglycosides	Amikacin Gentamicin Kanamycin Neomycin Netilmicin Streptomycin Tobramycin	Amikin Garamycin Kantrex, Klebcil Neomycin Netromycin Streptomycin Nebcin
Cephalosporins		
First generation	Cefazolin Cephapirin Cephalothin Cephradine	Ancef, Kefzol Cefadyl Keflin, Seffin Cephradine

Table 6-2   Aminoglycosides, cephalosporins, and penicillins—cont'd

	Generic Name	Trade Name
Second generation	Cefamandole	Mandol
	Cefonocid	Monocid
	Cefotetan	Cefotan
	Cefotiam	Ceradon
	Ceforamide	Precef
	Cefoxitin	Mefoxin
	Cefuroxime	Zinacef
Third generation	Cefoperazone	Cefobid
	Cefotaxime	Claforan
	Ceftazidime	Fortaz, Tazidime
	Ceftizoxime	Cefizox
	Ceftriaxone	Rocephin
	Moxalactam	Moxam
Penicillins		
Natural penicillins	Penicillin G	Pentids
	Penicillin V	Pen V, V-Cillin
Aminopenicillins	Amoxicillin	Amoxil, Larotid, Polymox, Sumox, Trimox
	Ampicillin	Omnipen, Polycillin, Principen, Supen, Totacillin
	Bacampicillin	Spectrobid
	Cyclacillin	Cyclapen
	Hetacillin	Versapen
Extended spectrum penicillins	Azlocillin	Azlin
	Carbenicillin (oral only)	Geocillin
	Mezlocillin	Mezlin
	Piperacillin	Pipracil
	Ticarcillin	Ticar
Penicillinase-Resistant	Cloxacillin	Tegopen cloxacillon
	Dicloxacillin	Dynapen, Pathocil
	Methicillin	Staphcillin
	Nafcillin	Nafcil, Nallpen, Unipen
	Oxacillin	Bactocill, Oxacillin, Prostaphilin

IV Narcotic Infusions

Although narcotics may be administered intravenously for severe pain as a bolus dose, the most effective analgesia is achieved when a consistent serum level of narcotic is maintained. IV narcotic administration allows predictable drug absorption through the use of an infusion that is titrated to achieve analgesia, or with a specialized, programmable pump that allows the patient to administer predetermined doses of the narcotic. The latter method is called patient-controlled analgesia, or PCA.

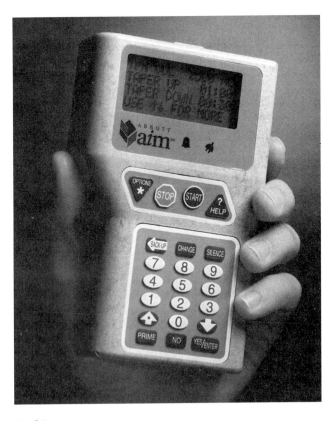

Fig. 6-8
The Abbott AIM-Pain Management.
Courtesy Abbott Laboratories, Abbott Park, IL.

Narcotic infusions are usually prepared as large-volume solutions and are regulated by a pump or controller to ensure accurate drug delivery. Patients require frequent monitoring for respiratory depression and the presence of other adverse narcotic effects such as nausea and vomiting. (Refer to *Chapter Resources* for morphine infusion rates.)

PCA doses are individualized for the patient and allow the patient to deliver a drug dose as needed for pain relief by pushing a button connected to the PCA pump. Frequently, patients use less medication than they are allowed and have accelerated recoveries following surgical procedures: The more consistent pain control is, the greater ease of movement the patient experiences.

Patients with terminal cancer pain are also frequent candidates for PCA. Often these patients are cared for at home. A small ambulatory pump is set at a basal level and then programmed to allow intermittent, patient-controlled bolus doses (Figure 6-8).

Successful PCA requires clear patient instruction. The patient should receive a complete explanation of the pump and an explanation of the lockout interval before surgery. Periodic doses of narcotic may be administered by the nurse when the patient is sleeping to allow prolonged rest periods.

PCA pumps are designed with safeguards, such as allowed doses and lockout intervals, to protect against tampering and misuse of the drugs. Physician orders for PCA include the following:

1. Drug to be administered—usually morphine or meperidine (Demerol)
2. Dose volume—the amount administered each time the PCA infusor is activated
3. Time lockout interval–-the period during which the pump cannot be activated and no analgesia can be delivered; this allows time for the dose to take effect before the patient receives another; the usual lockout interval is 6 to 10 minutes for postoperative pain, but it may be longer according to patient need
4. Volume limits—the maximum volume to be delivered over a prescribed period of time

Epidural Narcotic Infusions

Epidural narcotic infusions are used increasingly for the management of acute and chronic pain (Figure 6-9). Postoperative patients and oncology, trauma, and chronic pain patients all may benefit from epidural narcotics. The discovery of opiate receptors and

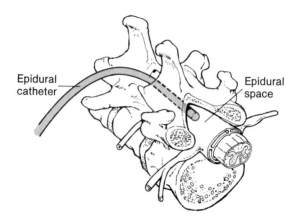

Fig. 6-9
Epidural catheter.

endorphins has led to the use of morphine in the epidural space for pain control. Opiates such as morphine have a direct spinal effect, acting at receptor sites in the dorsal horn of the spinal cord. The major mechanisms by which morphine is thought to gain entry to the dorsal horn are diffusion into and across the cerebrospinal fluid and venous entry along a nerve root sleeve.

The epidural catheter is placed between the dura mater and the vertebral arch, an area that contains fat, blood vessels, and nerves. Some contraindications to epidural catheter placement include the presence of infection, coagulopathy or current anticoagulation therapy, increased intracranial pressure, allergy to narcotics, and patient refusal.

Epidural analgesia brings the patient longer-lasting pain relief with smaller, less-frequent narcotic dosing than the IV route requires. The most intense analgesia is at the level of injection. Analgesia spreads along the dermatomes to provide site-specific pain relief with relatively low morphine doses. Systemic absorption by the epidural vasculature can result in blood levels similar to those provided by an intramuscular injection.

Morphine (duramorph) and fentanyl citrate are the most common narcotics administered. Meperidine and sufentanil citrate are occasionally used. Side effects of epidurally administered narcotics include respiratory depression, nausea and vomiting, urinary retention, and pruritus. Less commonly, catheter migration to the subarachnoid space can occur, causing profound respiratory depression and hypotension.

CLINICAL ALERT: Clearly label epidural catheters to prevent inadvertent administration of IV medications into the epidural space.

There are three different systems used to deliver morphine to the epidural space. The first system is a totally internal system in which an epidural catheter is connected to a reservoir placed in the abdomen. This reservoir's mechanism allows slow, continuous administration of morphine. It must be filled with the desired drug concentration on a weekly or biweekly interval by inserting a Huber needle into the reservoir septum. This system is permanently placed and used most often for the patient requiring long-term pain management.

In the second system, an epidural implantable port with a catheter connected to the portal chamber is anchored to muscle tissue over a bony surface. The catheter is tunneled subcutaneously and then threaded into the epidural space at the desired level, usually L1 or L2. A Huber needle is used to access the septum of the portal chamber,and medication is pumped continuously with an ambulatory, programmable pump. Like the first system, this system is permanently placed and used for the patient who requires long-term pain management.

The third system consists of an externally threaded catheter that is tunneled subcutaneously from the epidural space to an abdominal exit site. It is then connected to an injection cap and a 0.22 μm filter with extension tubing through which morphine can be administered intermittently by an IV infusion pump. This system may be used on a temporary or a permanent basis. Temporary catheters are placed for pain relief following operative procedures such as thoracic, abdominal, orthopedic, and vascular surgery. Temporary catheters may be used also to evaluate the efficacy of this treatment modality before placing a permanent catheter for the management of chronic pain.

Epidural morphine must be free of preservatives and additives and should be prepared under a laminar flow hood. Commercially prepared morphine is available in the following concentrations: 1 mg/ml, 2 mg/ml, 5 mg/ml, and 25 mg/ml. Preservative-free hydromorphone (Dilaudid) and fentanyl citrate are other medications that may be used for epidural analgesia. Many of the ambulatory infusion pumps can hold a 100-ml infusion bag that allows bag changes every 4 to 5 days for patients who receive epidural infusions for chronic pain management (Figure 6-10).

Adverse effects associated with epidural morphine include respiratory depression, urinary retention, pruritus, and nausea and

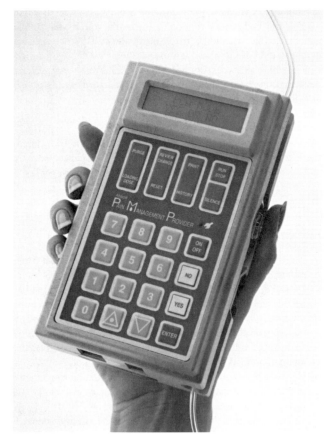

Fig. 6-10
The Abbott Pain Manager-APM.
Courtesy Abbott Laboratories, Abbott Park, IL.

vomiting. These effects are encountered most often with postoperative use of epidural analgesia and may be reversed by an IV naloxone (Narcan) infusion. Patients require ongoing monitoring for pain relief, sedation level, and adverse drug effects, especially respiratory depression. As with all catheters, the site should be assessed for pain or tenderness.

CLINICAL ALERT: Patients receiving epidural narcotic infusions require ongoing observation of their blood pressure and pulse and respiratory rates. Crucial times when the drug will have the most potent effect on the respiration are during the first 2 hours following catheter insertion and again after 6 hours.

Use *preservative-* and *additive-free* morphine for epidural analgesia; never administer IV solutions by the epidural route.

Check catheter placement before injecting a drug by aspirating for clear fluid with bubbles. If yellow- or blood-tinged fluid is aspirated, *stop* the procedure and notify the physician, because only clear fluid should be aspirated. Expect to feel some resistance as the medication is injected.

Documentation Recommendations

- Observation of the site before and after infusion or injection of a drug
- Medication name, dose, route, and time of administration
- All supplies used for medication administration
- Name and amount of all flush solutions (normal saline or heparin)
- Any patient complaints of discomfort symptoms experienced in conjunction with the medication; actions taken to alleviate symptoms (report to physician when applicable)
- With narcotic infusions: pain relief status, sedation levels, analgesia level, and respiratory rate; with PCA: the total dose delivered since the last notation and the number of doses delivered

Conscious Sedation

Combinations of local anesthetics with IV opioids and sedatives are used to cause conscious sedation of patients during diagnostic and minor surgical procedures. Conscious sedation is a depressed level of consciousness during which patients retain the ability to maintain their airway and to respond to physical and verbal stimulation. Advantages include maintenance of consciousness and cooperation, elevation of the pain threshold with minimal changes in vital signs, partial amnesia, and rapid recovery following the procedure.

Patient cooperation with the procedure is essential. Closely monitor the patient during the procedure and during recovery, because there is potential for rapid progression to a state of deep sedation or to general anesthesia. Both experienced personnel and equipment for airway management are essential in all settings where conscious sedation is used.

A position statement of the Association of Operating Room Nurses requires that the registered nurse managing a patient under IV conscious sedation have no other responsibilities during the procedure. Registered nurses require advanced training before working with conscious sedation and need to follow all procedures carefully when monitoring patients under conscious sedation.

Document the ongoing care, monitoring, and other information required by institutional policy, such as oxygen therapy, untoward reactions and subsequent treatment, vital signs, and level of consciousness.

 ## Nursing Diagnoses

- Infection, risk for, related to a break in sterile technique during drug preparation or administration
- Injury, risk for, related to adverse effect of medication
- Pain, related to infiltration or phlebitis

 ## Patient/Family Teaching for Self-Management

Education for home IV medication administration is most effective when a standardized content is developed and a standardized approach is taken to patient education. A learning assessment should include the following patient/family information:

- Reading skills
- Motivation
- Prior self-care experience
- Physical limitations that could interfere with the treatment, such as arthritis, neuropathy, diminished vision

Each skill requires a demonstration and a return demonstration by the patient or the responsible caregiver. Materials sent home with the patient for reference need to be easy to read and should contain pictures of all procedures for nonreaders.

Instruction for self-medication should include the following information:

- Name, dose,and frequency of the drug to be administered
- Aseptic technique
- Use and disposal of needles and syringes
- How to obtain medications and other supplies
- Medication storage requirements and medication preparation (if applicable)
- How to administer the drug
- Infusion pump operation (if applicable)
- Expectations for medical follow-up, such as physician visit, laboratory sampling
- Adverse drug effects and what should be done if these occur
- The importance of strict compliance with the medication regimen and how to recognize symptoms of a worsening condition
- Care of the IV access including problem recognition and troubleshooting techniques

Home Care Considerations

I. Home teaching
   A. Information taught at the initiation of IV therapy should be reviewed on subsequent home visits.
   B. The patient should demonstrate each self-care skill to the nurse.
   C. Inspect storage areas for adequacy.
   D. Teach acceptable thawing methods when frozen drugs are used (NOTE:) microwaves are *not* recommended for thawing antibiotics in the home).
II. Documentation recommendations
   A. Initial visit
      1. Record a detailed physical assessment of the patient, including manual dexterity and coordination.
      2. Document information on home adequacy and safety in relation to IV therapy.
      3. Assess and record the patient's or caregiver's ability to comply with the prescribed regime; include specific situations that indicate evidence of understanding.
      4. Inform the patient of 24-hour staff accessibility and instances when use of the emergency department is indicated.

B. Ongoing visits
 1. Record treatment compliance including storage of supplies; check the temperature of the home refrigerator if temperature is an important factor in drug stability.
 2. Evaluate and record the patient's response to the prescribed treatment, noting any adverse effects and the corrective action taken; include an assessment of vital signs and a review of equipment operation.
 3. Provide evidence of the review of appropriate laboratory data.
 4. Document all other care given.
 5. Record the periodic treatment review conducted with the patient's physician.
C. Dismissal visit
 1. Detail the assessment leading to termination of therapy.
 2. Record all discharge instructions.
III. Quality assurance issues for home IV medication administration—periodic audits should be conducted on topics that indicate safety and availability of all appropriate services; some items include the following:
 A. All educational topics were taught and documented.
 B. There is timely delivery of medications, supplies, and equipment.
 C. Medication information was provided to the patient.
 D. There is 24-hour availability of professional staff for problem solving.
 E. All nursing care providers have current certification for resuscitation, such as Basic Cardiac Life Support.
 F. When IV antibiotics are administered, there is documentation of infection by culture and sensitivity results; the patient is medically stable before home administration has begun; and there is evidence of acceptable infection cure rates in the home setting (it is desirable for a pharmacist to be available to provide pharmacokinetic dosages and drug information).

Geriatric Considerations

Both the use of many drugs (polypharmacy) and the physiologic changes that occur with aging place elderly people at high risk for adverse drug reactions. Some factors to consider include the following:

- Reduced lean body mass (an increased percentage of total body fat) alters the number of receptor sites available for drug binding. This phenomenon increases serum drug levels, so toxic levels can be achieved even using usual drug doses.
- Elderly people normally have a decreased cardiac output and decreased total body water. These conditions adversely affect both drug metabolism and drug excretion in older individuals and predispose this population to more adverse drug effects.
- When the elderly patient experiences disease in one part of the body, there is a reduced ability to maintain physiologic homeostasis. Renal function is frequently compromised in illness, and thus drug excretion is negatively affected.

Chapter Resources

MEDICATION INFUSION RATE

Many medications administered by continuous IV infusion require calculations involving several steps. To minimize these calculations, conversion charts are provided in the following boxes:

Aminophylline infusion rate 1000 ml solution with 1000 mg aminophylline concentration (1 mg/ml)

Volume	Infusion Rate (ml)	Mg/Hr
1000 ml	5	5
	10	10
	15	15
	20	20
	25	25
	30	30
	40	40
	50	50
	60	60

Heparin infusion rate 500 ml solution with 20,000 units heparin concentration (40 units/ml)

Volume	Infusion Rate (ml)	Units/Hr
500 ml	5	200
	10	400
	15	600
	20	800
	25	1000
	30	1200
	35	1400
	40	1600
	45	1800
	50	2000
	55	2200
	60	2400

Morphine infusion rate 500 ml solution with 100 mg morphine sulfate concentration (1 mg/5ml)

Volume	Infusion Rate (ml)	Mg/hr
500 ml	5	1
	10	2
	15	3
	20	4
	25	5
	30	6
	35	7
	40	8
	45	9
	50	10
	55	11
	60	12

Parenteral Drug Administration Audit

	Yes	No	NA
Critical Elements			
1. Checks medication orders with physician orders			
2. Verifies that the medication maTches the patient for whom it is ordered			
3. Verifies that the patient is not allergic to medication			
4. Administers medication in:			
a. Prescribed dose			
b. Prescribed time			
c. Prescribed route			
5. Documents:			
a. Name of medication			
b. Dose			
c. Route			
d. Time			
e. Nurse's name or initial, according to policy			
f. Response of the patient to the medication, if indicated			
g. Patient education regarding potential side effects of drugs			
h. Blood return status and frequency			
Routes of Drug Administration			
1. IV Push Medications:			
a. Checks IV site for infiltration and patency			
b. Administers medication without introducing contaminate			
c. Administers IV at prescribed rate			
d. Validates blood return before, during, and at the end of drug administration (when administering chemotherapy)			
e. Following IV push medication, locks the IV catheter according to agency policy			

Continued.

Parenteral Drug Administration Audit—cont'd

	Yes	No	NA
2. IV Piggyback Medications:			
a. Checks IV site for infiltration/patency			
b. Administers medication without introducing contaminate			
c. Administers IV at prescribed infusion rate			
d. Administers IV drug with prescribed dilution			
e. Flushes IV site in a timely manner following completion of infusion to ensure site patency			
3. Continuous IV Infusions:			
a. Checks IV site for infiltration/patency			
b. Administers medication without introducing contaminate			
c. Administers IV at prescribed rate			
d. Uses electronic-controlled devices to monitor and assist in administration of drug infusion			
e. Attaches time-tape label to IV solution			
f. Following completion of IV continuous infusion, locks IV catheter or discontinues peripheral IV site			
4. Intraperitoneal (IP):			
a. Checks IP site for patency			
b. Administers medication without introducing contaminate			
c. Administers IP drug at prescribed rate			
d. Following completion of drug administration, injects normal saline to maintain catheter patency			

Parenteral Drug Administration Audit—cont'd

	Yes	No	NA
5. Intraarterial (IA):			
a. Checks IA site for patency			
b. Administers medication without introducing contaminate			
c. Administers IA drug at prescribed rate			
d. Electronic pump is used to monitor and assist in drug administration			
e. Validates blood return q2hr with continuous IV			
f. Following completion of IA drug, injects normal saline or heparinized saline to maintain catheter patency			
6. Intrathecal:			
a. Prepares drug in 3-ml syringe and attaches 23-gauge butterfly needle with tubing to syringe			
b. *Physician* injects drug via Ommaya reservoir or lumbar puncture			
c. Following completion of intrathecal drug, the *physician* flushes device with preservative-free saline			
Management of Drug Extravasation of Antineoplastic Agents			
1. Can state signs and symptoms of drug extravasation			
2. Can state the procedure for drug extravasation			
3. Knows placement of supplies used in management of drug extravasation			

TOPICS FOR POLICY STATEMENTS CONCERNING IV INSTRUMENTATION
Indications for Use of Pumps or Controllers

1. Priority list for use during high patient census
2. Administration of medication, including the following:

    a. Statement regarding intermittent medications and heparin locks

    b. Central lines

    c. Arterial lines

    d. Special applications, such as double- or triple-lumen catheters, blood

    e. Administration of chemotherapy and treatment of infiltration (extravasation) of chemotherapeutic drugs

    f. Registering central venous pressure measurement

3. Tracking of accumulated volumes

4. Inspection of site when using an infusion pump

5. Pressure titrations

6. Use of volume limit feature

7. Transfer of patients, that is, unit to unit

8. Use of volumetric sets (burettes)

9. Responsibilities of users including registered nurses, licensed practical nurses, nurse's aides, ancillaries

10. Documentation of instrument use on patient record

11. Special sets required

SKILL CHECKLIST

IV Medication Administration

1. Checks for patient allergies.

2. Demonstrates 5 rights.
   a. Medication
   b. Dose
   c. Time
   d. Patient
   e. Route

3. Identifies type of IV line.
   a. Peripheral
   b. Midline
   c. PICC
   d. Central

4. Obtains correct flush supplies and solution.

5. Unclamps IV line when clamped.

6. Uses aseptic technique.

7. Checks for patency of IV site.

8. Flushes line with correct volume of normal saline.

9. Administers medication using correct IV push or IV piggyback procedure.
10. Demonstrates proper rate of administration.
11. Flushes IV after medication with normal saline at the same rate as the medication was administered to clear the IV line. Finishes with a locking flush.
12. Reestablishes IV flow rate of continuous IV solution if indicated.
13. Documents procedure.

Study Questions

1. The half-life of a drug refers to the following:
   a. Half of the loading dose
   b. A value measured after the third dose
   c. Time for plasma levels to fall to half original level
   d. A value that is not measured if a drug is given continuously

2. The following is true of drug peak levels:
   a. The level is measured prior to a drug dose
   b. The level is measured within 30 minutes of dose completion
   c. Must be drawn daily for the first two days
   d. Are measured if a toxicity is suspected

3. Which of the following is not true regarding adverse drug reactions?
   a. May be a side effect that is documented in the literature
   b. Is usually a predictable medical emergency
   c. Hypersensitivity occurs more rapidly with IV drug administration
   d. The very young and the elderly are at greatest risk

4. Which of the following is not true of drug incompatibility?
   a. Visual inspection will detect particulate formation in an IV solution.
   b. Chemical effects are often not detected with visual inspection of a solution.
   c. Drug incompatibility results in physical, chemical, and therapeutic changes.
   d. Refrigeration improves drug stability.

5. True or false: IV push medication administration provides a predictable drug response.
   a. True
   b. False

6. True or false: A major adverse effect of aminoglycosides is nephrotoxicity.
   a. True
   b. False

7. True or false: Urinary retention is a potential adverse effect of epidural analgesia.
   a. True
   b. False

ANSWERS: 1. c   2. b   3. b   4. a   5. a   6. a   7. a

Blood and Blood Component Administration

7

Objectives

1. List critical verification elements of blood product, donor, and recipient prior to initiating a blood product transfusion.

2. Discuss the nursing management process for initiating blood product transfusions related to equipment, patient monitoring, and documentation.

3. Recognize potential signs and symptoms for acute hemolytic transfusion reaction.

4. Describe the nursing management process for blood and blood product transfusion reaction.

5. List three national agencies that monitor blood and blood product transfusion practices.

General Principles of Blood Transfusion Therapy

Blood transfusions have been a major factor in restoring and maintaining quality of life for patients with cancer, hematological disorders, and trauma-related injuries and those who have undergone major surgical procedures. Although blood transfusions are significant for the return to homeostasis, they can be detrimental. Many complications can result from blood component therapy, such as potentially lethal acute hemolytic reactions, transmission of infectious disease (hepatitis, AIDS), and febrile reactions. Most life-threatening transfusion reactions result from incorrect identification of patients or inaccurate labeling of blood samples or blood components, leading to the administration of incompatible blood. Monitoring patients receiving blood and blood components and administration of these products are nursing responsibilities. Blood components should be administered by competent, experienced, well-prepared personnel following the guidelines of the accrediting organizations and agencies providing blood component therapy.

Blood Group Antigens, Antibodies, Rh Type, HLA Antigen

Blood is composed of several constituents that play a major role in blood transfusion therapy. These components—antigens, antibodies, Rh type, and HLA antigen—contribute greatly to the success of any transfusion.

An antigen is a substance that elicits a specific immune response when coming in contact with foreign matter. The body's immune system responds by producing antibodies to destroy the invader. This antigen (Ag) and antibody (AB) reaction is demonstrated by agglutination or hemolysis. The antibody in the serum responds to the invading antigen by clumping the red cells together and rendering them ineffective or by completely destroying the red cell. Blood typing systems are based on Ag-AB reactions that determine blood compatibility.

The ABO blood group is important in transfusion therapy. Blood type is determined by detection of both antigens on the red cells and corresponding antibodies in the plasma. The antigens on the red cells that are important in the ABO system are the A antigen and the B antigen. Individuals with type A blood have A antigen present on red blood cells; type B individuals have B antigen present; and type O individuals have neither antigen present.

Corresponding antibodies exist in the plasma for each of the antigens (A, B). These antibodies occur naturally in the blood. The antibodies, anti-A and anti-B, act against the antigen normally present. If the patient's ABO blood type is B, the B antigen is present on the red blood cells and the anti-A antibody occurs naturally in the plasma.

After the ABO system, the Rh type is the group of red cell antigens with greatest clinical importance. Unlike anti-A and anti-B, which occur in normal, unimmunized individuals, Rh antibodies do not develop without an immunizing stimulus. Persons whose red blood cells possess D are called Rh positive; those whose cells lack D are called Rh negative, no matter what other Rh antigens are present. The presence of this antibody (anti-D) may cause destruction of the red blood cell, as in the case of delayed hemolytic transfusion reaction.

Blood typing identifies the ABO and Rh groupings in the donor blood. Crossmatching then determines the compatibility of donor and recipient cells. ABO and Rh compatibility criteria are essential in blood transfusion therapy.

The HLA system is the next component to consider in transfusion therapy. It is based on antigens present on leukocytes, platelets, and other cells. HLA typing and crossmatching are sometimes necessary before repeated platelet transfusions. Granulocytes and platelets with HLA typing compatible with the patient have a longer life span when infused. HLA-matched granulocytes and platelets are *avoided* in patients who are expected to be candidates for a bone marrow transplant (BMT) to diminish potential graft-versus-host disease (GVHD).

Indications for Transfusion

The primary indications for transfusion are to provide adequate blood volume and prevent hemorrhagic shock, increase the oxygen-carrying capacity of blood, and replace blood platelets or clotting factors to maintain hemostasis. Numerous blood components are available, each with its own potential benefits and adverse effects.

Whole Blood

Transfusing a unit of whole blood (500 ml) over 30 to 60 minutes increases the blood volume by this amount. The six general rules for transfusion of whole blood are as follows:

1. Transfuse whole blood only for the treatment of acute, massive hemorrhage.
2. Do not give whole blood when the ABO group is unknown.
3. Use platelet concentrates and fresh-frozen plasma to correct documented impaired homeostasis when large volumes of whole blood have been transfused.
4. Administration of whole blood should be synonymous with multiple transfusion.
5. Whole blood is for treating patients who are actively bleeding and who have lost greater than 25 percent of total blood volume.

6. Whole blood is indicated only for patients with symptomatic deficit in O_2 carrying capacity combined with hypovolemia of such a degree to be associated with shock.

7. Whole blood is indicated for cardiopulmonary bypass patients, introperatively and during the first 6 hours postoperatively.

Red Blood Cells

Red blood cells (RBCs) are the component of choice to restore or maintain oxygen-carrying capacity. Transfusing red blood cells increases the oxygen-carrying capacity with minimal expansion of blood volume and therefore is indicated when chronic anemia and congestive heart failure exist. RBC transfusions may be administered for red cell loss (hemoglobin greater than 8 Gm/dl) or for losses related to obstetrical, surgery, trauma, or treatment-related side effects, such as losses incurred in chemotherapy, radiation therapy, or bone marrow transplantation.

Two major types of RBC products are available. The first is an RBC product with CPDA-1 anticoagulant with a final hematocrit value of 70 percent to 80 percent. Second is an RBC product with 100 ml additive solution (AS-1) containing RBCs with 90 percent of the plasma removed and 100 ml of a special solution containing necessary additional preservative to increase shelf life and decrease viscosity.

Leukocyte-poor red blood cells are given to multiparous women and previously transfused patients who develop antibodies to leukocytes or platelets. These products prevent recurrence of febrile, nonhemolytic transfusion reactions caused by donor white blood cell (WBC) antigens reacting with recipient WBC antibody.

Platelet Types

There are two types of platelet products: (1) single-donor platelets (obtained by apheresis), whereby a single donor's platelets are harvested while returning red cells, yielding a product of six to ten units of transfusable platelets; and (2) multidonor (random) platelets, which are obtained by centrifuging units of whole blood and expressing off the platelet-rich plasma. One unit of whole blood yields one unit of platelets; therefore, multiple platelet units must be pooled together to obtain a sufficient quantity for a transfusion.

Indications for platelet transfusion relate to the platelet count, the functional ability of the patient's platelets, and the patient's clinical condition. Individuals with platelet counts of 20,000/mm^3 or less and who do not have specific platelet-destroying disease benefit from prophylactic transfusion. Patients who are actively bleeding or require major surgery require a platelet count of 50,000/mm.^{3} Platelets are transfused to control or prevent bleeding associated with deficiencies in the number or function of a patient's platelets. The platelet unit will increase the recipient's platelet count by 5,000 to 10,000 mm.^{3} It is recommended to give one unit of random platelets for every 10 kg of body weight, or one platelet pheresis pack. Obtain a postplatelet count at 1 and 24 hours after platelet transfusion.

Granulocyte Transfusion

Only patients with documented granulocyte abnormalities in number or function should receive granulocyte transfusion. Examples are those with severe neutropenia with a granulocyte count of less than 500/mm^3 and evidence of significant infection or temperature greater than 38.3°C with lack of responsiveness to antibiotic to which the organism is known to be sensitive. The patient receiving granulocyte transfusions should have a good chance of recovering from the episode of neutropenia. Granulocytes should be transfused as soon as possible after collection but must be infused within 24 hours. The granulocyte concentrates are usually given daily for at least 4 to 6 days unless bone marrow recovers or severe reactions occur.

Febrile reactions often occur in patients receiving granulocyte concentrates. Antipyretics (nonaspirin) are administered for this reaction. Meperidine injection may be prescribed by the physician to stop shaking chills. Avoid infusion of amphotericin B at the same time; infuse 4 hours before and after granulocyte transfusion. Potential exists for pulmonary insufficiency and leukocytosis in lungs.

The use of granulocyte transfusions to treat neutropenia has decreased in recent years because of difficulties in collecting a sufficient number of granulocytes. The other significant issue is the availability and varied uses of the hematopoietic growth factors (e.g., granulocyte-colony-stimulating factor, granulocyte-macrophage-colony-stimulating factor, and interleukin-3). The hematopoietic growth factors provide a stimulus response to the bone marrow stem cells to produce more cells in the peripheral blood.

Massive Transfusion

Massive transfusion is the replacement of the patient's total blood volume within a 24-hour period. A blood volume is estimated as 75 ml/kg, or about 5000 ml (10 or more units of whole blood) in a 70-kg adult.

Complications that may result from massive transfusion include circulatory overload, microemboli, hypothermia, citrate toxicity, hypokalemia, hyperkalemia, and coagulation disorders. Patients receiving massive transfusions must be observed closely during the transfusion process. Replacement of blood volume requires rapid infusion (greater than 100 ml/min) of *warmed* blood components or isotonic saline solutions. Frequent laboratory testing is performed during and after the transfusion process to monitor critical values—hemoglobin, hematocrit, prothrombin time, platelet count, sodium, potassium, and calcium levels, and arterial blood gases.

Volume Expanders

Volume expanders such as Hespan, dextran, and Plasmonate provide expansion to the plasma volume and may be used in conjunction with blood product infusions. Volume expanders are recommended for use early in the management of shock or impending shock from burns, hemorrhage, surgery, sepsis, or trauma, as well as for maintenance of cardiac output. A physician's order is required to use the varied products. Adverse reactions may include circulatory overload, pulmonary edema, nephrotoxicity, hypotension, and hypersensitivity reactions. Because of the potential serious adverse reactions, prudent monitoring of the patient before, during, and after volume expander infusion is required.

Frequently Transfused Patients

Following frequent transfusions, alloimmunization to red cells, platelets, and leukocyte (HLA) antigens may occur. This results in crossmatching difficulty and febrile and allergic reactions. Alloimmunization risk may be decreased by limiting the number of transfusions or donors, using leukocyte-depleted components, and using irradiated blood products. The patient receiving frequent transfusions should be closely monitored throughout the transfusion process. Administration of the blood component is usually given over an increased infusion time.

Irradiated Blood Products

Viable lymphocytes (cells capable of division) present in all cellular transfusion products, including stored RBCs, are thought to be capable of triggering GVHD. This rejection reaction of the graft against seemingly "foreign" host tissues can occur in both allogenic and autologous patients. GVHD can occur in HLA-matched siblings, allogenic BMT recipients, and more frequently with lesser degrees of matches. Using irradiated blood products can avert GVHD produced by blood products transfusion. Blood products that have been exposed to a measured amount of radiation render the donor lymphocytes incapable of replication. The usual radiation dosage recommended is between 1.5 and 3.0 Gray (1500 to 3000 centiGray) of gamma radiation. The irradiation of blood products usually takes place at the regional blood center, at the hospital blood bank, or in the hospital radiation therapy department.

Irradiated blood products are used to prevent GVHD in immunocompromised patients who are receiving blood components containing viable WBCs. Irradiation destroys the donor lymphocytes' ability to engraft in the patient. Patients susceptible to transfusion-associated GVHD are those who have Hodgkin's or non-Hodgkin's lymphoma, aplastic anemia, acute leukemia, or congenital immunodeficiency disorder; low-birth-weight neonates; and patients undergoing bone marrow transplant or intrauterine transfusions.

A recent problem with directed donations is transfusion-associated graft-versus-host disease (TA-GVHD). Although exceedingly rare, TA-GVHD carries a mortality rate approaching 100%. This high mortality rate is associated with bone marrow failure. TA-GVHD has been associated most frequently with directed donations from first-degree relatives such as parents or siblings. TA-GVHD occurs when the transfusion recipient has two nonidentical HLA haplotypes and the transfusion (lymphocyte) donor is homozygous (identical) for either of the HLA haplotypes of the recipient. The recipient is unable to recognize the donor lymphocytes as "not-self" while the donor (transfused) lymphocytes *are* able to recognize the recipient as "not-self." The lymphocyte reaction is essentially the same as that seen following allogenic marrow transplantation. Because of the potential for

TA-GVHD following directed donation, it is recommended that all blood components from first-degree relatives be irradiated before transfusion.

Quality Control Measures

Blood bank responsibilities

Blood collection facilities have the responsibility for providing the safety and efficacy of each blood product it collects. The American Association of Blood Banks (AABB), American Red Cross, Food and Drug Administration, and Occupational Safety and Health Administration (OSHA) provide rules, regulations, and standards for operation to which all blood bank centers must comply.

Criteria for collection of donor blood are the following:

1. Detailed health history; especially related to high-risk activities associated with AIDS and hepatitis (hepatitis B and C, HIV 1 and 2)
2. Screening for diseases such as hepatitis B and C, HIV 1 and 2, human T-cell leukemia virus types I (HTLV-1—T-cell leukemia) and II (HTLV-II—hairy-cell leukemia), syphilis, and cytomegalovirus antigen when the blood product will be given to bone marrow and organ transplantation patients
3. A check for vital signs (blood pressure, temperature, pulse)
4. Minimum age of 17 years
5. Weight not less than 110 pounds
6. Freedom from any skin disease
7. Time since last blood donation at least 56 days
8. Hemoglobin level of at least 12.5 g/dl or higher (or hematocrit value at least 38% or higher) for female patients and 13.5 g/dl for male patients

Who can donate blood?

Some conditions may warrant temporary deferral from donation, such as colds, flu, and therapy with certain drugs, but the following groups are *permanently* ineligible as homologous donors:

- People who have AIDS or symptoms of AIDS or who have ever tested positive for AIDS or for the AIDS virus
- Men who have had sex with another man since 1977—even just one time
- Men and women who have ever taken illegal drugs by needle—even just one time
- Men and women who have had sex with a prostitute in the last 12 months

- People who have had sex with anyone who fits in the preceding categories
- People who have ever had hepatitis
- People who have a history of certain types of cancer (other than minor skin cancer)
- People who have hemophilia or who have received clotting factor concentrates

Procedure for blood collection

To prevent any potential contamination to the blood specimen, a thorough, skilled, sterile procedure is used. The skin is scrubbed with povidone-iodine solution, and the blood is collected into sterile, labeled tubes and bags. The donor's blood is tested for ABO grouping, Rh type (including D), antibody screening, rapid plasma reagin (RPR) syphilis, hepatitis B surface antigen, hepatitis C core antibody, alanine aminotransferase (ALT)—also called serum glutamic-pyrovi transaminase (SGPT)—hepatitis C antibody, HIV-1 and 2 antibodies, and HTLV-I and II antibodies.

To ensure accuracy in collecting blood samples for recipients of transfusions and for those providing blood donation, the following guidelines have been developed:

1. The intended recipient and the blood sample shall be identified positively at the time of the collection.
2. Blood samples shall be obtained in stoppered tubes, each identified with a firmly attached label bearing at least the recipient's first and last names, identification number, and the date.
3. The completed label shall be attached to the tube before leaving the recipient.
4. There must be a mechanism to identify the person who drew the blood.
5. Before a specimen is used for blood typing or compatibility testing, all identification information on the request form shall be confirmed by a qualified person as being in agreement with that on the specimen label; *in case of discrepancy or doubt, another specimen shall be obtained.* (See *Chapter Resources* for "Transfusion Resources")

Storage techniques

Red cell products are stored under temperature-controlled refrigeration in the range of 1° to 6°C. Platelets are usually stored at 22° to 24°C (room temperature) and require gentle agitation during storage. Plasma separated from whole blood shortly after collection can be frozen at −18°C or lower temperatures for use as coagulation factor-rich plasma (fresh-frozen plasma).

The blood bank cannot refrigerate and later reissue *any* blood component meant to be stored at 1° to 6°C if the temperature of the component exceeded 10°C (50° F) at any time. This will happen if the blood component is removed from the blood bank refrigerator for longer than 30 minutes.

CLINICAL ALERT: Refrigeration and freezing of blood products on the nursing unit does not ensure accurate temperature regulation and is never acceptable.

Release of blood products

Only qualified blood bank personnel may issue any blood components, and only after following all the guidelines for proper identification of the blood unit—ABO grouping, Rh type, antibody screening, and expiration date (Fig. 7-1). The ABO group and Rh type must match on the donor unit and the requested transfusion form. On some occasions, substitutions occur in the blood bank.

Group O packed red cells (not whole blood) may be substituted for any ABO group. Rh (D) negative red cells may be safely transfused to Rh (D) positive patients. Rh (D) positive red cells may *not* be safely transfused to Rh (D) negative patients. However, it is acceptable to transfuse Rh (D) positive plasma products to Rh (D) negative patients, because Rh (D) antigens are on the red cells only.

Separation techniques—apheresis

Apheresis is a process that removes whole blood from the donor and then separates it into component parts by centrifugation, harvesting the desired component. The remainder is returned to the donor, thus allowing collection of large amounts of a single component for an individual recipient. This technique is used for selective collection of platelets or white cells (granulocytes), and it provides human leukocytes and matched platelets in sufficient numbers for specific patients.

Currently apheresis is being used extensively for harvesting peripheral blood stem cells in autologous and allogenic peripheral stem transplantation. A large-bore double-lumen central catheter is placed to permit the collection of stem cells through apheresis. The patient's blood is circulated through a high-speed cell separator, and the peripheral stem cells are retained and stored. The plasma

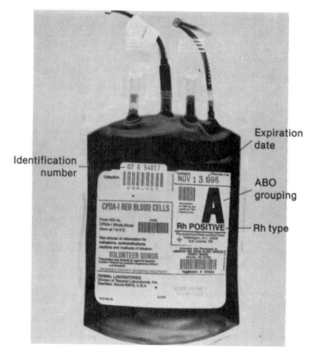

Fig. 7-1
Blood product identification.

and erythrocytes are returned to the patient. Approximately 9 to 14 liters of blood are processed over 2 to 4 hours. The number of apheresis procedures performed depends on the viability and number of the collected stem cells. Generally, 6 to 8 apheresis procedures are performed over a week to 10 days. Stem cell harvest is usually performed on an outpatient basis.

Autologous transfusions

Autotransfusion has become an accepted cornerstone in comprehensive blood conservation programs. Autologous transfusion is the reinfusion of a patient's own blood by various methods. There are several advantages to autologous transfusions: Because exposure to homologous red blood cell transfusions is minimized, there is no disease transmission (hepatitis, AIDS) or alloimmunization, and using the patients' own blood is sometimes an acceptable alternative for patients who object to receiving banked blood for religious reasons.

Preoperative autologous blood donation begins 4 to 6 weeks before surgery, with the last donation collected no later than 72 hours before the surgical procedure. The units are collected, properly labeled, and stored using the AABB guidelines. Bacteremia is the only absolute contraindication. A patient must have a hemoglobin level of at least 11 g/dl and a hematocrit level greater than 34 percent before each donation.

Perioperative blood salvage is collected during surgery (thoracic or cardiovascular surgery, ruptured ectopic pregnancy, liver transplantation, or repair of traumatic injuries). To remove blood from the wound, the surgeon uses a suction wand with a double-lumen catheter. The catheter delivers an anticoagulant CPDA-1 (citrate-phosphate-dextrose-adenine) or heparin to the tip of the wand. Blood mixes with the anticoagulant and is collected in a sterile plastic container with a flexible lining and filter. The salvaged blood is filtered and reinfused as whole blood or processed before the infusion. Salvaged blood must not be stored because neither filtering nor processing can remove bacteria completely from the blood.

Autotransfusion systems are regulated by the FDA and must meet safety and regulatory guidelines. Some features that are incorporated into the design of the devices include a preset suction control mechanism to regulate the vacuum and allow consistent suction throughout the collection period, a mechanism to protect tissue damage at the wound site and protect RBCs from potential hemolysis, a spill-proof bag and suction port to prevent spillage if the unit is tipped over, and a one-way valve to allow air-evacuation while preventing air reentry.

Blood collection for reinfusion must be completed within 6 hours of *initiating* the collection process if the blood is going to be used. Blood salvage is not attempted during procedures that involve spilled intestinal contents, bacterial peritonitis, intraabdominal abscess, osteomyelitis, or cancer resections.

Hemodilution is the process by which the patient's blood is withdrawn from the patient (immediately before surgery in the operative suite) and replaced with an IV infusion of a crystalloid or colloid solution to maintain volume for adequate circulation. The collected blood is reinfused after the bleeding has been controlled.

Reinfusing salvaged blood after surgery is accomplished by collection of the blood through a closed, sterile, plastic drainage system (Fig. 7-2). Collection techniques include carefully regulating suction (not to exceed 100 mm Hg), adding anticoagulant ACD-A per physician's order, monitoring the fluid level in the sterile container at least every hour, and keeping the system closed and free of air. Because of bacterial growth risks, the blood should not remain in the collection reservoir for more than 6 hours. The blood can be reinfused by gravity drip or infusion pump. The blood must be reinfused within 6 hours of *initiating* the collection process if it is going to be used. Use of microaggregate filter for reinfusion of the blood product is required.

CLINICAL ALERT: Follow all the AABB guidelines for patient identification: Correctly write the patient's name, identification number, date, time collection was initiated, and anticoagulant used on the space provided on the autotransfusion collection device. Consult the manufacturer's guidelines and instructions for setup and use of postoperative autotransfusion systems.

Time of blood production administration

Identification of the patient and the proper blood component are the most important procedures in transfusion safety. The correct blood product must be verified, and all labels must be read carefully. All information on the blood product (donor number, ABO group, Rh type, and expiration date) must be compared and matched with the patient's identification bracelet and the transfusion requisition. Discrepancies in spelling, identification numbers, or expiration dates should not exist. All the identification steps must be confirmed by licensed nursing personnel or blood bank personnel before the transfusion is initiated. Baseline vital signs must be obtained, and the patient must be monitored throughout the transfusion process. On completion of the infusion, the date and time the blood unit was initiated and infusion completed must be documented on the transfusion requisition. Signatures of the personnel confirming all identification information and initiating the transfusion must also be recorded on the requisition.

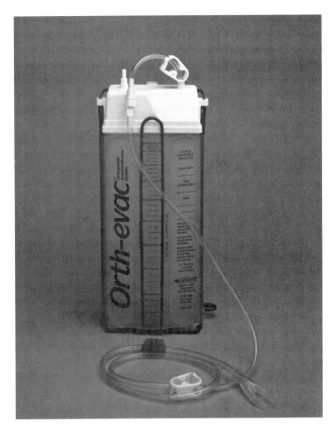

Fig. 7-2
Orthopedic Autotransfusion System.
Courtesy Deknatel Snowden Pencer, Fluid Management Systems, Tucker, GA.

Equipment and Supplies Used for Transfusions
Equipment
Blood warmers

The warming of the blood to the body temperature is necessary during transfusions in certain clinical situations. Research indicates that rapid or massive administration of cold blood has a hypothermic effect on the patient and could have lethal consequences. Patients with cold agglutinin disease (cold-type autoimmune hemolytic anemia in which unexpected antibodies in the patient's serum react at temperatures below 20°C) need to have the blood warmed before transfusion to diminish potential adverse effects. Exchange transfusions in neonates and children receiving rapid or massive transfusions must always be warmed, especially when given through a central line. Hypothermia produced by the rapid infusion of cold blood may lead to dysrhythmia and cardiac arrest. For patients requiring extensive operative procedures, a 2°C body temperature loss is not uncommon, reducing the normal body temperature to 35°C. In these situations blood must be infused at this temperature (35°C) to prevent further heat loss.

An effective blood warmer provides a constant temperature between 32° and 37°C and flows to 150ml/min. Because warm blood dilates veins, reduced resistance helps to offset flow loss that may result when a warmer is attached. Commercial blood warmers may use a warm bath or dry incubator through which blood passes in sterile, disposable plastic coils to warm the blood. Safety mechanisms include thermostats and audible and visual alarm systems for close monitoring of the blood temperature. Follow the prescribed manufacturer's directions for appropriate use and the specific tubings and supplies required.

CLINICAL ALERT: Heating blood under hot-water faucets, in incubators, or in microwave ovens can cause hemolysis and is never acceptable.

Pressure cuffs

A pressure cuff is the most commonly used device for increasing the flow rate during transfusion. To increase flow rate, the pressure cuff sleeve is secured snugly around the blood bag. The pressure cuff is then filled by a pressure manometer (similar to a blood pressure cuff) that inflates the sleeve with air. As the blood unit empties, the pressure sleeve decreases. Agency guidelines for use of pressure cuffs should be followed. Use only cuffs specifically designed for blood infusion. Do *not* exceed 300 mm Hg when pressure-transfusing components containing red blood cells.

Electronic infusion devices

The use of an electronic infusion pump is strongly advised for all pediatric transfusions, although the flow rate is difficult to regulate when small volumes are administered. Gravity flow administration (as used in the adult) is contraindicated because of its potential for allowing too much blood flow over a short period of time. Whenever electronic infusion devices are used, the nurse should be knowledgeable of the features of the device used—for example, alarm operation and rate consistency, rate and volume of infusion, memory, power supply, and maintenance—and the manufacturer's recommendations for the types of solutions the device is capable of delivering. Not all electronic infusion devices are acceptable for use in transfusing blood products.

Supplies

Filters

Blood and components must always be transfused through a filter designed to retain blood product debris. Standard filters have a pore size of about 170μm. To use a blood filter properly, the tubings and filter must be primed adequately. The filter needs to be completely covered with blood or component, and the drip chamber in the tubing should be approximately half full. Incomplete priming can result in air being trapped in the filter, thus causing an inaccurate drop rate. Damage to blood cells may occur if they fall on the exposed filter. Priming procedures differ slightly from one brand of filter and tubing to another; therefore, it is important to follow the manufacturer's instructions included with each set.

Microaggregate filters with a pore size of 20 to 40μm are used occasionally for massive transfusions, open-heart surgery, and preparation of leukocyte-poor blood. These filters trap the smaller particles that have potential for causing microemboli. For routine blood transfusions, microaggregate filters are used more often with children than with adults. The manufacturer's guidelines for the correct procedure in priming the filter and (if applicable) for flushing the filter after the transfusion should be followed.

 CLINICAL ALERT: Do not use a blood filter set for more than 4 hours. If the flow rate decreases after more than 1 unit has been transfused, you may have to change the filter set.

High-efficiency leukocyte depletion filters

Considerable data link nonhemolytic febrile transfusion reactions, HLA alloimmunizations, and CMV transmission of infection to white cells in homologous transfusions. In many high-risk populations, leukocyte filtration is a standard of care and has been demonstrated to be cost-effective. The new information concerning leukocyte-associated viral reactivation and postoperative infections suggests that a wider population of patients would benefit from leukocyte reduction. Surgical procedures such as cardiac procedures, joint replacement, transplants, transurethral resection of the prostate, and vascular surgery are the major consumers of blood and blood products. Patients undergoing these surgical procedures should be evaluated for leukoreduction blood and blood products.

High-efficiency leukocyte removal devices use a surface modification that is permanently integrated into the microfibrous filter medium (Figs. 7-3 and 7-4). These fibers have an affinity for leukocytes, so as the blood component passes through the filter,

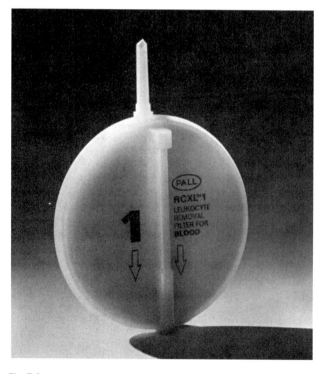

Fig. 7-3
Pall RCXL 1 High Efficiency Leukocyte Removal Filter for Red Cell Transfusion.
Courtesy Pall Biomedical Product Co, Port Washington, NY.

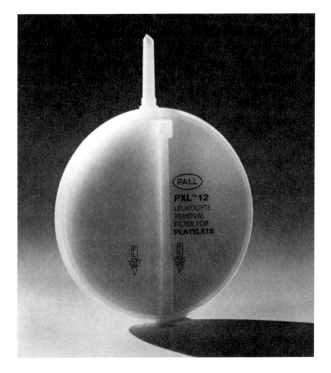

Fig. 7-4
Pall PXL 12 High Efficiency Leukocyte Removal Filter for Platelet Transfusion.
Courtesy Pall Biomedical Product Co, Port Washington, NY.

greater than 99.9% of the leukocytes are removed. When used according to the manufacturer's instructions, these filters provide consistent performance; however, when used improperly, they can cause difficulties during the transfusion. For example, not properly priming a leukocyte depletion filter according to the manufacturer's directions can create an air lock. To avoid misuse and to achieve the manufacturer's stated claims, platelets and red blood cells should be given through a leukocyte removal filter designed for that specific transfusion. Filters used for more than the manufacturer's recommended number of units will no longer remove the desired number of leukocytes.

CLINICAL ALERT: High-efficiency leukocyte removal filters for red blood cells and platelets are *not* interchangeable. For example, it is not recommended to use a leukocyte-depleting RBC filter to transfuse platelets or a leukocyte-depleting platelet filter to transfuse RBCs. Follow the manufacturer's instructions. Leukocyte depletion filters are *not* indicated for transfusion of granulocytes.

Tubings

Filtered IV tubings may contain a single line from the blood bag to the patient or a Y-type (dual) line. The Y-type set allows the infusion of normal saline while the blood component bags are being initiated or changed. This dual line offers the availability of normal saline to be used as a diluent for red blood cells that are too viscous to flow properly. However, AS-1 RBCs are already diluted with 100 ml of the adenine saline preservative. Therefore, additional saline is *not* needed to increase flow. CPDA-1 RBCs are the type of RBCs that would flow better with the addition of normal saline. In the event of a blood transfusion reaction, the dual line provides an immediate IV access for isotonic solutions (Fig. 7-5).

Only normal saline (0.9% USP) may be administered with blood. Solutions such as 5% dextrose in water or Ringer's lactate solution can cause in vivo hemolysis or initiate coagulation of the donor blood. Medications should *never* be added to a unit of blood.

Blood and Blood Components

Table 7-1 lists blood and many blood components with the approximate volume of each unit, the recommended filter, and the administration rate. The comment section refers to ABO and Rh compatibility and specific product preparation for infusion. The agency blood bank or blood center should be referred to for blood product information.

Protocol for Blood and Blood Component Administration
Pretransfusion

1. Verify prescribed physician order for specific blood or blood component with the appropriate date of transfusion administration.
2. Verify patient's informed consent (see guidelines for obtaining informed consent in *Chapter Resources*).

Text continued on p. 199.

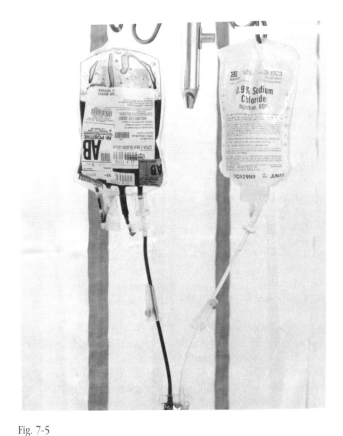

Fig. 7-5
Blood administration with normal saline. Note that the RBC is a CP-DA-1 RBC.

From Perry AG, Potter PA: *Clinical nursing skills and techniques,* ed 3, St Louis, 1994, Mosby.

Table 7-1 Blood and blood components

Product	Infusion Guidelines
Red Blood Cells *Volume* AS-1 RBC 375–425 ml CPDA-1 RBC 300–350 nl *Filter* Standard 170 μm blood filter or micro-aggregate filter	Infuse over 1½–2 hours; maximum: 4 hr/unit; if blood loss, transfuse as rapidly as the patient can tolerate; if the patient is in unstable cardiovascular balance (chronic severe anemia, congestive heart failure, very small, or young) and circulatory overload is a concern, rate should be 1 ml/kg/hr; average pediatric dose and rate: 10 ml/kg, 2–4 ml/kg/hr
High-Efficiency Leukocyte Depletion Filter	*Comments* Must be ABO and Rh compatible; occasionally RH_O negative will be transfused to an Rh_O positive patient, but *never* an Rh_O positive to an Rh_O negative; group O packed red cells may be given to *any* blood group, provided the Rh type is appropriate; crossmatch is required
Washed Red Cells (WRCs) (Leukocyte-Poor) *Volume* 200 to 280 ml *Filter* Standard 170 μm blood filter	Infuse over 1½–2 hours *Comments* Same as RBCs; blood bank requires notification to prepare WRCs; cells expire 24 hours after washing

Continued.

Table 7-1 Blood and blood components—cont'd

Product	Infusion Guidelines

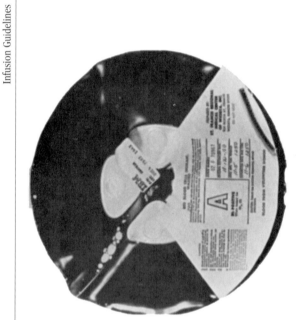

Washed red cells.

Frozen-Deglycerolized Red Cells (FDRCs)

Volume
200–250 ml
Filter
Standard 170 µm blood filter

Infuse over 1½–2 hours

Comments
Same as RBCs; blood bank will not deglycerolize until requested; required time to deglycerolize, approximately 1 hour; used primarily for transplant patients or patients who have multiple antibodies; expires 24 hours after deglycerolizing; frozen must be thawed and washed before administration to remove glycerol

Whole Blood

Volume
450–500 ml
Filter
Standard 170 µm blood filter

Infuse over 2–3 hours; maximum: 4 hr/unit; average pediatric dose: 20 ml/kg initially, followed by volume required for stabilization

Comments
Must be ABO and Rh exact

Fresh-Frozen Plasma (FFP)

Volume
200–250 ml
Filter
Special component filter; standard blood filter may be used

Infuse over 15–20 minutes when given for bleeding or clotting factor replacement; 1–2 hours when given for other reasons; average pediatric dose and rate: acute hemorrhage, infuse 15–30 ml/kg as indicated; clotting deficiency, 10–15 ml/kg, infuse 1–2 ml/min

Continued.

Table 7-1   Blood and blood components—cont'd

Product	Infusion Guidelines
	Comments
	Must be ABO compatible; Rh$_O$ antigens not in plasma; no crossmatch required; group AB plasma may be given to any blood group; blood bank does not thaw until required to do so; required time to thaw, 20 minutes; expires 24 hours after thawing
Albumin—25% salt poor	Infuse within 1 hour at 1 ml/min; average pediatric dose and rate: 1 g/kg, infuse 4 ml/kg
Volume	
12.5 g/50 ml	*Comments*
Filter	Dosage based on BSA requirements (estimating blood and plasma volume); refer to manufacturer's package insert; very hypertonic
Special tubing comes with this product	
Albumin—5%	Infuse within 1 hour at 2–4 ml/min; average pediatric dose and rate: 1 g/kg, infuse 10 ml/kg
Volume	
12.5 g/250 ml	*Comments*
Filter	Dosage based on BSA requirements (estimating blood and plasma volume); refer to manufacturer's package insert
Special tubing comes with this product	

Plasma Protein Fraction (PPF)
Volume
Varies according to scheduled dose
Filter
Special tubing comes with this product

Infuse no more than 1 to 10 ml/min
Comments
No typing or crossmatching required; used for volume expansion

RhO Immune Globulin (RhoGam)
Volume
1 ml
Filter
None

Given intramuscularly (IM)
Comments
Usually ordered from blood bank; to achieve optimal effect, must be administered within 72 hours to Rh negative patients who have been exposed to Rh(D) antigens through transfusion or pregnancy
Usually given prenatally 28–30 weeks to protect during delivery exposure after a negative coomb's is drawn

Immune Serum Globulin (ISG)
Gamimune N 100–400 mg/kg administered monthly
Gammagard 200–400 mg/kg administered monthly

May be given IV or IM *(Recommended IV infusion rates)*
Gamimune (Miles Inc.) 0.01 to 0.02 ml/kg initial 30 minutes; increase to maximum of 0.08 ml/kg/min
Gammagard (Baxter) 0.5 ml/kg/ increase to maximum of 4 mg/kg/hr
Gammar (Amour) 0.01 ml/kg/hr; increase to 0.2 ml/kg/min after 15–30 minutes
Iveegam (Immuno-US Inc.) 1 ml/min up to 2 ml/min

Continued.

Table 7-1 Blood and blood components—cont'd

Sandoglobulin 200 mg/kg administered monthly Venoglobulin 200 mg/kg administered monthly *Volume* Up to 1.2 ml/kg body weight *Filter* IV immunoglobulin (IVIG) filter supplied with product	*Sandoglobulin* (Sandoz) 0.5–1 ml/min (10–15 drops); increase after15–30 minutes to 1.5–2.5 ml/min (30–50 drops) *Venoglobulin* (Alpha Therapeutic Corp) 0.01–0.02 ml/kg/min for first 30 minutes *Comments* Compatible with D5W only; incompatible with any other drug in syringe or solution IV infusion should begin within 2 hours after reconstituting; usually ordered from pharmacy; supplies IgG antibodies; patients with severe allergic reactions to plasma should not receive ISG
Purified Factor VIII Concentrate (Hemofil, Hyland) *Volume* Freeze-dried Reconstitute with diluent provided *Filter* Filter needle or IV drip using component recipient set provided with product	Administered intravenously as fast as tolerated by patient to a maximum of 6 ml/min; monitor pulse rate while infusing Dose is calculated according to body weight and designated level of factor activity *Comments* Use for hemophilia A patient (classical hemophilia or Factor VIII deficiency); usually ordered from pharmacy; preheat diluent to 37° C before reconstituting, and use within 3 hours

Purified Factor IX Concentrate (Complex, Hyland)

Volume
Freeze-dried
Reconstitute with diluent provided

Filter
Filter needle provided with product

Same as Purified Factor VIII

Comments
Use for hemophilia B patient (Christmas disease, factor IX deficiency); usually ordered from pharmacy; preheat diluent to 37°C before reconstituting, and use within 3 hours

Fibrinogen
Use cryoprecipitate

Comments
Each unit of cryoprecipitate contains approximately 250 mg fibrinogen per 15 ml of plasma; average pediatric dose: 1 unit/7–10 kg

Platelets (Random)

Volume
60–70 ml/unit; minimum order for adult: 1 unit per 10 kg body weight, usual order: 6–10 units

Filter
Special component filter use of microaggregate filter may be controversial
High-efficiency leukocyte depletion filter

Administer intravenously as rapidly as patient can tolerate; recommend 150–200 ml/hr; may be given more usual order of 6–10 units slowly if danger of circulatory overload exists; maximum transfusion time 4 hours

Comments
ABO and Rh compatible preferred but not necessary; no crossmatch required; request blood bank to pool (combine units); required cooling time: 20 minutes; blood bank will not pool until ready to infuse product

Continued.

Table 7-1   Blood and blood components—cont'd

Platelets (Apheresis)

Volume
200–400 ml

Filter
Same as Platelets (Random); dose: 1 platelet
pheresis pack

Same as Platelets (Random)

Comments

Arrangements must be made with blood center apheresis
department before need; must be ABO and Rh compatible;
crossmatch required unless red cell–free product is provided

Granulocyte Pheresis

Volume
200–400 ml

Filter
Same as Platelets (Random)

Give *slowly* over 2- to 4-hour period; reactions are
common—check vital signs every 15 minutes throughout
transfusion; granulocytes should be transfused as soon as
possible after collection but must be infused within 24 hours;
premedicate with antihistamines, acetaminophen, steroids, or
meperidine hydrochloride to prevent reaction; pediatric dose:
10 ml/kg wt (volume of infusion is usually 200 ml)

Comments

Same as Platelets (Apheresis) except red cell–free product;
observe patient for a severe reaction indicated by cyanosis,
shortness of breath, temperature above 104°F, and drop in
blood pressure; febrile reactions occur in approximately two-
thirds of patients receiving leukocytes; the following
laboratory work is usually ordered 1 hour after transfusion;
WBC, differential, platelet count

Continued.

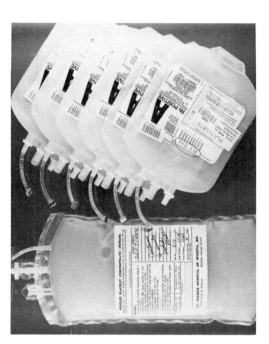

Pooled platelets.

Table 7-1 Blood and blood components—cont'd

Product	Infusion Guidelines
Cryoprecipitate	Rapid infusion: recommend 30–60 minutes
Volume	*Comments*
10–20 ml/unit; total of 10 ml normal saline is added in the blood bank; usual order 8-10 units	Crossmatch not required; need not be ABO of Rh specific; each unit contains approximately 150 grams of fibrinogen and 80 units of Factor VIII; blood bank does not thaw and cool until requested; required preparation time; 20 minutes; expires 6 hours after pooling
Filter	
Special component filter	

3. Obtain the patient's transfusion history, and report any incidence of previous adverse reaction during or after previous blood transfusion.
4. Follow agency-prescribed procedure for type and crossmatching for blood and blood component therapy.
5. Establish patent peripheral or central line site. To ensure safety of blood product administration for patients with multilumen catheters, reserve one lumen of the catheter for blood and blood component infusions. This technique minimizes the potential of infection for patients with these catheters.
6. Select appropriate tubing. All blood and components must be administered through a filter designed to retain blood clots and other debris. Follow agency policy for use of appropriate filter.
7. Blood bank personnel issuing the blood unit and nursing personnel administering the transfusion must identify the blood product, the identification number on the transfusion request, and the identical information on the recipient's medical record.
   a. The identification number and name on the patient's wrist band must be identical with the name and number on the transfusion unit and on the compatibility label.
   b. Donor's ABO group and Rh type must be present on donor unit and transfusion request.
   c. Patient's (recipient) ABO group and Rh type must be present on the transfusion request. Verify ABO and Rh compatibility between the patient (recipient) and donor.
   d. Check the expiration date on the blood bag.
   e. Inspect the blood product for any abnormalities.
   f. Ask patients to identify themselves by giving their complete name. If a patient is unable to state name, follow appropriate agency procedure in validating patient identification. *Never* administer blood to a patient without correct, appropriate identifying bracelet or tag.
   g. Explain the procedure to the patient.
   h. Obtain written consent form if required by the agency.
   i. Inform the patient of potential adverse effects of blood transfusion (see Table 7-2) and instruct the patient to report symptoms experienced promptly to nurse or physician.
   j. Encourage the patient to ask questions about the procedure and potential adverse effects.
   k. On completion of the identification process, the person starting the transfusion and the other licensed person

Table 7-2   Adverse effects of blood transfusion

Reactions	Symptoms
Air Embolism Cause: Improper maintenance of a closed administration system	Shortness of breath, chest pain, cough, hypotension, cyanosis
Anaphylaxis Cause: Previous sensitization by IgA-deficient patients who develop anti-IgA antibodies	Shock, respiratory distress (wheezing, cyanosis), nausea, hypotension, abdominal cramps; absence of fever; occurs quickly following only a few milliliters of blood or plasma
Circulatory Overload Cause: Excessive or rapid volume of blood or blood component	Dyspnea, tightness in chest, dry cough, restlessness, severe headache, increased pulse, respiration, and blood pressure
Citrate Toxicity Cause: Citrate anticoagulant accumulates; toxic effects of ionized calcium in the blood, for example, hypocalcemia	Tingling in fingers, hypotension, nausea and vomiting, cardiac arrhythmias
Febrile Nonhemolysis Cause: Recipient anti-HLA antibodies react to transfused leukocyte or platelet antigens	Fever, flushing, chills, absent RBC hemolysis, lumbar pain, malaise, headache
Hemolysis Immediate Cause: Antibodies in recipient's plasma react to donor's antigens on red cells	Anxiety, increased pulse, respiration, and temperature, decreased blood pressure, dyspnea, nausea and vomiting, chills, hemoglobinemia, hemoglobinuria, abnormal bleeding, oliguria, back pain, shock; reactions may occur when as little as 10–15 ml of incompatible blood have been infused

Table 7-2   Adverse effects of blood transfusion—cont'd

Reactions	Symptoms
Delayed Cause: Recipient becomes sensitized to foreign RBC antigens not in the ABO system	Occurs 2 or more days after transfusion; continued anemia, hemoglobinuria, fever, lumbar pain, and mild jaundice
Hyperkalemia Cause: Prolonged storage of blood; releases potassium into the cell plasma	Onset within few minutes; ECG changes, peaked T-wave and widening of QRS, weakness of extremities, abdominal pain
Hypokalemia Cause: Associated with citrate-induced metabolic alkalosis but may be affected by respiratory or tissue alkalosis	Onset gradual; ECG changes, flattened T-wave, depressed ST segment, polyurea, muscle weakness, decreased bowel sounds
Hypothermia Cause: Rapid administration of cold blood components or when cold blood is administered through a central venous catheter	Shaking chills, hypotension, cardiac arrhythmias, cardiac arrest
Urticaria Cause: Allergy to soluble product in the donor plasma	Local erythema, hives, and itching, usually without fever
Infections Transmitted by Transfusions	
Acquired Immune Deficiency Syndrome (AIDS) Cause: Donor blood HIV seropositive	Can be asymptomatic for up to several years or develop flulike symptoms within 2–4 weeks. Later signs and symptoms include fever, night sweats, fatigue, weight loss, adenopathy, and skin lesions; seropositive for HIV virus

Continued.

Table 7-2   Adverse effects of blood transfusion—cont'd

Reactions	Symptoms
Bacterial Contamination Cause: Contamination at time of donation or preparation; gram-negative bacteria release endotoxins	Onset within 2 hours of transfusion; chills, fever, abdominal pain, shock, marked hypotension
Cytomegalovirus (CMV) CMV virus can exist in healthy adult	Immunosuppressed patients are at high risk (bone marrow transplant, open-heart surgery, newborn positive heterophil); fatigue, weakness, adenopathy, low-grade fever
Graft-Versus-Host Disease (GVHD) Cause: Immunocompetent donor; lymphocytes engraft and multiply in immunodeficient recipient; GVHD may occur in recipients of transfusions from first-degree family members (parents, children, siblings) due to shared specificities at the major histocompatibility complex; irradiation of cellular blood components before administration is useful in reducing the risk of GVHD	Bone marrow-suppressed patients at risk; fever, skin rash, diarrhea, presence of infection, jaundice
Hepatitis Hepatitis B, hepatitis A extremely rare; chronic liver disease more common with hepatitis C than hepatitis B	Occurs in a few weeks to months after transfusion; nausea and vomiting, fever, dark orange urine, jaundice, weakness, malaise, elevated liver enzyme levels (serum glutamic-oxaloacetic transaminase [SGOT], SGPT)

Table 7-2   Adverse effects of blood transfusion—cont'd

Reactions	Symptoms
Malaria	Spiking fever after receiving transfusion containing red cells, platelets, or fresh-frozen plasma; malaria organism isolated in the blood
Syphilis	Rare; blood test positive for syphilis
Thrombocytopenia Purpura	Occurs most often in women; decreased platelet count; generalized purplish rash

verifying the correct product must record date, time, and their signatures on the transfusion requisition.

Initiating the Transfusion

After following protocol to obtain the blood product from the blood bank, begin to administer the blood product within 30 minutes, since blood can deteriorate and become rapidly contaminated at room temperature. (A blood product cannot be returned to the blood bank if the product is not initiated in appropriate time.)

The transfusion should be initiated slowly and then maintained at an administration rate appropriate for the patient's condition. All blood components should be infused within 4 hours; time the transfusion accurately.

During the first 15 minutes of initial transfusion, remain and observe the patient for adverse reactions. Note any adverse or unusual symptoms. The earlier these symptoms are detected, the more promptly the infusion can be discontinued and treatment instituted. (See Table 7-2 for effects and symptoms of blood transfusion.) Assess the patient on an ongoing basis. Take baseline vital signs (temperature, pulse, respirations, and blood pressure) before the transfusion and throughout the transfusion process.

Use only compatible IV fluids. Never inject any drug into a blood bag; only normal saline solution may be added to or run simultaneously with blood or components before or during transfusion.

Prevent damage to the blood cells. For infusing most blood

components, an 18-gauge catheter is appropriate. For patients with small veins (small children and the elderly), a thin-walled, 23-gauge "scalp vein" needle may be used. Also, consider use of a blood warmer for massive transfusions and transfusions in the neonate, child, or immunosuppressed patient.

Pitfalls to Avoid

- *Do not* store component in nursing unit or other unmonitored refrigerator.
- *Do not* keep blood out of a monitored refrigerator for more than 30 minutes before beginning transfusion.
- *Do not* warm blood in an unmonitored water bath or sink or in a microwave oven.
- *Do not* administer blood component without a blood filter.
- *Do not* use the same blood filter for more than 4 hours.
- *Do not* transfuse a unit of blood for more than 4 hours.
- *Do not* add any medications, including those intended for intravenous use, to blood or components or infuse through the same administration set as the blood component.
- *Do not* allow any solution other than *0.9 percent normal saline* to come in contact with the blood component or the administration set.

Troubleshooting Tips

Sluggish IV lines and clogged filters that decrease the flow rate may be encountered during transfusion. Investigative questions to ask include the following:

- Is there a kink in the administration set?
- Is the correct gauge of needle or catheter being used?
- Has irrigation with normal saline been attempted?
- Has the filter been used for more than 2 units?
- Has the blood bag been rotated to distribute contents evenly?
- Is the blood bag 36 to 48 inches above the venipuncture site?
- Does the roller clamp need to be adjusted?

If all the preceding points are negative or problems have been corrected, consider use of pressure cuff according to agency policy.

Posttransfusion

1. Complete posttransfusion documentation.
2. Return completed transfusion form to blood bank.
3. Continue to observe the patient, and monitor vital signs according to agency policy.

4. Dispose of used supplies in a puncture-proof, leakproof container. NOTE: If transfusion reaction occurs, return discontinued bag of blood and blood component with all attached solutions to the blood bank.

5. Follow up with prescribed, scheduled posttransfusion laboratory tests, such as complete blood count (CBC), hemoglobin, hematocrit, platelet count, prothrombin time, or Factor VIII level.

CLINICAL ALERT: Wear gloves while initiating and discontinuing a blood transfusion to protect from blood-borne infections (hepatitis, AIDS). Immediately and thoroughly wash hands and other skin surfaces contaminated with blood, body fluids containing visible blood, or other body fluids to which universal precautions apply.

Adverse Effects of Blood Transfusion

Hemolytic (immediate and delayed) reactions, febrile non-hemolytic reactions, and allergic reactions are the most frequent in occurrence of all the adverse effects listed in Table 7-2. To provide immediate intervention for a transfusion reaction, the most common symptoms of a transfusion reaction and the appropriate interventions need to be studied. The greatest risk of exposure to infectious disease from blood transfusions is a 1% to 2% incidence of posttransfusion hepatitis. If the patient is suspected of having posttransfusion hepatitis, the blood bank service should be notified so that the donor can be investigated.

Consider avoiding concurrent infusions of blood components and amphotericin-B. Similar adverse reactions to these products may include fever, chills, nausea, vomiting, hypotension, decreased urine output, dyspnea, and anaphylaxis. It may be difficult to determine the source (blood component or amphotericin-B) of the reactions. Additionally, there is the potential deleterious effects of amphotericin-B on blood cell survival posttransfusion. Further studies are needed to clearly evaluate the differences between adverse reactions and the effects of amphotericin-B on the blood components.

Management of Transfusion Reactions

The time between suspicion of a transfusion reaction and the initiation of appropriate therapy should be as short as possible. The nurse administering blood component therapy is responsible for obtaining baseline vital signs and monitoring the patient for any changes that may develop during and after any transfusion. An accurate assessment of clinical symptoms and reporting of this information is crucial in life-threatening reactions. Nursing staff should be skilled in blood component therapy, and policies and procedures for management of transfusion reactions should be readily available.

Guidelines established by the American Association of Blood Banks for reactions to blood transfusions include the following:

1. *Stop* the transfusion to limit the amount of blood infused.
2. Notify the physician.
3. Keep the IV line open with an infusion of normal saline.
4. Check all labels, forms, and patient identification to determine if the patient received the correct blood or component.
5. Report the suspected transfusion reaction to blood bank personnel immediately.
6. Send required blood samples, carefully drawn to avoid mechanical hemolysis, to the blood bank as soon as possible, together with the discontinued bag of blood, the administration set, attached IV solutions, and all the related forms and labels.
7. Send other samples—for example, urine for evaluation of acute hemolysis—as directed by the blood bank director or patient's physician.
8. Complete agency report or "Suspected Transfusion Reaction" form (if appropriate).
9. Medication and supplies to have nearby:
   a. Injectable: aminophylline, diphenhydramine hydrochloride (Benadryl), dopamine, epinephrine, heparin, hydrocortisone, furosemide (Lasix)
   b. Oral: acetaminophen, aspirin
   c. Oxygen setup, tubing, cannula and/or mask, and airway device
   d. Foley catheterization kit
   e. Blood culture bottles
   f. IV fluids (isotonic solution)
   g. IV tubings

CLINICAL ALERT: The nurse must become familiar with all the equipment used in the employing agency so that intervention for a transfusion reaction can be administered promptly and safely.

Documentation Recommendations

- Location of patent peripheral or central line IV site
- Baseline vital signs before transfusion

- Time transfusion was started
- Type of product and identification number
- Signature of person initiating the transfusion and signature of second licensed person verifying correct product
- Total number of units infused and their identification numbers
- Total volume of blood component, saline infused, and filters used
- Time transfusion was completed
- Premedication or postmedication supplies (tubings) used for blood component therapy
- Patient's response to transfusion, especially any symptoms of an adverse reaction (chills, fever, urticaria, sweating, nausea, blood in urine, shortness of breath, dyspnea, hypotension, or anxiety)
- All nursing interventions initiated and performed in response to an adverse reaction

Nursing Diagnoses

- Fluid volume excess, potential, related to infusion of the product or volume of the infusion
- Infection, risk for, related to contamination of supplies or blood product
- Fluid volume deficit, actual or risk for, related to loss of blood volume
- Cardiac output, decreased
- Body temperature, altered: hypothermia/hyperthermia
- Knowledge deficit related to side effects of transfusion reaction
- Injury, risk for, related to allergy, air embolism, hemolytic transfusion reaction related to blood products

Patient/Family Teaching for Self-Management

- Describe purpose, schedule, and procedure for blood component administration.
- Explain the potential blood transfusion reactions (fever, chills, urticaria, back pain, pain at infusion site, chest pain, dyspnea, and nausea) and the importance of reporting the reactions promptly to the nurse or physician.
- Instruct the patient or caregiver regarding potential delayed reactions to transfusions, which may occur several hours, days, or a week after transfusion; examples are jaundice and generalized purplish rash (purpura); advise to notify the physician promptly.
- If blood component therapy is to be administered in the home setting, assess availability of the caregiver to be present in the home during administration of the blood product.

Home Care Considerations

- The patient must be *homebound* (unable to drive self or leave home without assistance).
- The patient should be alert, cooperative, and able to respond appropriately to body symptoms.
- The patient must have been previously transfused without difficulty.
- A responsible adult must be present in the home to participate in the identification process and to summon assistance (physician or paramedic) if necessary.
- A usable telephone must be available during the transfusion.
- Whole blood must not be administered in the home.
- The blood specimen for type and crossmatch should be drawn 24 to 48 hours before blood product administration.
- Each unit of the blood component therapy must be checked by a registered nurse and blood bank personnel before administration.
- The registered nurse must work under the direction of a physician in accordance with federal, state, and local regulations and the standards of the American Association of Blood Banks.
- The registered nurse should be knowledgeable and skilled in the procedure of blood product administration.
- The nurse must remain in attendance throughout the blood transfusion process and for at least 30 minutes after transfusion.
- Blood should be transported in insulated containers with ice packets that maintain the temperature between 1°C and 10°C for 24 hours.
- The container, empty bags, and tubing should be returned to the blood bank on completion of the transfusion.
- Posttransfusion instructions must be given in writing, and the patient or caregiver must be given the names and phone numbers of individuals available at all times to be called in the event of a delayed problem.
- The nurse should arrange for prescribed posttransfusion laboratory tests to be completed; examples are red blood cells (hemoglobin, hematocrit), within 24 hours; platelets, 18 hours after transfusion.

CLINICAL ALERT: Home care nursing personnel should be alert and prepared for possible transfusion reactions. The drugs and supplies necessary to manage these potential reactions must be readily available for use. Protocols for management of transfusion reactions should be clearly defined and easily accessible to home care nursing staff.

Geriatric Considerations

- Previous history of homebound status may include anemia with bone-marrow failure, anemia associated with malignancy, chronic gastrointestinal bleeding, chronic renal failure.
- There is potential for cardiac, renal, and respiratory systems compromise: Adjust flow rate if the patient cannot tolerate the prescribed flow rate. Flow rate should be 1 ml/kg/hr in the patient at risk for circulatory overload.
- Sensory deficits may occur: Consult medical records or family members for previous blood transfusion reactions.
- The patient may require assistance with elimination needs before the blood product transfusion.
- Premedications may cause drowsiness; encourage the patient to use transportation resources (family, public, American Cancer Society, American Red Cross) if receiving blood transfusions on an outpatient basis.
- Venous integrity may be compromised; ensure catheter or needle patency before transfusion.
- Consult with community resources if homebound situation becomes compromised.

Chapter Resources

Blood Product Administration Audit

	Yes	No	NA
1. Verify the physician order for specific product to be given on a stated date.			
2. Check appropriate laboratory data.			
3. Review transfusion history of the patient.			
4. Select correct tubing and filter for the blood and blood product.			
5. Explain the procedure to the patient.			

Continued.

Blood Product Administration Audit

	Yes	No	NA
6. Obtain baseline vital signs (BP, T, P, R).			
7. Identify the patient by name and by written ID number on the patient bracelet.			
8. Confirm blood unit number, ABO group, Rh type, expiration date of product on donor unit, patient transfusion request form, and patient identification number on patient bracelet with another licensed professional.			
9. Prime blood tubing and filter, taking care to cover the entire filter.			
10. Initiate the transfusion slowly (5 ml/min for initial 15 minutes).			
11. Readjust the transfusion rate after 15 minutes to the desired infusion rate.			
12. Use only normal saline for flushing of IV line.			
13. Take the patient's vital signs throughout the transfusion according to agency policy.			
14. Document the procedure according to agency policy.			
15. Return completed posttransfusion request to blood bank.			

PATIENT AND PROFESSIONAL INFORMATION BOOKLETS

The American Red Cross and the Public Health Service have made available the following publications regarding the blood supply and AIDS:

- AIDS and the Blood Supply
- AIDS and the Health Care Workers
- AIDS and Your Job
- Caring for the AIDS Patient at Home
- AIDS and Your Children
- If Your Antibody Test is Positive
- AIDS, Sex and You

TRANSFUSION RESOURCES

American Association of Blood Banks
1117 N. 19th, Suite 600
Arlington, VA 22209

Centers for Disease Control and Prevention (CDC)
1600 Clifton RD NE
Atlanta, GA 30333

Food and Drug Administration
Office of Consumer Action
HFE-88
5600 Fishers Lane
Rockville, MD 20857

National Blood Resource Education Program
  Information Center
4733 Bethesda Avenue, Suite 530
Bethesda, MD 20814-4820

U.S. Department of Labor Occupational Safety
  and Health Administration (OSHA)
Directorate of Technical Support
200 Constitution Avenue NW
Washington, DC 20210

American Red Cross
National Headquarters
1730 E. Street NW
Washington, DC 20006

Council of Community Blood Donors
725 15th Street NW, Suite 700
Washington, DC 20005

Intravenous Nurses Society
Fresh Pond Square
10 Fawcett Street
Cambridge, MA 02138

Oncology Nursing Society
501 Holiday Drive
Pittsburgh, PA 15220-2749

GUIDELINES FOR OBTAINING INFORMED CONSENT

I. What do you convey?
   A. The reason for the transfusion.
      1. The benefits and risks of the transfusion.
      2. What to expect during and after the transfusion.
   B. The transfusion options available to the patient.
   C. The message that we do not have a completely risk-free blood supply.
      1. The assurance that every step is being taken to make the blood supply as safe as possible.
      2. Risk information that can be put into reasonable perspective (numbers and percentages are not always useful by themselves).
      3. Comparisons to other risks in life the patient may have taken.

II. How do you obtain consent?
   A. When possible, do not schedule a teaching session for the night before surgery.
   B. When possible, get the consent several days before the transfusion.
      1. Evaluate comprehension by asking the patients to tell you what they heard you say and what they understand from the written consent.
      2. Try to arrange more than one opportunity for discussion.
      3. Arrange supplemental support (transfusion-service staff, educational videos, health educators).
      4. Provide reading material.
      5. Give the patient a copy of the consent form.
   C. Respect the patient's religious and cultural beliefs about transfusion, especially any that preclude the receipt of blood.

? Study Questions

1. Select *one* best answer.
   Chills, fever, headache, hypotension, tachycardia, and lower back pain are symptoms for:
   a. Circulatory overload
   b. Iron overload
   c. Acute hemolytic reaction
   d. Delayed transfusion reaction

2. Platelet products should be administered at what rate?
   a. Slow infusion at 15 ml/hr
   b. Slowly over 2 to 3 hours
   c. Usual rate, 1 to 1 ½ hours
   d. Rapid infusion (150–200 ml/hr) based on patient tolerance

3. Which intravenous solution is compatible with blood/blood products?
   a. Lactated Ringer's
   b. 0.9% normal saline
   c. 5% dextrose water
   d. 0.45% saline

4. If the scheduled blood product infusion is delayed, the blood or blood products should be:
   a. Stored in nursing unit medication refrigerator
   b. Frozen in the nursing unit refrigerator
   c. Returned to the laboratory collection center
   d. Returned to the agency blood bank

5. Which information must be verified by two licensed professional nurses prior to blood or blood product administration?
   a. Patient's name, agency/hospital/blood unit number, blood expiration date, and verification of blood order
   b. Patient's name, agency/hospital insurance number, blood expiration date, and verification of blood order
   c. Patient's name, agency/hospital/blood unit number, physician, and ID number
   d. Patient's name, social security number, blood expiration number, blood order, and date

6. At what rate are blood or blood products administered during the initial 15 minutes?
   a. 2–5 ml/min
   b. 10 ml/min
   c. 15 ml/min
   d. 20 ml/min

7. Viral diseases that may be transmitted via blood product transfusions include:
   a. Leukemia, measles, AIDS, CMV
   b. Measles, AIDS, CMV, hepatitis D

    c. AIDS, CMV, hepatitis D, hepatitis E
    d. AIDS, CMV, hepatitis B, hepatitis C

8. Patient and family education for blood or blood product administration include:
    a. Signs and symptoms of transfusion reaction, blood product administration, and documentation requirements
    b. Signs and symptoms of transfusion reaction, rationale for all supplies used, donor supply for blood product, and physician's home phone number
    c. Signs and symptoms of transfusion reaction; nursing assessment and management process before, during, and after the transfusion; follow-up laboratory tests, to whom/where/when/how to report delayed reactions and or symptoms
    d. Signs and symptoms of transfusion reaction, blood bank collection and storage of blood products, blood product supplies and equipment

9. Which agencies monitor blood and blood product transfusion practices?
    a. American Association of Blood Banks, Centers for Disease Control, American Red Cross, Federal Bureau of Investigation
    b. American Association of Blood Banks, Centers for Disease Control, American Red Cross, Food and Drug Administration
    c. American Association of Blood Banks, Federal Bureau of Investigation, American Red Cross, Occupational Safety and Health Administration
    d. American Association of Blood Banks, Centers for Disease Control, Federal Bureau of Investigation, Occupational Safety and Health Administration

10. Guidelines established by the American Association of Blood Banks for transfusion reactions include these *sequential:*
    a. Call the physician, stop the transfusion, keep the IV open with normal saline, check all the ID forms, send the required blood/urine specimens to lab, and document the occurrence.
    b. Call the physician, start a second IV with normal saline, check all the ID forms, send the required blood/urine specimens to lab, and monitor the patient's vital signs.
    c. Stop the transfusion, call the physician, keep the IV open

with normal saline, check all ID forms, send the required specimens to the lab, and document the occurrence.

d. Stop the transfusion, keep the IV open with normal saline, send the required specimens to the lab, check all ID forms, and document the occurrence.

ANSWERS: 1. c   2. d   3. b   4. d   5. a
6. a   7. d   8. c   9. b   10. c

Chemotherapy Administration

8

Objectives

1. Identify the phases of the cell generation cycle and explain the primary activity occurring at each phase.

2. Describe the principles of cancer cells' tumor growth.

3. List at least 5 considerations used in combination chemotherapy.

4. Correlate safe drug administration with the routes of chemotherapy administration: oral, subcutaneous, topical, intraarterial, intracavity, intraperitoneal, intrathecal, and intravenous.

5. Describe precautions that should be taken by the nurse during preparation, administration, and disposal of chemotherapy drugs.

6. List the sequential steps for chemotherapy drug extravasation management.

7. Identify the major system toxicities associated with chemotherapy drugs.

8. Discuss the use of test dosing and premedication sequence for chemotherapy drugs' potential for anaphylaxis.

9. State the appropriate nursing interventions used in chemotherapy drug anaphylaxis management.

10. Design a patient plan of care for side effects: anorexia, nausea/vomiting, constipation, diarrhea, pain, and stomatitis.

Chemotherapy is the use of cytotoxic drugs in the treatment of cancer. It is recognized as one of the four modalities—surgery, radiation therapy, chemotherapy, and biotherapy—that provide cure, control, or palliation as a goal of therapy. Chemotherapy may be used separately or in conjunction with other modalities.

Nursing has major responsibilities in caring for patients who receive chemotherapeutic agents. It is important that nurses know treatment goals, drug classification with modes of action, principles of tumor growth and cell kill, and administration protocol. Chemotherapeutic agents should be administered only by nurses who have been educated and are skilled in the various procedures. Patient and family education on the many aspects of chemotherapy (for example, procedure, potential side effects and toxicities, and follow-up care) requires competent nursing assessment and intervention. The nurse should encourage the patient and family to participate and become an integral part in planning and implementing care. These responsibilities offer many challenges for the nurse administering chemotherapy.

Principles of Chemotherapy

Cell Generation Cycle

Normal cells and cancer cells go through the same division cycle characterized by a sequential series of phases or steps (Fig. 8-1). The length of time that it takes for a cell to complete the phase or cycle varies. This time is called generation time. Chemotherapeutic drugs are most active against frequently dividing cells. Normal cells with rapid growth changes most commonly affected by chemotherapeutic agents include bone marrow (platelets and red and white blood cells), hair follicles, mucosal lining of the gastrointestinal tract, skin, and germinal cells (sperm and ova).

CLINICAL ALERT: Chemotherapy is given according to scheduled sequences or cycles that are planned to allow recovery of the normal cells. Anticipate changes, such as low blood counts and hair loss, and incorporate these in the patient care plan.

Drug Classification

Chemotherapeutic agents are classified according to their pharmacologic action and their interference with cellular reproduction. The basic groups are cell cycle phase specific and cell cycle phase nonspecific. Their potential actions are the following.

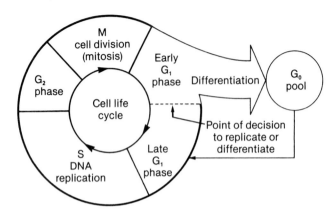

Fig. 8-1
Cell generation cycle.
Courtesy Adria Laboratories, Columbus, OH.

Cell cycle phase–specific drugs

These drugs are active on cells undergoing division in the cell cycle. Cell cycle phase–specific drugs are given in minimal concentration via continuous dosing methods.

G_1 Phase	G_2 Phase
Asparaginase	Bleomycin
Prednisone	Etoposide (VP-16)

S Phase M Phase	
Cytarabine (ara-C)	*Vinca* Alkaloids
Floxuridine (FUDR)	Vinblastine
Fludarabine	Vincristine
5-Fluorouracil	Vindesine
Hydroxyurea	Vinorelbine (Navelbine)
Idarubicin (Idamycin)	
6-Mercaptopurine	
Methotrexate	

Teniposide (Vumon)

6-Thioguanine

Cell cycle phase–nonspecific

These drugs are active on cells in either a dividing or resting state. Drugs of this nature are often given as single bolus injections.

Alkylating Agents	Nitrosureas
Busulfan (Myleran)	Carmustine (B:CNU)
Carboplatin (Paraplatin)	Lomustine (CeeNu)
Chlorambucil (Leukeran)	Semustine (MeCCNU)
Cisplatin (Platinol)	Streptozocin (Zanosar)
Cyclophosphamide (Cytoxan)	
Ifosfamide (IFEX)	
Mechlorethamine (Mustargen)	
Melphalan (Alkeran)	
Thioplex (Thiotepa)	

Antibiotics	Miscellaneous
Dactinomycin (Actinomycin, Cosmegen)	Cladribine (Leustatin)
	Dacarbazine (DTIC-Dome)
Daunorubicin (Daunomycin, Cerubidine)	Docetaxel (Taxotere)
	Hexamethylmelamine
Doxorubicin (Adriamycin)	Mitoxantrone (Novantrone)
Mithramycin	Paclitaxel (Taxol)
Mitomycin-C (Mutamycin)	Pentostatin (2'deoxycoformycin)
	Procarbazine (Matulane)
	Topotecan

Hormone and steroid drugs

The remaining group of drugs that affect tumor cell growth by altering the intracellular environment is hormone and steroid drugs. The mechanism of action for each drug is different. Steroidal drugs provide an antiinflammatory effect on the body tissues. These drugs all recruit malignant cells out of G^0 phase, making them vulnerable to damage, caused by cell cycle–phase specific agents. Hormones are cell cycle phase–nonspecific. These chemicals, secreted by the endocrine glands, alter the environment of the cell by affecting the cell membrane permeability. By manipulating hormone levels, they can suppress tumor growth. Antihormonal agents derive their antineoplastic effect from their ability to neutralize the effect of or inhibit the production of natural hormones used by hormone-dependent tumors.

Hormones	Corticosteroids
Androgens	Dexamethasone (Decadron)
Fluoxymesterone (Halotestin)	Hydrocortisone Sodium Succinate (Solu-Cortef)
Testosterone	Prednisone (Deltasone)
Progestins	Prednisolone (Prelone)
Medroxyprogesterone acetate (Depo-Provera intramuscular; Provera oral)	
Megestrol acetate (Megace)	

Estrogens	Antihormonal Agents
Diethylstilbestrol (DES)	Finasteride (Proscar)
Conjugated estrogens (Premarin)	Flutamide (Eulexin)
Chlorotrianisene (TACE)	Leuprolide (Lupron)
	Mitotane (Lysodren)
	Tamoxifen (Nolvadex)
	Goserelin (Zoladex)

 CLINICAL ALERT: Become familiar with the potential side effects and toxicities associated with chemotherapeutic drugs in all categories.

Tumor Growth

The regulatory mechanism controlling the growth of cancer cells differs from that of normal cells. Unlike normal cells, cancer cells grow via a pyramid effect; however, they grow at the *same rate* as the tissue from which they originated. The time required for a tumor mass to reach a certain size is called doubling time. During early stages of tumor growth, doubling time is more rapid than later stages. This pattern of growth is called the Gompertzian growth curve (Fig. 8-2).

CLINICAL ALERT: Tumor cells are more sensitive to chemotherapeutic agents that are toxic to rapidly dividing cells. Treatment protocols for patients with leukemia and lymphoma may include interventions for rapid cell destruction. A protocol may include fluid hydration and administration of allopurinol to minimize renal toxicity 24 hours before the initial chemotherapeutic drug dose is given.

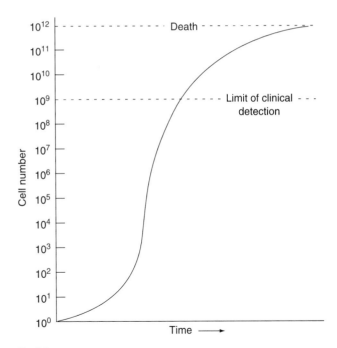

Fig. 8-2

The Gompertzian growth curve.

Reprinted with permission, *The American Cancer Society textbook of clinical oncology,* Atlanta, 1995, American Cancer Society.

Cell Kill Hypothesis

A single cancer cell is capable of multiplying and eventually killing the host. The last tumor cell needs to be killed to achieve a cure in the treatment of cancer. With each course of the drug therapy a given dose of chemotherapeutic drug kills only a *fraction* and *not all* of the cancer cells present. Repeated courses of chemotherapy must then be used to reduce the total cancer cell number (Fig. 8-3).

 CLINICAL ALERT: Repeated courses of chemotherapeutic drugs require anticipation of potential drug cumulative effects.

Factors Considered in Drug Selection

1. Patient's eligibility for chemotherapy (confirmed diagnosis; age; bone marrow, nutritional, cardiac, hepatic, and renal

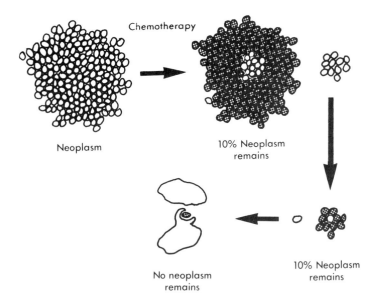

Fig. 8-3
Cell kill hypothesis.
From Goodman MS: *Cancer chemotherapy and care,* part 1, Evansville, IN, 1995, Bristol Laboratories, Division of Bristol-Myers Co.

status; expectation of longevity; previous history of chemotherapy and radiation therapy)

2. Cancer cell type (for example, squamous cell, adeno-
   carcinoma)
3. Rate of drug absorption (for example, treatment interval and
   routes—oral, IV, intraperitoneal)
4. Tumor location (for example, many drugs do not cross the
   blood-brain barrier)
5. Tumor load (for example, larger tumors are generally less
   responsive to chemotherapy)
6. Tumor resistance to chemotherapy (for example, tumor cells
   can mutate and produce variant cells distinct from the tumor
   stem cell of origin)

Combination Chemotherapy

Chemotherapeutic drugs are most frequently given in combination.
This process enhances the effect of the drugs on the tumor cell
kill. Consideration for drugs used in combination include effectiveness as a single agent, results in increased tumor cell kill,
increased patient survival, presence of a synergistic action, varied
toxicities, different mechanisms of action, and administration in
repeated courses to minimize the immunosuppressive effects that
might otherwise occur. Table 8-1 lists combination chemotherapy
regimens.

Combination chemotherapy provides additional benefits not
possible with single drug treatment, such as maximal cell kill within
the range of toxicity tolerated by the host for each drug, a broader
range of coverage of resistant cell lines in a heterogeneous tumor
population, and prevention or slowing of the development of new
resistant cell lines. Because numerous cellular variants exist within
a metastasis by the time it is detected, therapy for metastatic disease
is often directed toward characteristics of the secondary tumor
rather the primary tumor. Combination chemotherapy rather than
single sequential therapy maximizes therapeutic response by
addressing the diversity of cellular response.

Chemotherapy Administration
Drug Dosage Calculation

Drug dosage for cancer chemotherapy is based on body surface area
(BSA) in both adults and children. Drug calculations should be

Table 8-1   Combination chemotherapy regimens

Breast

CMF: *C*yclophosphamide, *M*ethotrexate, *5-F*luorouracil
CMFVP: *C*yclophosphamide, *M*ethotrexate, *5-F*luorouracil,
  *V*incristine, *P*rednisone
FUVAC: *5-Fl*uorouracil, *V*inblastine, *A*driamycin,
  *C*yclophosphamide

Hodgkins

ABVD: *A*driamycin, *B*leomycin, *V*inblastine, *D*acarbazine
MOPP: *N*itrogen *M*ustard, *O*ncovin, *P*rednisone, *P*rocarbazine

Lung

CAV: *C*isplatin, *A*driamycin, *V*inblastine
CAMP: *C*yclophosphamide, *A*driamycin, *M*ethotrexate,
  *P*rocarbazine

Lymphoma

CHOP-BLEO: *C*yclophosphamide, *A*driamycin, *O*ncovin,
  *P*rednisone, *Bleo*mycin
PROMACE-Cyta-BOM: *Pr*ednisone, *O*ncovin, *M*ethotrexate,
  *A*driamycin, *C*yclophosphamide, *E*toposide, *C*ytarabine,
  *B*leomycin, *L*eucovorin, *D*examathasone, *T*rimethoprim *S*ulfa

verified by a second person to ensure dose accuracy. The dosage range of one drug may vary with different drugs regimens. (See Chapter 12 for specifics of drug calculations.)

Drug Reconstitution

Prepare and reconstitute drugs using aseptic technique in accordance with the manufacturer's current recommendations. Label all syringes of reconstituted drugs immediately with the name of the drug. Many of the chemotherapeutic agents are colorless and cannot be distinguished from one another after reconstitution. (See Safe Handling Recommendations for Drug Preparation Guidelines on page 228.)

Route of Administration Guidelines

  I. *Oral*—emphasize importance of patient compliance with
     prescribed schedule.

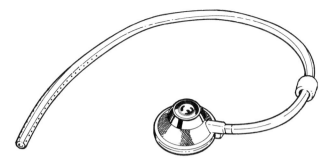

Fig. 8-4
Implantable intraperitoneal port.
Courtesy CR Bard, Inc, Cranston, RI.

II. *Subcutaneous and intramuscular*—may require demonstration with a return demonstration if the patient is receiving prescribed self-injections. Be sure to rotate injection sites for each dose.

III. *Topical*—cover surface area with thin film of medication; instruct the patient to wear loose-fitting, cotton clothing. Wear gloves and be sure to wash hands thoroughly after procedure. Caution the patient not to touch area of topical ointment application.

IV. *Intraarterial*—requires catheter placement in artery near tumor site; because of arterial pressure, administer the drug in a heparinized solution by means of an infusion pump. Throughout the infusion, monitor vital signs, color and temperature of extremity, and potential for bleeding at the site with temporary catheter placement. Instruct the patient and family on care components of catheter and infusion pumps if chemotherapy is given in home setting.

V. *Intracavity*—instill the drug into the bladder through a catheter and/or through a chest tube into the pleural cavity. Follow prescribed premedication dosage to minimize potential local irritation caused by drugs given through the intracavity route.

VI. *Intraperitoneal*—warm the infusate solution (with dry heat) to body temperature of 38°C before administration.

Deliver the drug into the abdominal cavity through the implantable port or external suprapubic catheter (Fig. 8-4). Monitor the patient for abdominal pressure, pain, fever, and electrolyte status. Measure and record abdominal girth for 48 hours.

VII. *Intrathecal*—reconstitute all intrathecal medications with preservative-free, sterile normal saline or sterile water. Infusion of medication may be given through an Ommaya reservoir, if available, through lumbar puncture procedure or through both mechanisms. Usual volume of medication instilled is 15 ml or less (Fig. 8-5). The medication should

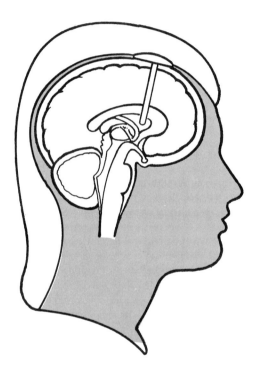

Fig. 8-5
The Ommaya reservoir.
From Brager B, Yasko J: *Care of the client receiving chemotherapy,* Reston, VA, 1984, Reston.

be injected *slowly.* If chemotherapy drugs ara-C or methotrexate are given in high doses, monitor the patient closely for potential neurotoxicity. Only a physician may administer intrathecal drugs.

VIII. *IV*—may be given through central venous catheters or peripheral venous access. Methods of IV administration include the following:

    A. *Push* (bolus): medication is administered through syringe by direct IV method.

    B. *Piggyback* (secondary setup): drug is administered using a secondary bag (bottle) and tubing; primary infusion is concurrently maintained throughout drug administration.

    C. *Side arm:* drug is administered through syringe and needle into side port of a running (free-flowing) IV infusion.

    D. *Infusion:* drug is added to prescribed volume of fluid IV bag (bottle); continuous or intermittent flow.

CLINICAL ALERT: Check for blood return before, during, and after infusion of chemotherapeutic drugs. Follow the agency guidelines for frequency of monitoring continuous chemotherapeutic infusions. For vesicant drug continuous infusion, suggestions include validating blood return every 2 hours; for nonvesicant drug continuous infusion, validate blood return every 4 hours.

Vein Selection and Venipuncture

Many chemotherapeutic agents can be irritating to veins and surrounding tissues. Peripheral sites should be changed daily before administration of vesicants. (See "Extravasation Management.") The number of available veins may be limited as a result of previous therapy. (See Chapter 2.)

Procedure for Chemotherapeutic Drug Administration

1. Verify patient identification, drug, dose, route, and time of administration with the physician's order.
2. Review drug allergy history with the patient.
3. Review appropriate laboratory data and other tests.
4. Verify informed consent for treatment.
5. Select the appropriate equipment and supplies.
6. Calculate the dose and reconstitute the drug using aseptic technique (follow safe handling guidelines).

7. Explain the procedure to patient and family. (See Patient/Family Teaching for Self-Management.)
8. Administer prescribed antiemetics or other medications.
9. Initiate the peripheral IV site or prepare a central venous access site.
10. Administer chemotherapeutic agents.
11. Monitor the patient at scheduled frequencies throughout the course of drug administration.
12. Anticipate and plan interventions for potential side effects or major system toxicity. (See Tables 8-2 and 8-3.)
13. Dispose of all used supplies and unused drugs into approved puncture-proof, leakproof containers outside of the patient area.
14. Document the procedure according to agency policy and procedure. (See Documentation Recommendations.)

Chemotherapeutic Toxicities

Chemotherapeutic drugs have the potential for causing adverse side effects and major system toxicity and dysfunction in patients receiving these agents. Each side effect and toxicity varies in severity according to the patient's individual response to the drug therapy. Nursing responsibilities include evaluating individual patient response to the drugs, teaching the patient or caregiver management interventions, and monitoring various laboratory data and symptoms observed or reported by the patient.

The information listed in Tables 8-2 and 8-3 may be referred to in developing the plan of care for the patient receiving chemotherapeutic drugs.

Safe Handling of Chemotherapeutic Agents

The number and usage of chemotherapeutic agents have increased considerably in recent years. A concern among health care workers has emerged regarding the potential occupational hazard associated with the handling of these drugs. Clinical studies have indicated that many agents are carcinogenic, mutagenic, and teratogenic or any combination of the three. The exposure to these chemotherapeutic agents can occur from inhalation, absorption, and digestion. Recommended safe handling practice guidelines should be referred to when establishing policies and procedure within each agency that

Text continued on p. 244.

Table 8-2 Patient teaching for self-management of most common side effects from chemotherapeutic drugs

Side Effects	Points to Cover
Aches and Pains	Pain medication should be taken on a regular schedule
Nursing action	Side effects of pain medicine are constipation, dry mouth, and drowsiness
Assess location, intensity, quality, and duration of pain	Rest and relaxation strategies include music, progressive relaxation exercise, distraction, and positive imaging
Alopecia	Hair loss occurs 10–21 days after drug treatment
Hair loss	Hair loss is temporary, and hair will regrow when drug is stopped
Cyclophosphamide, dacarbazine, dactinomycin, daunorubicin, doxorubicin, idarubicin, mechlorethamine, mitomycin, paclitaxel, topotecan, vinblastine, and vinorelbine	Hair loss may occur suddenly and in large amounts; select wig, cap, scarf, or turban before hair loss occurs
	Avoid use of hair dryers, curling irons, and harsh or frequent shampoos
Hair thinning	Keep the head covered in summer to prevent a severe sunburn and in winter to prevent heat loss
Bleomycin, etoposide, 5-fluorouracil, floxuridine, and vincristine	
Anorexia	Eating is a social event; eat with others in a pleasant area with soft music and attractive settings
Nursing action	Freshen up before meals, with mouth care and exercise, for example
Assess dietary history, monitor serum transferrin levels and weight loss	

Continued.

Table 8-2 Patient teaching for self-management of most common side effects from chemotherapeutic drugs—cont'd

Side Effects	Points to Cover
	Small, frequent meals (five to six meals daily); avoid drinking fluids with meals to prevent feeling of fullness
	Concentrate on eating foods high in protein, such as eggs, milk products, peanut butter, tuna, beans, peas
	Breakfast may be the most tolerable meal of the day; try to include one-third of daily calories at this time
	Monitor and record weight weekly; report weight loss
Constipation	Increase intake of high-fiber foods, such as whole grain products, bran, fresh fruit, raw vegetables, popcorn
Drugs associated with potential: vinblastine, vincristine, vindesine, vinorelbine, and narcotics	Increase fluid intake to 2–3 quarts of liquids daily; encourage fresh fruit juices, prunes, hot liquids on waking
Nursing action	Follow prescribed schedule for use of stool softener; follow prescribed physician orders if no bowel movement for 3 days or more
Determine normal bowel habits; advise the patient not to strain with bowel evacuation, and to respond immediately to the urge to defecate	
Cystitis	
Drug associated with potential; cyclophosphamide and ifosfamide	

Nursing action
Observe urine for color and amount, and assess frequency of voiding; advise patient to take oral cyclophosphamide early in the day

Increase fluid intake to 3 quarts daily
Empty bladder at least every 4 hours, especially at bedtime and at least once during the night
Report increasing symptoms and frequency of bleeding, burning, pain, fever, and chills promptly to the physician
Set small goals that are achievable daily

Depression

Nursing action
Assess for changes in mood, affect

Participate in enjoyable and diversionary activities, such as music, reading, outings
Share feelings and concerns with someone

Diarrhea

Nursing action
Monitor serum fluid and electrolytes and number, color, frequency, and consistency of diarrhea stools

Avoid eating high-roughage, greasy, and spicy foods; avoid using milk products or use boiled skim milk
Avoid caffeine and alcoholic products and beverages
Eat a bland diet
Increase fluid intake to 3 quarts of liquids daily (weak, tepid tea, bouillon, grape juice)
Record number and consistency of daily bowel movements; report information to the physician
Follow prescribed medication schedule if problem persists beyond 1 day
Cleanse rectal area after each bowel movement

Continued.

Table 8-2 Patient teaching for self-management of most common side effects from chemotherapeutic drugs—cont'd

Side Effects	Points to Cover
Fatigue	Conserve energy; rest when tired; plan rest periods
Nursing action	Plan for gradual accommodation of activities into lifestyle
Assess for possible causes (anemia, chronic pain, stress, depression, and insufficient rest or nutritional intake)	Monitor dietary and fluid intake daily
Hematopoietic Changes	Avoid sources of infection, such as people with bacterial infections, colds, sore throats, flu, chickenpox, measles, or cold sores or people recently vaccinated with live vaccines such as measles-mumps-rubella (MMR) or diphtheria-pertussis-tetanus (DPT)
Leukopenia	
Most myelosuppressive agents produce WBC nadir 7–14 days after drug administration; myelosuppression will be severe and prolonged with increased dosages: for example, with cytarabine 3–6 g; busulfan 2–6 g, cyclophosphamide 2–3 g, methotrexate 6–8 g, etoposide 2–3 g	Avoid having fresh fruit, plants, and flowers at or near bedside
	Avoid eating raw vegetables, fruits and eggs
	Avoid cleaning animal litter boxes since feces contain high levels of bacteria and fungi
Nursing action	Maintain good personal hygiene—for example, bathe daily, wash hands before eating and preparing food, clean carefully after bowel movements, and keep nails clean and clipped short and straight across; maintain adequate fluid intake
Monitor white blood count and differential; change equipment as indicated—for example, O₂ set up, denture cups, IV supplies; teach sexual hygiene	

Conserve energy; get adequate rest and exercise

Prevent trauma to the skin and mucous membranes

Avoid elective dental work or surgery

Avoid enemas, rectal suppositories and temperatures, and catheterizations

Use toothettes or nonabrasive dental cleaning devices

Report signs and symptoms of infection immediately to the physician; for example, report fever of 38°C or greater, cough, sore throat, a shaking chill, painful or frequent urination, or vaginal discharge

Avoid use of straight-edge razor, power tools, and physical activity that could cause injury

Avoid use of drugs containing aspirin

Humidify the air; use lotion and lubricants on skin and lips; use a soft bristle toothbrush

Avoid invasive procedures; no intramuscular injections, rectal or vaginal exams, enemas, suppositories, or the use of rectal thermometers

Discourage bare feet when ambulatory

Use sanitary pads instead of tampons

Report the following signs and symptoms immediately to the physician: bleeding gums, increased bruising, petechiae, purpura, hypermenorrhea, tarry-colored stools, blood in urine, or coffee-ground emesis

Thrombocytopenia

Drugs associated with a delayed cumulative effect: mitomycin and all nitrosureas

Nursing action

Monitor platelet counts; observe bleeding precautions; apply firm pressure to venipuncture site for 3–5 minutes; monitor pad count on menstruating females; monitor environment for sharp objects

Continued.

Table 8-2   Patient teaching for self-management of most common side effects from chemotherapeutic drugs—cont'd

Side Effects	Points to Cover
Anemia *Nursing action* Monitor hematocrit and hemoglobin, especially during drug nadir	Check with the physician before any dental work Adjust physical activity to accommodate periods of rest Report the following signs and symptoms promptly to the physician: fatigue, dizziness, shortness of breath, and palpitations
Mucositis, Rectal Symptoms occur 3–5 days after chemotherapy *Nursing action* Monitor for electrolyte imbalance and granulocyte count; monitor number, consistency, and amount of bowel movements and urine output; assess for rectal bleeding	Report weight loss to physician Eat low-residue and easily digestible foods Increase intake of liquids to replace fluid loss Follow prescribed medication schedule, such as antidiarrheal and pain control drugs Wash rectal area with soap and water following each bowel movement; pat or air dry
Mucositis, Vaginal Symptoms occur 3–5 days after chemotherapy and subside in 7–10 days after therapy	Report pain, ulceration, or bleeding of mucous membranes lining the perineum and vagina to physician Sitz bath with warm salt water may provide relief of vaginal itching and odor

Use hydrogen peroxide (one-quarter strength) with warm water after voiding to rinse perineal area

Avoid commercial douches, tampons, and vaginal pads or liners containing deodorants

Nausea and Vomiting

Nursing action

Premedicate with antiemetic before nausea begins, for example, one-half hour before meals; patient may require routine antiemetics for 3–5 days following some chemotherapy protocols; monitor fluid and electrolyte status

Drugs with high emetic potential: cisplatin, dacarbazine, dactinomycin, daunorubicin, doxorubicin, mechlorethamine, paclitaxel, and high-dose cytarabine, cyclophosphamide, and methotrexate

Eat frequent, small meals

Avoid greasy or fatty foods and very sweet foods or candies

Avoid unpleasant sights, odors, and tastes

Cold foods, salty foods, dry crackers, and dry toast may be more tolerable

If vomiting is severe, restrict diet to clear liquids and notify the physician

Consider diversionary activities, such as music therapy and relaxation techniques

Recall strategies that were successful during pregnancy, illness, or other times of stress, for example, sipping on a flat cola drink

Continued.

Table 8-2   Patient teaching for self-management of most common side effects from chemotherapeutic drugs—cont'd

Side Effects	Points to Cover
Pharyngitis and Esophagitis	Eat a soft pureed or liquid diet
Symptoms are often first noted by difficult or painful swallowing	Follow prescribed scheduled medication to relieve discomfort
	Report to the physician symptoms that persist more than 3 days
Skin Changes	Maintain good personal hygiene
	Use topical preparations to minimize itching, such as creams or lotions containing vitamins A, D, or E
	Avoid use of perfume and perfumed lotion, wearing fabrics such as wool or corduroy, and wearing tight-fitting clothes such as jeans or pantyhose
Stomatitis (Oral)	Continue brushing regularly; use soft toothbrush
Symptoms occur 5–7 days after chemotherapy and persist up to 10 days	Use nonirritant mouthwash, such as salt, soda, and water solution (¼ tsp salt, pinch of soda, 8 oz water) at least four times daily
	Avoid irritants to the mouth, such as tobacco, alcoholic beverages, spices, and commercial mouthwashes
	Avoid wearing dentures until mouth soreness heals

Maintain good nutritional intake; eat soft or liquid foods high in protein; add sauces or gravies in foods to make food soupier

Points to Cover

Follow prescribed medication schedule, such as scheduled drugs for oral candidisis

Report persistent symptoms promptly to physician, and report if white patches occur on tongue, back of throat, or gums

Table 8-3 Major system toxicity or dysfunction and nursing management

Toxicity/Dysfunction	Nursing Management
Cardiac Toxicity	
Drugs associated with potential: chlorambucil, cyclophosphamide, daunorubicin, doxorubicin, mitoxantrone, and high-dose ifosfamide	Verify baseline cardiac studies (for example, ECG, ejection fraction, cardiac enzymes) before drug admininstration
	Monitor cardiac status and report symptoms regarding tachycardia, shortness of breath, distended neck veins, gallop heart rhythm, and ankle edema
	Monitor and record total cumulative dose of drug in the patient's medical record; doxyrubicin approximate maximum lifetime dose is 500 mg/m^2
Hematopoietic Toxicity (See Table 8-2)	
Hepatic toxicity	
Drugs associated with potential: asparaginase, busulfan, carmustine, chlorambucil, cytarabine, doxorubicin, lomustine, mercaptopurine, methotrexate, mithramycin, and streptozocin	Monitor liver function studies, such as lactic dehydrogenase (LDH), bilirubin, prothrombin time, and liver function tests (SGOT, SGPT)
	Report to the physician signs of jaundice, tenderness over the liver, and urine and stool color changes

Hypersensitivity Reaction

Drugs associated with potential: asparaginase, bleomycin, docetaxel, doxorubicin (local erythema), etoposide, paclitaxel, and teniposide

Review the patient's allergy history

Monitor for symptoms of hypersensitivity and anaphylaxis, such as agitation, urticaria, rash, chills, cyanosis, bronchospasm, abdominal cramping, and hypotension; onset may be rapid or delayed; advise the patient to report subjective symptoms promptly

Ensure proper medical equipment is nearby and in good working condition

Emergency drugs for intervention should be readily available

When administering a drug with potential for a reaction, give a test dose, monitor vital signs, and observe for allergic response

If allergic response occurs, stop drug administration and notify the physician immediately

Metabolic Alterations

Hypercalcemia

Monitor serum level; observe for anorexia, constipation, nausea, vomiting, polyuria, and mental status change

Hyperglycemia

Monitor serum and urine levels; observe for symptoms of thirst, hunger, glucosuria, and weight loss

Continued.

Table 8-3   Major system toxicity or dysfunction and nursing management—cont'd

Toxicity/Dysfunction	Nursing Management
Hyperkalemia	Monitor serum level: observe for symptoms of confusion, complaints of numbness or tingling, weakness, and cardiac arrhythmias
Hypernatremia	Monitor serum level and weight loss; observe for symptoms of thirst, dry mucous membranes, poor skin turgor, rapid thready pulse, restlessness, lethargy
Hyperuricemia Potential with treatment of highly proliferative tumors, such as leukemia and lymphoma	Monitor serum and urine levels; daily intake and output Initiate prescribed drug therapy (for example, allupurinol) to inhibit the formation of uric acid before administration of chemotherapy drug Provide vigorous hydration, such as oral and IV fluid intake (2000 to 3000 ml), beginning 12–24 hours after initiation of chemotherapy Alkalize urine to pH ≥ 7.0 by administration of IV Na HCO₃ (sodium bicarbonate) Report symptoms of pain, chills, fever, and diminished urinary output
Hypocalcemia	Monitor serum level; observe for symptoms of muscle cramping, tingling of extremities, depression, and tetany

Hypomagnesemia	Monitor serum level; observe for symptoms of personality changes, anorexia, nausea, vomiting, lethargy, weakness, and tetany
Hyponatremia	Monitor serum level; observe for symptoms of rales, shortness of breath, distended neck vein, weight gain, edema of sacrum or lower extremity, increasing mental status changes
Neurotoxicity Drugs associated with potential: ifosfamide, vinblastine, vincristine, high peak plasma levels of etoposide, 5-fluorouracil; high-dose and/or intrathecal administration of cytarabine, cisplatin, and methotrexate	Monitor and report symptoms of weakness, numbness, and tingling sensation of hands, arms, and feet; also monitor and report symptoms of hoarseness, jaw pain, hallucinations, mental depression, decreased or absent deep tendon reflexes, slapping gait or foot drop, severe constipation, and paralytic ileus
Ototoxicity Drug associated with potential: cisplatin	Verify baseline audiogram Monitor and report symptoms of tinnitus, hearing loss, and vertigo

Continued.

Table 8-3 Major system toxicity or dysfunction and nursing management—cont'd

Toxicity/Dysfunction	Nursing Management
Pulmonary Toxicity Drugs associated with potential: bleomycin, busulfan, carmustine	Verify baseline respiratory function Individuals older than age 70 years have increased risk Monitor respiratory status and report symptoms of dyspnea, dry cough, rales, tachypnea, and fever
Renal System Toxicity Drugs associated with potential: cisplatin, cyclophosphamide, ifosfamide, methotrexate, mithramycin, streptozocin, and thioplex (thiotepa)	Assess 24-hr urine creatinine clearance before treatment, 2–3 liters for 24 hours before and after therapy Verify baseline renal function Encourage adequate fluid intake, such as 2–3 liters for 24 hours before and after therapy Monitor intake and output, weight changes Report diminished output to physician—for example, less than 500 ml in 24 hours Administer drug MESNA concomitant with ifosfamide, high-dose cyclophosphamide, and thiotepa
Reproductive System Dysfunction Drugs associated with potential: busulfan, chlorambucil, cyclophosphamide, mechlorethamine, thiotepa, vincristine	Assess for nature and frequency of sexual dysfunction Counsel patients regarding avoidance of pregnancy and sperm banking before chemotherapy administration; provide information on contraceptives

Antihormonal agents: finasteride, flutamide, luprolide, tamoxifen, goserelin, zoladex	Birth control practices are recommended by most practitioners for 2 years following chemotherapy to provide for evaluation of disease response, avoidance of possible teratogenic drug effects, and in male patients, recovery of spermatogenesis
	Inform the patients of potential for temporary or permanent infertility and loss of libido
	Women may experience symptoms including amenorrhea, "hot flashes," insomnia, dyspareunia, and vaginal dryness; estrogen therapy may be helpful in management of these symptoms

prepares, administers, stores, or disposes of supplies of unused chemotherapeutic agents.*

Safe handling practice guidelines include the following:

- Drug preparation
- Drug administration
- Disposal of supplies and unused drugs
- Management of chemotherapy spill
- Caring for patients receiving chemotherapy, such as handling of linen contamination, patient excreta
- Staff education
- Employment practice regarding reproductive issues

Drug Preparation

To ensure safe handling, all chemotherapeutic drugs should be prepared according to the package insert in a class II biological safety cabinet (BSC). Venting to the outside is preferable where feasible. Personal protective equipment includes disposable surgical latex gloves and a gown made of lint-free, low-permeability fabric with a closed front, long sleeves, and elastic or knit cuffs. Wear eye-protective splash goggles or face shield when preparing drugs if not using a biological safety cabinet.

Suggestions to minimize exposure:

- Wash hands before and after drug handling.
- Limit access to the drug preparation area.
- Keep a labeled drug spill kit near preparation area.
- Apply gloves before drug handling.
- Prepare drugs using aseptic technique.
- Avoid eating, drinking, smoking, chewing gum, applying cosmetics, or storing food in or near the drug preparation area.
- Place an absorbent pad on the work surface.
- Use Luer-Lok equipment.
- Open drug vials or ampules away from the body.
- Vent vials with a hydrophobic filter needle or pin to prevent spray of the drug.
- Wrap an alcohol wipe around the neck of the ampule before opening it.

---

* Recommendations for safe handling of chemotherapeutic drugs are available from OSHA, National Cytotoxic Study Commission, and American Society of Hospital Pharmacists.

- Prime lines containing drugs inside the BSC using the original drug vial or a sealable bag.
- Cover the tip of the needle with sterile gauze or an alcohol wipe when expelling air from the syringe.
- Label all chemotherapeutic drugs with a chemotherapy hazard label.
- Clean up any spills immediately.
- Transport drugs to the delivery area in a leakproof container.

CLINICAL ALERT: Change gloves between drug preparation and administration and at least every 30 minutes during drug preparation or administration to ensure maximum protection.

Drug Administration

1. Wear protective equipment (gloves, gown, and eyewear) as mentioned in "Drug Preparation."
2. Inform the patient that chemotherapeutic drugs are harmful to normal cells and that protective measures used by personnel minimize their exposure to these drugs throughout their workday.
3. Administer drugs in a safe and unhurried environment.
4. Place a plastic-backed absorbent pad under the tubing during administration to catch any leakage.
5. Do not dispose of any supplies or unused drugs in patient care areas. (See "Disposal of Supplies and Unused Drugs.")
6. Avoid hand-to-eye or hand-to-mouth contact when handling chemotherapeutic drugs.

CLINICAL ALERT: High dose etoposide (≥60 mg/kg) should be given via glass bottle with non poly-vinyl chloride (NON PVC) tubing to prevent chemotherapy spill. (High dose etoposide will melt routine chemo tubing.)

Disposal of Supplies and Unused Drugs

1. Avoid clipping or recapping needles and breaking syringes.
2. Place all supplies used *intact* in a closable, leakproof, puncture-proof, appropriately labeled container.
3. Place all unused drugs in containers into a leakproof, puncture-proof, appropriately labeled container; position these containers in every area where drugs are prepared or administered so that waste materials need not be moved from one area to another.
4. Disposal of containers filled with chemotherapeutic supplies and unused drugs should be in accordance with regulations regard-

ing hazardous wastes, including use of a licensed sanitary landfill or incineration at 1000°C.

Management of Chemotherapy Spills

Chemotherapy spills should be cleaned up immediately by properly protected personnel trained in the appropriate procedures. A spill should be identified with a warning sign so that other persons in the area will not be contaminated. Recommended supplies and procedures to manage a chemotherapy spill on hard surfaces, linens, personnel, or patients include the following:

 I. Supplies
  A. Chemotherapy spill kit:
   1. Respirator mask for airborne powder spills
   2. Plastic safety glasses or goggles
   3. Heavy-duty rubber gloves
   4. Absorbent pads to contain liquid spills
   5. Absorbent towels for clean-up after spill
   6. Small scoop to collect glass fragments
   7. Two large waste disposal bags
  B. Protective disposable gown (see "Drug Preparation")
  C. Containers of detergent solution and clear tap water for postspill cleanup
  D. Approved chemotherapy waste disposal closable, puncture-proof, and leakproof container
  E. Approved, specially labeled, impervious laundry bag
  F. Eye wash faucet adapters or fountain available in or near work area
 II. Procedure for a spill on a hard surface
  A. Restrict the area of the spill.
  B. Obtain a drug spill kit.
  C. Put on protective gown, gloves, and goggles (respirator mask if powder spill).
  D. Open waste disposal bags (double bag).
  E. Place absorbent pads gently on the spill; be careful not to touch spill.
  F. Place saturated absorbent pads into the waste bag.
  G. Cleanse the surface with absorbent towels using detergent solution; wipe clean with clean tap water.
  H. Place all contaminated materials (for example, gown, gloves, saturated absorbent pads, and towels) into double-bagged waste disposal bags.

    I. Discard the waste bag with contents into an approved waste disposal container.

    J. Wash hands thoroughly with soap and water.

III. Procedure for a spill on linen

    A. Restrict the area of the spill.

    B. Obtain a drug spill kit.

    C. Obtain a specially marked, approved laundry bag, and a labeled, impervious bag.

    D. Put on protective gown, gloves, goggles.

    E. Remove soiled, contaminated linen from the patient's bedside.

    F. Place linen in an approved, specially marked, impervious laundry bag.

    G. Contaminated linen should be washed two times in laundry; laundry personnel should wear surgical latex gloves and gown when handling this material.

    H. Clean the contaminated area with absorbent towels and a detergent solution.

    I. Place all contaminated supplies used for management of spill into a waste disposal bag and discard it in an approved waste disposal container.

    J. Wash hands thoroughly with soap and water.

IV. Procedure for a spill on personnel or a patient

    A. Restrict the area of spill.

    B. Obtain a drug spill kit.

    C. Immediately remove the contaminated protective garments or linen.

    D. Wash the affected skin area with soap and water.

    E. Eye exposure; immediately flood the affected eye with water for at least 5 minutes; obtain medical attention promptly.

    F. Properly care for contaminated linen. (See "Procedure for a Spill on Linen.")

    G. Notify the physician if the drug spills on the patient.

V. Documentation

    A. Document in the patient's medical record management of drug spill and notification of the patient's physician.

    B. Document on the agency's approved forms management of any spill occurring on hard surface, linen, or personnel.

Caring for Patients Receiving Chemotherapeutic Drugs

Personnel handling blood, vomitus, or excreta from patients who have received chemotherapy within the previous 48 hours should wear disposable surgical latex gloves and gowns to be discarded after use. (See "Disposal of Supplies and Unused Drugs.") Linen contaminated with chemotherapeutic drugs, blood, vomitus, or excreta from a patient who has received these drugs up to 48 hours before should be placed in a specially marked, impervious laundry bag. (See "Procedure for a Spill on Linen.")

Staff Education

All personnel involved in any aspect of the handling of chemotherapeutic agents should receive an orientation to chemotherapy drugs, including their known risks, relevant techniques and procedures for handling, the proper use of protective equipment and materials, spill procedures, and medical policies; this personnel category includes those who are pregnant or actively trying to conceive children (per OSHA requirements). Evaluation of staff compliance may be achieved by quality monitoring on a regular basis. (See "Chapter Resources" for an example of an audit tool.) When possible, use a peer review system. Peer pressure often induces improved compliance.

Employment Practices Regarding Reproductive Issues

The handling of chemotherapeutic agents by women who are either pregnant or actively trying to conceive and by those who are breast-feeding remains a sensitive and unsettled issue. Suggestions have been made to offer these personnel the opportunity to transfer to areas that do not involve chemotherapeutic agents. All safe handling guidelines should be practiced with utmost care by all pregnant personnel.

Extravasation Management

Definition

Extravasation is the accidental infiltration of vesicant or irritant chemotherapeutic drugs from the vein into surrounding tissues at the IV site. A vesicant is an agent that can produce a blister, tissue destruction, or both. An irritant is an agent that is capable of producing venous pain at the site of and along the vein with or

Table 8-4   Chemotherapeutic drugs, nonvesicants

Generic Name	Trade Name
Asparaginase	Elspar
Bleomycin	Blenoxane
Carboplatin	Paraplatin
Cisplatin	Platinol
Cladribine	Luestatin (2-cdA)
Cyclophosphamide	Cytoxan
Cytarabine (ara-C)	Cytosar-u
Docetaxel	Taxotere
Floxuridine	FUDR
Fludarabine	Fludara
Fluorouracil	Efudex
Ifosfamide	IFEX
Methotrexate	Methotrexate
Mitoxantrone	Novantrone
Paclitaxel	Taxol
Pentostatin	Deoxycoformycin
Thioplex	Thiotepa
Topotecan	

without an inflammatory reaction. Injuries that may occur as the result of extravasation include sloughing of tissue, infection, pain, and loss of mobility of an extremity. The degree of tissue damage is related to several factors such as drug concentration, the quantity of drug extravasated, individual tissue responses, and anatomic location (e.g., dorsum of hand, wrist, or antecubital fossa). (See Tables 8-4 to 8-6 for a list of the nonvesicant drugs and drugs with irritant and vesicant potential.)

Clinical Studies

Because of the harmful effect of vesicants on tissues, studies using patients as subjects are ethically and morally prohibitive. As a result, controlled clinical trials demonstrating effectiveness of treatment have been difficult to attain. Most extravasation interventions have been based on preclinical studies using animal model systems including mice, pigs, rabbits, and dogs. Treatment strategies for extravasation management include the use of specific antidotes based on their mechanism of action and guidelines for immediate intervention to minimize the tissue damage. Prevention of the extravasation and prompt intervention are the key elements for successful extravasation management.

Controversial Issues*

The management of extravasation of chemotherapeutic drugs involves some controversial issues. These issues include the following:

I. Use of antecubital fossa for drug administration
   A. Favoring antecubital fossa access
      1. Larger veins permit more rapid infusion of drug.
      2. Larger veins permit potentially irritating drugs to reach the general circulation sooner, with less irritation.
   B. Opposing antecubital fossa access
      1. Arm mobility is restricted.
      2. Infiltration could cause extensive reconstructive efforts.
      3. Early infiltration may be difficult to assess.
      4. Potential for venous fibrosis; blood drawing from antecubital fossa may be more difficult.
II. Methods of drug sequencing
   A. Favoring the administration of vesicants first
      1. Vascular integrity decreases over time.
      2. Initial assessment of vein patency is most accurate.
      3. There is a potential for diminishing patient awareness of symptoms related to drug infiltration.
   B. Favoring the administration of vesicants last
      1. Vesicants are irritating and may increase vein fragility.
      2. Venous spasm may occur at onset of drug administration and alter assessment of venous access.
III. Needle or catheter size
   A. Favoring the use of larger gauge, such as 18 or 19 gauge
      1. Potentially irritating chemotherapeutic agents can reach circulation sooner, with less irritating effect on the peripheral veins (see Table 8-5).
   B. Favoring the use of smaller gauge, such as 20 or 23 gauge
      1. Smaller-gauge devices are less likely to puncture the wall of a small vein.

* Adapted from Oncology Nursing Society Task Force: *Cancer chemotherapy guidelines and recommendations for nursing education and practice,* 1996 guidelines, Pittsburgh, 1996, The Society.

Table 8-5   Chemotherapeutic drugs with irritant potential

Generic Name	Trade Name
Carmustine (BCNU)	BiCNU
Dacarbazine	DITC-Dome
Etoposide	VePesid
Mitoguazone	Methyl-GAG, MGBG
Streptozocin	Zanosar
Teniposide	Vumon

2. Increased blood flow around a smaller-gauge device increases dilution of chemotherapeutic agents.
3. Phlebitis may be minimized with a smaller-gauge device.

Prevention of Extravasation

Nursing staff responsibilities for the prevention of extravasation include the following:

- Knowledge of drugs with vesicant potential (see Table 8-6)
- Skill in drug administration
- Identification of risk factors, such as multiple vein punctures, previous treatment
- Anticipation of extravasation and knowledge of approved management protocol
- Establishment of a new venipuncture site daily if peripheral access is used
- Consideration of central venous access for difficult peripheral access
- Administration of drug in a quiet, unhurried environment
- Testing of vein patency *without* using chemotherapeutic agents
- Adequate drug dilution, such as side port infusion via free-flowing IV infusion
- Careful observation (visualization of access site, extremity) throughout the procedure
- Validation of blood return from IV site before, during, and after vesicant drug infusion
- Education of patients regarding symptoms of drug infiltration, such as pain, burning, and stinging sensations at IV site

Table 8-6   Chemotherapeutic drugs with vesicant potential

Generic Name	Trade Name
Dactinomycin	Actinomycin D, Cosmegen
Daunorubicin	Cerubidine, Daunomycin
Doxorubicin	Adriamycin
Epirubicin	Pharmorubin
Esorubicin	4-Deoxydrorubicin
Idarubicin	Idarmycin
Mechlorethamine	Nitrogen Mustard, Mustargen
Mitomycin-C	Mutamycin
Menogaril	Tomasar
Piroxantrone	Oxantrazole
Plicamycin	Mithracin
Vinblastine	Velban
Vincristine	Oncovin
Vindesine	Eldisine
Vinorelbine	Navelbine

Protocol for Extravasation Management (Peripheral Site)

Agency policy and procedure guidelines for management of extravasation with the responsible physician's prescription should be easily accessible to the staff. The approved antidote should be readily available, and the following procedure should be initiated with a physician's prescription as soon as extravasation of a vesicant or irritant agent is suspected or occurs:

1. Stop the administration of the chemotherapeutic drug.
2. Leave the needle or catheter in place.
3. Aspirate any residual drug and blood in the IV tubing, needle or catheter, and suspected infiltration site.
4. Instill the IV antidote (see Table 8-7).
5. Remove the needle.
6. If unable to aspirate the residual drug from the IV tubing, remove needle or catheter.
7. Inject the antidote subcutaneously clockwise into the infiltrated site using a 25-gauge needle; change the needle with each new injection.
8. Avoid applying pressure to the suspected infiltration site.
9. Photograph the suspected area of extravasation according to agency's policy and procedure for documentation and follow-up.

Table 8-7   Chemotherapeutic vesicant drugs with recommended antidotes

Drug	Antidote
Alkylating Agent	
Mechlorethamine (Mustargen, Nitrogen Mustard), Mitomycin-C (Mutamycin)	Isotonic Sodium thiosulfate 1/6-molar–4.4 g/10 ml Dilute 1.6 ml of sodium thiosulfate 25% with 8.4 ml of sterile water for injection; apply cold compresses
Antibiotics	Apply *Ice cold* compresses immediately for 30–60 minutes
Daunorubicin (Daunomycin, Cerubidine), Doxorubicin (Adriamycin)	
Amsacrine	Alternate protocol: Topical dimethyl sulfoxide (DMSO) 1–2 ml of 1 mmol DMSO 50%–100%; apply topically one time at the site; apply *cold* compresses
Bisantrene	Sodium bicarbonate 1 mEq/ml Mix equal parts of sodium bicarbonate with sterile normal saline (1:1 solution); resulting solution is 0.5 mEq/ml Inject 2–6 ml (1.0–3.0 mEq) IV through existing IV line and sub.q. into the extravasated site; apply cold compresses

Table 8–7   Chemotherapeutic vesicant drugs with recommended antidotes—cont'd

Drug	Antidote
Vinca Alkaloids	Hyaluronidase (Wydase) 150 u/ml
Teniposide	Add 1 ml sterile sodium chloride
Vinblastine	Inject 1–6 ml (150 to 900 u) sub.q. into the extravasated
Vincristine	site with multiple injections; apply warm compresses;
Vindesine	DO NOT inject corticosteroids
Vinorelbine	
These drugs have no known specific antidotes	
Dactinomycin	
Epirubicin	
Esorubicin	
Idarubicin	
Menogaril	
Mitoxantrone	
Piroxantrone	

10. Apply topical ointment if ordered.
11. Cover lightly with an occlusive sterile dressing.
12. Apply cold or warm compresses as indicated (see Table 8-7).
13. Elevate the extremity.
14. Observe regularly for pain, erythema, induration, and necrosis.
15. Document the following elements of extravasation management:
    a. Date
    b. Time
    c. Needle or catheter size and type
    d. Insertion site, location, and description
    e. Number and location of previous venipuncture attempts and any difficulty in venipuncture
    f. Drug sequence
    g. Approximate amount of drug extravasated
    h. Nursing management of extravasation
    i. Photo documentation
    j. Patient complaints and statements
    k. Appearance of site
    l. Physician notification
    m. Follow-up measures
    n. Nurse's signature

CLINICAL ALERT: The process of tissue destruction resulting from drug extravasation may be subtle and progressive. Initial symptoms include pain or burning at IV site, progressing to erythema, edema, and superficial skin loss. Tissue necrosis may not develop until 1 to 4 weeks after the drug extravasation.

Anaphylaxis

Nursing personnel administering chemotherapy should be alert and prepared for the possible complications of anaphylaxis. The drugs and supplies necessary to manage these complications must be readily available.

Emergency medications and supplies for management of anaphylaxis include the following:

Injectable aminophylline, diphenhydramine hydrochloride
    (Benadryl), dopamine, epinephrine, heparin, hydrocortisone
Oxygen setup, tubing cannula or mask, and airway device

IV fluids (isotonic solutions)

IV tubings and supplies for venous access

All or some of these symptoms may be present: anxiety, hypotension, urticaria, cyanosis, respiratory distress, abdominal cramping, flushed appearance, chills. The calm and reassuring presence of the nurse will facilitate in the management of these symptoms; management proceeds as follows:

1. Immediately stop the drug infusion.
2. Maintain an intravenous line with isotonic saline.
3. Position the patient for comfort and to promote perfusion of the vital organs.
4. Notify the physician, nursing agency, and emergency medical services.
5. Maintain the airway and anticipate the need for cardiopulmonary resuscitation.
6. Monitor the vital signs according to agency policy.
7. Administer the appropriate medications with the approved physician's order.
8. Follow the nursing agency's protocol for follow-up care (for example, evaluation of the patient by physician).
9. Document the incident in the patient's medical record.

CLINICAL ALERT: Prompt and effective nursing interventions for anaphylaxis decrease complications. The nurse must be alert to the signs and symptoms of an anaphylactic response to a chemotherapeutic drug. Table 8-8 lists Chemotherapy Drugs' potential for anaphylaxis.

Documentation Recommendations

- Site assessment before and after infusion or injection of chemotherapeutic drug
- Establishment of blood return before, during, and after IV and intraarterial infusion of chemotherapy
- Needle or catheter size and type
- Establishment of catheter or device patency before, during, and after infusion of chemotherapy—for example, intraperitoneal, intrathecal
- Drug sequence and administration technique
- Patient/family education regarding chemotherapy protocol—potential side effects and toxicities, self-management of side effects, and schedule of follow-up blood counts, tests, and procedures

- Chemotherapeutic drug, dose, route, time, and date
- Premedications or postmedications, flushing solutions, other infusions, and supplies used for chemotherapy drug regimen
- Any patient complaints of discomfort and symptoms experienced before, during, and after chemotherapeutic infusion

Nursing Diagnoses

- Knowledge deficit, related to chemotherapeutic side effects
- Oral mucous membrane, altered, related to side effects of drugs
- Injury, risk for, related to alteration in immune system
- Injury, risk for, related to alteration in clotting factors
- Sexual dysfunction, related to effects of chemotherapeutic drugs (alkylating agents)
- Nutrition, altered: less than body requirements, related to nausea and vomiting
- Anxiety, related to bone marrow transplant rejection and use of a new drug for treatment

Patient/Family Teaching for Self-Management

- Assess patient's ability and willingness to learn, availability of caregiver, environment at home, ability to assume self-care, and compliance with treatment regimen.
- Describe purpose, schedule, and procedure of chemotherapeutic regimen.
- Explain to the patient the potential side effects from chemotherapeutic drugs (nausea and vomiting, anorexia, stomatitis, constipation, diarrhea, alopecia, and skin and hemopoietic changes).
- Instruct the patient or the caregiver on self-management interventions specific to each of the side effects.
- Review symptoms such as temperature elevation over 38°C, severe constipation or diarrhea, persistent bleeding from any site, sudden weight gain or loss, shortness of breath, pain not relieved by prescribed medications, and severe nausea and vomiting more than 24 hours after treatment, and reporting of these symptoms promptly to the physician.
- Instruct the patient or the caregiver regarding management of infusion devices of patient receiving chemotherapy in the home.
- Validate the aseptic technique and skills of the patient or the caregiver for prescribed self-administration and discontinuation of chemotherapeutic drugs.

Table 8-8   Chemotherapy drugs' potential for anaphylaxis

Drugs	Signs and Symptoms	Precautions
Asparaginase (Elspar)	Respiratory distress, increased pulse, respirations, hypotension, facial edema, anxiety, flushed appearance, hives, itching; risk for anaphylaxis increases with each dose	Test dose before initial IV/IM dosing; monitor 30 minutes IM or 60 minutes IV after drug administration; keep vein open with IV normal saline before, during, and 30/60 minutes after IV administration of asparaginase. Initiate drug infusion slowly (mg/m2/titrate infusion). Code Care; O₂; suction; drugs for anaphylaxis at or near patient's bedside
	Test Dose Procedure: Prepare 10,000 IU asparaginase with 5 ml N/S; inject 0.1 ml of this solution (200 IU) into 9.9 ml NS; inject intradermally 0.1 ml of this concentration (2 IU) to make a wheal in inner aspect of arm; observe wheal for 60 minutes for erythema, swelling, itching before doing infusion.	
Bleomycin	Dyspnea, hypotension, increased pulse and respiration, rash	Test dose prior to initial IV dosing; initiate drug infusion slowly (10–20 ml/15 min); monitor vital signs and auscultate breath sounds Q4hr during and for 24 hours postinfusion and/or on scheduled basis in outpatient setting
	Test Dose Procedure: Inject 2 units of bleomycin intradermal to make a wheal in inner aspect of arm; observe for erythema or edema itching before first 2 doses of bleomycin infusion	

Etoposide (VP-16)	Hypotension, bronchospasm, chest pain, increased pulse, respirations, facial flush, fever, chills, diaphoresis	Initiate drug infusion slowly(10–20 ml/15 min). Infuse total volume over at least 60 minutes. Monitor vital signs Q15 min. × 4; Q30 min. × 2 and Q4hr, during and 24 hours after infusion
Teniposide (VM-26)	Severe hypotension, anxiety, increased pulse, respirations, fever	Initiate drug infusion *slowly* (10–20 ml/30 min). Total infusion time 60–120 minutes. Monitor vital signs Q15 min. × 4; Q30 min. × 2, during and postinfusion; then monitor Q4hr × 24 hours
Paclitaxel (Taxol) (Fig. 8-6) Docetaxel (Taxotere)	Increased or decreased BP; increased temperature and pulse; restlessness, dyspnea, bronchospasm, facial flushing, hives *If any of these symptoms occur, stop the drug infusion and notify the physician immediately*	Premedicate with the following before Taxol or Taxotere infusion: Dexamethasone 10–20 mg PO/IV 12 to 16 hrs; diphenhydramine 50 mg IV push 30–60 mins; cimetidine 300 mg IV over 30 mins; infuse taxol/taxotere in a glass bottle with non-pvc tubing and a 0.22 micron filter; Obtain baseline VS: then monitor Q15 mins. × 4; Q1 hr. × 4; Q4 hrs. × 4 during the infusion. Ensure emergent medications: benadryl 50 mg; hydrocortisone 100 mg; adrenalin (Epinephrine) 1:1000—all IV bolus; oxygen, suction, equipment assembled and ready for use

- Explain safe handling precautions for administration and disposal of chemotherapy.
- Provide information and a list of resources for obtaining, storing, and disposing of drugs and supplies, and schedule of follow-up tests and care.
- Discuss requirements for scheduled physician and diagnostic appointments.
- Provide patient teaching materials from the National Cancer Institute and American Cancer Society (titles such as *Chemotherapy and You, What Are Clinical Trials All About, When Someone in Your Family Has Cancer*).
- Consider culture-sensitive materials and interventions.

Home Care Considerations

- Store drugs in a safe, recommended environment, such as refrigeration, away from sunlight.
- Follow procedures for preparation and administration of chemotherapy as in agency or hospital.
- Record drug, dose, route, and time given in home and provide this information to agency responsible for care management.
- Discard all unused drugs and used supplies into a recommended closable, puncture-proof, leakproof container, and return this container to appropriate agency for disposal.
- Provide prompt linen and clothing change with meticulous skin care for the patient with incontinence.
- Use plastic sheeting to protect bedding or furniture if incontinence is possible.
- Carefully handle linen contaminated from chemotherapeutic drugs and excreta, and wash two times separately from all other linen.
- The patient should receive the first dose of the drug(s) in an acute care or outpatient setting.

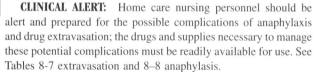

   CLINICAL ALERT: Home care nursing personnel should be alert and prepared for the possible complications of anaphylaxis and drug extravasation; the drugs and supplies necessary to manage these potential complications must be readily available for use. See Tables 8-7 extravasation and 8–8 anaphylasis.

Geriatric Considerations

- Potential for increased toxicities to drugs exist, as do related compromised cardiac, respiratory, renal systems; endocrine and liver functions; and neuromuscular deficits.

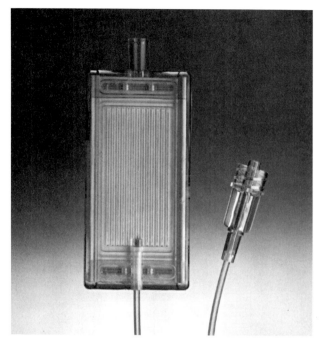

Fig. 8-6
Pall ELD-96P filter for Taxol administration.
Courtesy Pall Biomedical Product Co, Port Washington, NY.

- Anticipate potential sedation effects related to antiemetic therapy and analgesics.
- Monitor serum electrolyte values closely: Potential exists for alterations related to concomitant diseases such as arthritis, diabetes, and hypertension.
- Query the patient or caregiver about other current medications (prescribed and over-the-counter), which may interfere or increase toxicities related to the chemotherapy drugs.
- Age-related neuromuscular sensory deficits may include but are not limited to visual, hearing, fine motor skills, and mobility status deficits and changes to patterns of bowel and bladder elimination. Assess potential for changes and deficits and plan for appropriate intervention. Follow these basic guidelines:

- Introduce yourself and face the patient while speaking.
- Provide simple, step-by-step instructions for tasks.
- Include caregiver in the instructions.
- Monitor bowel and bladder function; for example, increased fluid intake may require limits due to bladder toxicity.
- Provide for rest or naps; reduce mental activity late in day.
- Assess and monitor skin integrity; for example, plan and provide body position changes on a scheduled frequency for the activity-compromised patient.
- Consult with community resources for patient health maintenance management. For example, consult social services (financial, housing, companion care), home health-care agencies (physical care), Meals on Wheels programs (nutrition), and senior citizen programs (recreation, socialization).
- Consider and plan developmental age-related interventions for sexuality issues such as dry vaginal mucous membrane and impotence related to side effects of chemotherapy drugs.

Chapter Resources

Safe Handling of Antineoplastic Agents—Process Audit
Agency Name _____

Nurse's Name _____
Monitor's Name _____
Date _____

	Yes	No	N/A
Preparation and Administration of Antineoplastic Drugs			
1. Hands are washed before preparing drug.			
2. Eye-protective splash goggles are to be worn with: no glasses, contacts, and/or glasses during drug preparation and administration.			
3. Polyethylene gown is worn during drug preparation.			
4. Polyethylene gown is worn during drug administration.			
5. Gown is changed between patients.			

	Yes	No	N/A
6. Gown is removed before leaving unit for errands.			
7. Latex gloves are worn during drug preparation.			
8. Latex gloves are worn during drug administration.			
9. Latex gloves are changed approximately every 30 minutes during drug preparation.			
10. Latex gloves are changed approximately every 30 minutes during drug administration.			
11. Luer-Lok fitting syringes are used for drug preparation.			
12. Luer-Lok fitting syringes are used for drug administration.			
13. Chemo-stick pin is used when withdrawing drug from a multi- or single-dose vial.			
14. A sterile alcohol wipe is used when breaking the cap off a glass ampule.			
15. Caution is used when removing air bubbles from filled syringe; sterile alcohol wipe is placed at needle, syringe, or IV tubing tip.			
16. All IV tubings are preprimed and tubing connection is checked for secure fitting of syringe or needle.			
17. Caution is used when inserting needle, syringe, or IV tubing containing antineoplastic drugs and when injecting drug into the patient's IV site (for example, Hickman catheter, Port-a-Cath, or heparin lock).			
18. Work area is kept clean and organized.			
Disposal of Antineoplastic Agents/Supplies Linen/ Excreta			
1. Contaminated needles and syringes are disposed of intact into chemotherapy waste box.			

Safe Handling of Antineoplastic Agents—Process Audit—cont'd

	Yes	No	N/A
2. Gown and gloves are removed and disposed into chemotherapy waste box.			
3. All antineoplastic drug supplies—syringes, IV tubings, IV bags, used alcohol wipes—are disposed of into chemotherapy waste box.			
4. Hands are washed after disposing of waste products and removing gloves.			
5. Chemotherapy waste box is properly labeled with expiration date.			
6. Chemotherapy waste box is properly secured for disposal pickup.			
7. Linen soiled with chemotherapy spill is handled appropriately.			
8. Procedure for disposal of patient excreta is handled appropriately.			
Management of Antineoplastic Drug Spillage			
1. Chemotherapy spill kit is accessible; use is understood.			
2. Management of antineoplastic drug spill on hard surface, such as countertop or floor is understood.			
3. Management of antineoplastic drug spill on soft surface such as linen or clothing is understood.			
4. Management of antineoplastic drug spill on person such as patient or nurse is understood.			
5. Use of eye wash adapters is demonstrated.			
Notification Caution Label for Chemotherapy			
1. Caution label for chemotherapy is attached to IV solution to remind hospital personnel not to alter IV rate and to report immediately to unit if there is an IV disconnection or a chemotherapy spillage.			

Study Questions

1. A patient experiencing chemotherapy drug anaphylaxis may have the following symptoms:
   a. Tachycardia, hypertension, dyspnea, back pain
   b. Bradycardia, hypotension, chest pain, fever
   c. Chills, constipation, diaphoresis, facial flushing
   d. Dyspnea, hypotension, hives, tachycardia

2. Which chemotherapy vesicant drugs have extravasation potential?
   a. Dactinomycin, daunorubicin, doxorubicin, Dilantin
   b. Carboplatin, cisplatin, cladribine, cyclophosphamide
   c. Methotrexate, mitoxantrone, mitotane, mustargen
   d. Vinblastine, vincristine, vindesine, vinorelbine

3. Nursing practice guidelines to prevent/diminish chemotherapy drug extravasation include the following:
   a. Knowledge of drugs with vesicant potential, testing of the vein with the chemotherapy drug, validation of blood return, monitoring of the drug during bolus/continuous infusion
   b. Knowledge of drugs with vesicant potential, testing of the vein with normal saline, validation of blood return after drug administration, monitoring of the drug during bolus/continuous infusion
   c. Knowledge of drugs with vesicant potential, testing of the vein with normal saline, validation of blood return during drug administration, monitoring of the drug during bolus/continuous infusion
   d. Knowledge of drugs with vesicant potential; testing of the vein with normal saline; validation of blood return before, during, and after drug administration; monitoring of the drug during bolus/continuous infusion

4. Recommended nursing practice guidelines for safe handling of chemotherapy drugs include the following:
   a. Physician's order to use gown, gloves, goggles
   b. Use of gown and goggles only when administering intrathecal chemotherapy drugs
   c. Use of gown, gloves, and goggles during preparation and administration only

d. Use of gown, gloves, and goggles during preparation, administration, and disposal; washing of hands before and after handling chemotherapy drugs

5. A visitor reports to the nurse at the desk that "my mother's chemotherapy tubing came apart and the drug is leaking." The nurse should do the following:
    a. Obtain a chemotherapy drug spill kit and designate the spill cleanup to housekeeping.
    b. Obtain a chemotherapy spill kit, apply gloves, clean up the chemotherapy drug spill, and document the occurrence.
    c. Obtain a chemotherapy spill kit, apply gown, gloves, and goggles; clean up the drug spill; and document the occurrence.
    d. Obtain a chemotherapy spill kit; apply gown, gloves, and goggles; clean up the drug spill; wash hands; and document the occurrence.

6. The following chemotherapy drugs have potential for cardiac toxicity:
    a. Chlorambucil, daunorubicin, doxorubicin, mitoxantrone
    b. Cyclophosphamide, etoposide, ifosfamide, teniposide
    c. Bleomycin, mitomycin-C, mithramycin, methotrexate
    d. Carboplatin, carmustine, cisplatin, cyclophosphamide

7. The following chemotherapy drugs have potential for neurotoxicity:
    a. Cladribine, vinblastine, vincristine, vinorelbine
    b. Chlorambucil, cisplatin, cytarabine, lomustine
    c. Etoposide, ifosfamide, vinblastine, vincristine
    d. Vinblastine, vincristine, vinorelbine, prednisone

8. Patient/family education strategies for anorexia include the following:
    a. Eating alone, freshening up before meals, small frequent feedings, concentration on low-calorie foods
    b. Eating with others, freshening up before meals, small frequent feedings, concentration on high-calorie foods
    c. Eating with others, freshening up before meals, large frequent feedings, concentration on high-calorie foods
    d. Eating alone, freshening up before meals, small frequent feedings, concentration on high-calorie foods

9. Myelosuppression from chemotherapy drugs increase the potential for infection; practices to diminish infection potential include the following:

   a. Avoid sources of infection, maintain good personal hygiene, get adequate rest and exercise, and report signs and symptoms of infection immediately.

   b. Avoid sources of infection, maintain good personal hygiene, omit all exercise, and report signs and symptoms of infection immediately.

   c. Avoid sources of infection, maintain good personal hygiene, get adequate rest and exercise, and report signs and symptoms of infection at the next scheduled appointment.

   d. Avoid sources of infection, maintain good personal hygiene, get lots of exercise, and report signs and symptoms of infection immediately.

10. Match the term in the left column with the correct definition in the right column.

Intraarterial chemotherapy	_____	a. Requires preservative-free diluent, volume less than 15 ml
Intraperitoneal chemotherapy	_____	b. May be administered bolus, continuously, intermittently, or by peripheral or central venous access
Intrathecal chemotherapy	_____	c. Warm infusate to 38°C prior to infusion; monitor abdominal pain, pressure, girth
Intravenous chemotherapy	_____	d. Monitor catheter placement site: circulation, warmth, color, bleeding

ANSWERS: 1. d   2. d   3. d   4. d   5. d
6. a   7. c   8. b   9. a   10. Intraarterial—d; intraperitoneal—c; intrathecal—a; intravenous-b

Parenteral Nutrition

9

Objectives

1. Identify indications for parenteral nutrition.

2. List conditions frequently treated with total parenteral nutrition (TPN).

3. Describe indicators of nutritional status.

4. Contrast peripheral and central administration of parenteral nutrition.

5. Discuss complications of TPN and information to be reported to the physician.

Parenteral nutrition is the IV form of nutritional support. Because this treatment is expensive and can cause significant risks to the patient, IV methods are used only when a catabolic (starvation) state is present or when the patient's digestive system does not function. The goal of parenteral nutrition is to provide all essential nutrients in adequate amounts to sustain an individual in nutritional balance during periods when oral or enteral routes of feeding are impossible or insufficient to meet the patient's needs. TPN maintains lean body mass, promotes tissue function, and maintains nitrogen balance.

Indications for Parenteral Nutrition

TPN is used as adjunctive therapy in patients with severe intestinal disease who would otherwise starve (Fig. 9-1). Much research, often with conflicting results, has been conducted on the effective-

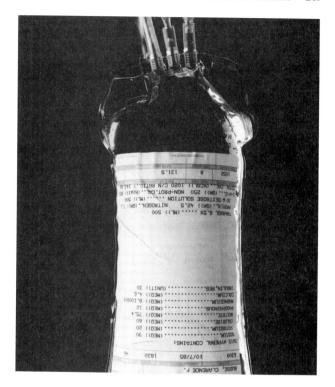

Fig. 9-1
Parenteral nutrition infusion.
From Perry AG, Potter PA: *Clinical nursing skills and techniques,*
St Louis, 1994, Mosby.

ness of parenteral nutrition as supplemental therapy. Exactly which
conditions are improved demonstrably by TPN is controversial. As
a rule of thumb, parenteral nutrition is indicated for patients who
are severely malnourished and cannot be fed adequately using the
oral or enteral route.

The following conditions are often treated with TPN:

1. Gastrointestinal dysfunctions, such as inflammatory bowel
   disease, short bowel syndrome, pancreatitis, colitis, fistulas,
   radiation enteritis, ileus, intractable diarrhea, bowel obstruction, gastric carcinomas, or entesocutaneous fistulas

2. Hepatic failure
3. Hypermetabolic states, such as sepsis, severe burns, long bone fractures, peritonitis
4. Anorexia secondary to patient's medical condition, as in renal failure
5. Severe hyperemesis during pregnancy
6. Severe gastrointestinal candida in patient with acquired immunodeficiency syndrome (AIDS)
7. Multisystem trauma

Nutritional Requirements

Both energy and nutrient sources are required by all persons, in health and in illness. Without adequate nonprotein calories, the body uses its own protein from muscles, from visceral stores, and from the amino acids provided in the parenteral nutrition solution. An objective of parenteral nutrition is to meet energy needs through nonprotein calorie sources so that the infused amino acids can be directed toward protein synthesis. (Protein breakdown for energy is a catabolic process; protein synthesis is an anabolic process.)

Parenteral nutrition solutions contain energy sources in the forms of dextrose and lipids, as well as nitrogen sources in the form of amino acids, vitamins, and trace elements. Research in the area of parenteral nutrition is focusing on the pharmacologic role of individual nutrients. In the future it is hoped that precise nutrient prescriptions may be used to treat specific diseases. The amounts of the various components of parenteral nutrition vary according to patient condition; however, the combinations of components tend to be standard. Each of the basic components of parenteral nutrition is discussed in the following sections.

Energy

Energy required by the body for metabolic processes, heat production, and physical activity can be provided by carbohydrates, protein, or fat. Energy needs are met in parenteral nutrition through dextrose (carbohydrate) and lipid (fat) administration. The greater the intake of carbohydrates and fat, the less protein is needed to achieve nitrogen balance. Even though basal levels of glucose and fat are required for normal body processes, there is not a fixed recommendation for the ratio of glucose to fat that should be provided (see Table 9-1 for a summary of the disadvantages of

Table 9-1   Disadvantages of either glucose or fat as the sole nonnitrogen energy source in TPN

Glucose	Fat
Increase of basal metabolic rate	Limited elimination capacity
Increased release of catecholamines	Reduced tolerance in premature infants
Increased release of insulin	Risk of fat overload
Increased release of glucagon	Immune functions—possible impairment
Hyperglycemia	
Increased CO_2 production	Increased gluconeogenesis—nitrogen losses
Essential fatty acid deficiency	Ketone body formation—acidosis
Lipid deposition in the liver	

From Ekman L, Wretlind A: The glucose-lipid ratio in parenteral nutrition. *Nutr Support Serv* 5(9):26, 1985.

using only dextrose or only fat as the nonnitrogen energy source). The energy expenditure of healthy individuals depends mostly on the basal metabolic rate and the level of physical activity. In illness a greater amount of energy is often required because the individual's metabolic rate is increased. For example, prolonged fever increases energy requirement by 7% per Fahrenheit degree and 13% per centigrade degree. A widely used method for calculating resting energy expenditure is the Harris-Benedict equations (see Chapter Resources). During illness, caloric (energy) needs vary according to age, sex, height, weight, activity, and the presence of catabolic states such as sepsis, severe injuries, and burns.

Carbohydrates

Carbohydrates, in the form of glucose, are the major energy source for humans and are the only energy source for the central nervous system. The CNS requires about 150 g of glucose per day. Dextrose is the least expensive source of glucose and is available in concentrations of 5% to 70% dextrose in water. Concentrated dextrose is the primary calorie source in TPN.

Fat Emulsion

Fat is the chief storage source of energy in the body. Fat emulsions, also called lipid solutions, provide a concentrated source of energy during parenteral nutrition. Fat emulsions are available in 10% and 20% concentrations. Fat may be administered to provide 40% to 60% of total daily calories. Only 140 calories are provided by 1 liter of 5% dextrose in water solution, although 1100 calories are provided by 1 liter of 10% fat.

In addition, lipids are a source of essential fatty acids and thus can prevent or correct fatty acid deficiencies. Because use of fatty acids can provide fuel for most tissues, glucose can then be made available for use by the (CNS) and protein for anabolic processes. Finally, the addition of lipids to a parenteral nutrition solution has a buffering effect and may provide some protection to the vein during an infusion of peripheral parenteral nutrition.

Protein

A patient experiences a greater improvement in weight gain and wound healing with the use of IV amino acids than with the use of only IV dextrose. Although protein can provide energy, the continued breakdown of protein for energy adversely affects body functioning, growth, and tissue repair. Enough protein must be administered to replace essential amino acids; otherwise the body will convert its own protein to glucose to meet energy requirements. If body protein is converted to glucose, the patient experiences a persistent loss of protein primarily from muscle tissue, causing a negative nitrogen balance. Because excess protein is metabolized and not stored in the body, maintenance of adequate protein stores is a major objective of nutritional support.

Protein is provided in parenteral nutrition in the form of amino acids, but optimal amino acid levels have not been established. Available preparations containing varying amounts of essential and nonessential amino acids are available in concentrations of 3.5% to 10%. The nitrogen from protein metabolization is excreted principally through urine, so nitrogen loss is measured through urine sampling. Because a small amount of nitrogen is lost through hair, skin, saliva, and stool, a correction factor for these losses is added to the Harris-Benedict equation. (See Chapter Resources.)

Vitamins

Vitamins function as essential cofactors in a number of enzymatic processes and cannot be manufactured within the body. Although actual IV vitamin requirements are unknown, IV requirements are considered greater than oral requirements because of increased renal excretion and absorption of vitamins to IV bags and tubings. Other factors considered in calculating vitamin dosages are the degree of stress experienced by the patient and the extent of depletion present.

Vitamins are classified as either water soluble or fat soluble. Water-soluble vitamins are vitamin C, folate, and the B-complex vitamins: thiamine, riboflavin, niacin, pyridoxine, cobalamin, and biotin. Fat-soluble vitamins are A, D, E, and K. Vitamin K is not included in most commercially prepared IV vitamin solutions because of possible adverse effects in patients taking oral anticoagulants.

Trace Elements

Trace elements are those elements present in the body in extremely small amounts. Like vitamins, trace elements must be provided in long-term parenteral therapy for normal metabolism to take place. All trace elements participate in enzymatic reactions and act as cofactors for other metabolic processes. Currently 15 trace elements have been identified; however, the exact requirements for each element are unknown. Among those thought to be essential are iron, iodine, cobalt, zinc, copper, chromium, and manganese. Commercially prepared trace element combinations are available.

Vitamin	Function	Deficiency
Vitamin A	Retinal function Prevents night blindness Bone metabolism	Night blindness Reproductive failure
Vitamin C	Wound healing	Scurvy
Vitamin D	Calcium absorption	Rickets

Vitamin E	Protects cellular mem-
	  brane
	Prevents oxidation of
	  vitamins A and C
		May contribute to
		  hemolytic anemia
		  and liver necrosis

Vitamin	Function	Deficiency
Vitamin K	Prothrombin formation	Prolonged clotting time and bleeding
Iron	Oxygen transport	Anemia
Zinc	Cofactor of many enzymes	Poor wound healing Growth retardation Diminished taste/smell Gonadal dysfunction
Copper	Hemoglobin synthesis	Associated with neutropenia
Calcium	Bone metabolism Neuromuscular function	Neuromuscular irritability
Phosphate	Found in bone Serum levels regulated by kidney reabsorption	Skeletal and cardiac muscle dysfunction
Potassium	Principal cation in intracellular fluid (ICF)	Critical cardiac dysrhythmias
Sodium	Principal cation in extracellular fluid (ECF) Regulates acid–base balance Neuromuscular function	Alteration in balance of ICF and ECF
Sulfate	Protein synthesis	Wasting
Iodine	Thyroid function	Hypothyroidism

Fluids and Electrolytes

Because they are determined by the patient's condition, fluid and electrolyte needs vary widely. Fluid needs vary when a condition causing fluid loss, fever, or renal or cardiac impairment is present. The amount of water provided in parenteral fluids depends on the patient's fluid needs. Water needs are determined by closely monitoring the patient's weight and intake and output. The greater the dextrose and amino acid concentration of the infusion, the less water will be delivered. For example, 70% dextrose solutions are used when fluid restriction is desired.

Electrolytes are adjusted by the physician according to serum levels. More potassium may be needed as glucose metabolizes.

Other Additives

Sometimes other agents are added to parenteral nutrition fluids. Medications such as regular insulin, heparin, and corticosteroids may be prescribed by the physician when a patient need exists.

Also, some antibiotics, antiemetics, and analgesics are able to be piggybacked to parenteral nutrition admixtures. A pharmacist should determine the compatibility of all additives and piggyback medications.

CLINICAL ALERT: All additives must be mixed in a pharmacy under a laminar flow hood to reduce the risk of infection.

Nutritional Assessment

Assessing the nutritional status of the patient is important when deciding whether parenteral nutrition is necessary and also when monitoring therapy. The first component of this assessment is an evaluation of the effect of the patient's underlying medical condition on nutritional status. Most patients receive TPN because of a gastrointestinal (GI) tract obstruction or inflammation. A diet history, anthropometric measurements, and laboratory tests are all used in the assessment. Each method currently used to assess the extent of malnutrition experienced by a patient has limitations. Currently there is no single, best test for evaluating nutritional status, because many factors influence an individual's nutritional condition. Ultrasonography, magnetic resonance imaging, and computed tomography scans are among the assessment tools that are the focus of current nutritional research.

Nutritional Status Indicators	Comments
Diet history	Includes 24-hour recall, special diets, food allergies or intolerances, appetite, chewing and swallowing difficulties, changes in food intake, and diarrhea associated with eating
Height and weight	Compared to standard height and weight tables; actual body weight is calculated as a percentage of ideal weight

Nutritional Status Indicators	Comments
Basal energy expenditure (BEE)	Estimate of the energy requirements at rest (Harris-Benedict equation)
Anthropometric measurements	Measurements of the midarm circumference, skinfold thickness, and arm muscle are are compared to standard values as a way of inferring patient body mass
Creatinine/height index	Indicates status of muscle stores in patients with normal renal function; creatinine is released from muscle at a constant rate in proportion to muscle mass; patient's index is compared to standards to determine the degree of impairment 5–15%—mild impairment 15–30%—moderate impairment >30%—severe impairment
Serum transferrin	Indicates a combination of protein depletion and iron deficiency 150–200 mg/dl—mild depletion 100–150 mg/dl—moderate depletion <30 mg/dl—severe depletion
Albumin levels	Indirect measures of visceral protein mass; low values are associated with reduced dietary protein or excessive losses; does not reflect immediate changes—20-day half-life; normal range 3.5–5 g/dl
Prealbumin	Short half-life; provides an analysis of protein changes during previous two days; 17–42 mg/dl—normal

Nutritional Status Indicators	Comments
Total lymphocyte count	Used for screening immune function; obtained from the CBC and differential 1200–200/mm^3—mild depletion 800–1200/mm^3—moderate depletion <800/mm^3—severe depletion
T-cell counts	Measure cellular and humoral immune function; normal $T_4:T_8$ ratio is 2
Skin antigen tests	Commonly used antigens include purified protein derivative (PPD), streptokinase-streptodornase (SKSD), *Candida,* mumps, and *Trichophyton;* positive response if 5 mm induration at 72 hours; used to measure response to nutritional therapy
Nitrogen balance	Nitrogen is an essential element of protein required for tissue building; measured as the total nitrogen excreted in urine, plus a correction factor for unmeasured losses, minus the total nitrogen consumed in the form of protein; *positive* nitrogen balance exists when nitrogen intake is greater than nitrogen loss; *negative* nitrogen balance is found in persons who are inadequately fed relative to protein needs; protein is broken down to meet their metabolic needs, and thus these persons excrete more nitrogen than they take in

Administration of Parenteral Nutrition

Central Venous Administration

Parenteral nutrition may be administered through a peripheral vein or through a central vein, depending on the osmolality of the solution. Dextrose concentrations greater than 12.5% need to be given through a large central vein, usually the subclavian. (See Chapter 3 for guidelines on managing central venous catheters.)

Peripheral Parenteral Nutrition

Parenteral nutrition may be administered through peripheral veins as maintenance nutrition for patients who are nutritionally compromised and unable to receive sufficient calories through oral or enteral routes. Maintenance parenteral nutrition is administered both preoperatively and postoperatively to surgical patients with a nutritional deficit in an effort to minimize the adverse effects of malnutrition. Usually the patient's serum albumin will be less than 3.5 g/dl, or it is expected that the patient will have no oral intake for at least 1 week, or both.

The major disadvantage of the peripheral route of administration is that a large fluid volume per gram of dextrose is required to deliver acceptable osmolalities. For example, a 10% dextrose solution provides only 340 calories per liter. To deliver 2000 calories each day would require 6 liters of 10% dextrose. Additional calories are added through the administration of fat emulsions. A 10% fat emulsion provides 550 calories per 500 ml of solution. Another disadvantage of peripheral parenteral nutrition is irritation and sometimes sclerosing of the patient's veins. This is due to the high osmolarity of the solutions.

CLINICAL ALERT: Use the largest rapid blood flow vein available. Hemodilution helps to minimize vein sclerosing by diluting the solution to a more isotonic state.

Total Parenteral Nutrition

TPN is administered over an extended period to maintain or increase a patient's lean body mass. Because hypertonic concentrations of dextrose and amino acids are necessary to provide adequate energy without fluid overload, a large central vein is required to provide rapid dilution of the fluid.

Cycling therapy

Usually TPN is initiated over a 24-hour period. Patients who receive continuous TPN over a prolonged period are often switched to an overnight schedule before returning home. This process is usually accomplished over a 2- to 3-day period with careful monitoring for fluid and glucose overload. Cycling allows administration of the same volume of solution over 8 to 12 hours and allows patients more freedom during daytime hours. Cycling may also be used to stimulate the patient's appetite when a transition from TPN to oral intake is occurring. During the last 30 to 60 minutes of the cycling, the rate of administration is gradually cut to allow the pancreas to adjust to the glucose load.

Initiating therapy

To ensure glucose tolerance, TPN infusions are initially increased at a rate that allows endogenous insulin production to handle the extra glucose load. Until the patient is in a stable state, daily weights, intake and output, blood glucose tests, electrolytes, and all other laboratory reports require close monitoring.

Discontinuing therapy

There are many methods recommended for discontinuing parenteral nutrition. Tapering of the infusion rate over at least several hours is usually recommended to prevent severe hypoglycemia.

Total Nutritional Admixture, or 3-in-1 Admixture

Total nutritional admixtures (TNAs) combine a 24-hour supply of parenteral nutrition in a 3-liter container. Research on the chemical stability of TPN solutions, growth of microorganisms, and compounding techniques has led to procedures that make TNAs safe and convenient. Lipids are mixed with the dextrose and amino acid solution in the pharmacy. TNA solutions are solid white and have a nonreflecting surface, making precipitation difficult to observe. This form of TPN is usually reserved for patients in a stable state, because the components are adjusted only once daily.

Advantages of TNA

1. Risk of contamination is reduced, because the TPN system is manipulated only once every 24 hours.
2. Fat emulsions do not need to be piggybacked.

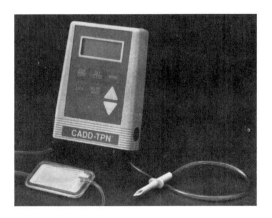

Fig. 9-2
Ambulatory infusion pump.
Courtesy Pharmacia Deltec Inc., St. Paul, MN.

3. Pharmacy compounding time is reduced, because only one bag is prepared every 24 hours.
4. Nursing time associated with setting up infusions is reduced.
5. Fewer supplies are required (Fig. 9-2).

Disadvantages of TNA

1. It is costly to adjust components of TNA more frequently than every 24 hours, because a new admixture is required.
2. Some infusion pumps do not accurately deliver the large admixture volume.

Equipment considerations

TNA solutions cannot be filtered with standard IV tubing filters. Where agency policy requires the filtering of all solutions, a large (1.2 µm) filter, not a 0.22 µm filter, should be used (Fig. 9-3).

Verify that infusion pump can deliver this product accurately.

 CLINICAL ALERT: Examine TNA admixtures before hanging for evidence of an unstable solution. Unstable solutions have small, clear, or slightly yellow pools of oil floating on the surface.

Considerations When Administering Parenteral Nutrition

1. If possible, do not use the parenteral nutrition catheter for other purposes. If using a multilumen catheter, dedicate one lumen to

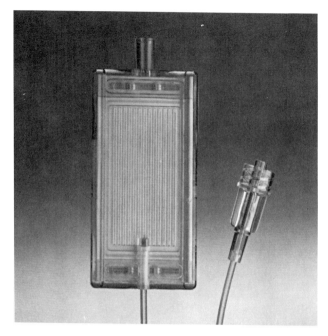

Fig. 9-3
New PALLTNA1 Intravenous Filter for total nutrient admixtures
containing lipid.

only the TPN solution. Never use this lumen to administer
piggyback medications, blood, or blood products. Do not draw
laboratory samples from the TPN lumen, and do not use this
lumen for measuring central venous pressures.
2. Refrigerate admixed solutions at 4° C. Remove solutions from
refrigeration approximately 30 minutes before use.
3. A volumetric pump will provide greater accuracy of administration than a controller.
4. Do not allow TNA bags (3-in-1) to hang longer than 24 hours.
5. Suspect catheter sepsis if a previously afebrile patient has a
fever. Notify the physician.
6. Solutions that have changed color are unacceptable for infusion,
because color changes result from decomposition of carbohydrates and amino acids during long-term storage.

7. Follow strict aseptic technique at all times when handling the catheter, dressing, tubing, or solution.
8. If the infusion falls behind schedule, do not attempt to catch up. Readjust the rate to the prescribed infusion rate. If the rate is too rapid, hyperglycemia will result. If the rate is too slow, hypoglycemia may result. The patient will not receive adequate calories or nitrogen.

Considerations when administering fat emulsions

1. Use unfiltered tubing, because the fat molecules are too large to pass through a filter smaller than 1.2 μm.
2. Monitor blood lipid levels and liver function tests.
3. When administering lipids by the piggyback method, use the Y-tube injection site closest to the catheter hub.
4. Do not use the solution if oil has separated.
5. Administer fat emulsions by peripheral vein, because the solution is isotonic.

Information to report to the physician

1. Blood glucose levels above 200 mg/dl
2. Hypoglycemia—blood glucose levels below 60 mg/dl
3. Urine glucose level above 1+ on test strip
4. Abnormal electrolyte results
5. Weight gains or losses—the goal for most patients is 1 pound/week

Monitoring during TPN

1. Daily weight: if the patient is monitored at home, may be reduced to a weekly weight check
2. Vital signs
3. Routine blood glucose monitoring
4. Catheter condition including exit site infection, break or tear, development of a fibrin sheath, catheter dislodgment
5. Laboratory results to screen for metabolic complications: electrolytes, CBC, liver enzymes, bilirubin, BUN, creatinine, calcium, magnesium, phosphorus, cholesterol, prothrombin time, serum albumin
6. Intake and output
7. Dietary intake
8. Adjustment to decreased oral intake

Complications of Parenteral Nutrition

Many serious complications may occur during parenteral nutrition. Contamination of some part of the infusion system is a major concern. A break in sterile technique at any point during manufacture, compounding, or infusion may cause contamination. Avoidance of contamination requires strict observance of sterile technique. Complications of parenteral nutrition are as follows.

Type of Complication	Examples
Catheter	Technical problems at the time of insertion: pneumothorax, hemothorax
	Problems after placement: thrombus formation, dislodgment, fibrin clot formation, vessel problems, and catheter tear (See Chapter 3)
Infusion equipment	Separation of tubing junctions; malfunction of infusion pump
Metabolic	Hypoglycemia or hyperglycemia, other blood chemistry abnormalities, vitamin and mineral imbalances, hematologic complications (Fig. 9-4)

Documentation Recommendations

Documentation of the patient's and caregiver's ability to perform all procedures and their understanding of troubleshooting measures, potential complications, and appropriate interventions is essential. Points to include in documentation are the following:

- Site assessment before and during the infusion
- Observation of catheter or device patency before, during, and after infusion
- Components of parenteral nutrition solution
- Infusion rate and any equipment used for regulation
- All supplies used; date and time of tubing changes
- Any complaints of discomfort and symptoms experienced before, during, or after infusion; action taken to correct problems

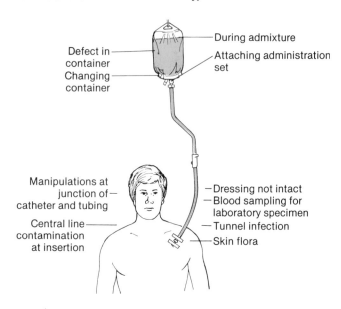

Fig. 9-4
Sites for contamination of parenteral nutrition system.
From Williams WW: Infection control during parenteral nutrition therapy, *JPEN J Parenter Enternal Nutr* 9:736, 1985.

- Patient weight; fluid intake and output record
- All patient and caregiver education for home care

 Nursing Diagnoses

- Knowledge deficit, regarding home care management of nutrition and venous catheter
- Nutrition, altered: less than body requirements, related to inadequate intake or absorption of foods
- Infection, risk for, related to high dextrose content of parenteral solution, break in sterile technique when managing catheter, or contamination of supplies
- Self-esteem disturbance, related to body image, placement of vascular access device
- Coping, ineffective family compromised: related to inadequate financial resources, family role changes, or stressors associated with parenteral nutrition management

Support Needs of Patients and Caregivers

The disruption of normal eating patterns and the intensity of long-term self-management required of persons who need parenteral nutrition place significant pressure on the patient and the family. Dependence on TPN leads to feelings of loss of control over many aspects of normal daily life and often progresses to periods of depression.

Food and eating are associated with many positive feelings such as security, acceptance, and belonging. Disruption of normal eating patterns, particularly over long periods of time, removes a major source of pleasure for the patients. The patient who is not eating is deprived of the sense of taste and of participating fully in social occasions involving food. The patient and family should be assisted in developing alternatives to food-related functions and in discovering ways of participating in social events designed around food.

Support and encouragement from the family are required as new procedures are learned and as adaptations in daily schedules are made around infusions. Encourage patient and family discussion of questions and feelings with the nursing staff and the physician. Acknowledge that patient and family feelings and concerns are commonly experienced by persons who require parenteral nutrition; occasional feelings of discouragement are to be expected. Reassure them that help is available when it is needed, and that they will be able to readjust successfully and return to normal activities.

CLINICAL ALERT: Frequent mouth care such as brushing teeth and using mouthwash and lip gloss is often helpful for the patient who is not eating. If the patient is allowed to eat but is experiencing anorexia, encourage small, frequent meals with others present.

Patient/Family Teaching for Self-Management

Extensive, formalized education is required for successful self-management of parenteral nutrition. Good communication of every aspect of management is required. Supervised practice with return demonstration is as important as written and visual materials that are easily understood by the patient and family. Initial teaching may take place in either the hospital or home setting. If the patient has difficulty reading, consider making an audiotape describing each procedure in a step-by-step fashion.

Initial Teaching

1. Assess ability and willingness to learn, availability of the caregiver, home environment, ability to assume self-care, and compliance with treatment regimen.
2. Describe purpose and procedures for the parenteral nutrition regimen.
3. Explain and demonstrate aseptic technique; stress that sterile technique is essential, and be consistent in all demonstrations and instructions to the patient and family; allow patients and families to handle equipment as much as possible.
4. Break each procedure into small tasks and guide the patient through each task; have the patient and the caregiver talk each other through each procedure to enhance learning.
5. Validate aseptic technique and skills of both the patient and the caregiver for initiation and discontinuation of therapy.
6. Instruct the patient and caregiver in signs, symptoms, and self-management interventions specific to each complication, such as lethargy, fluid retention, increased urine output, catheter complications.
7. Instruct the patient and caregiver in the management of infusion devices.
8. Provide information and list of resources for obtaining homecare services.
9. Ensure that follow-up care has been scheduled.

Home-Based Teaching

Because home and hospital environments are different, the patient and family need assistance transferring information learned in the hospital to the home setting. Written materials are required, and checklists should be provided for each procedure to be performed by the patient and for all necessary supplies. Equipment and supplies used in the hospital often are different from those available through the home care agency; specific instructions will be needed. Provide the patient with telephone numbers for 24-hour assistance.

1. Teach use of all home equipment; include troubleshooting tips for infusion pump alarms and malfunctions.
2. Validate aseptic technique and skills.
3. Evaluate home refrigeration and supply storage areas.
4. Teach the patient and caregiver how to order supplies.
5. Advise the patient and caregiver on disposal of used supplies.

6. Review symptoms and implications of infection and all other complications; ensure that what is to be done in case of a complication is known by both the patient and the family.
7. Provide a list of emergency phone numbers.

Home Care Considerations

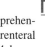

Medical stability, a motivated patient and family, and comprehensive agency support are required for successful home parenteral nutrition. Home TPN is scheduled usually over 10 to 14 hours during the night. This allows the patient to assume a more normal daytime schedule.

Although equipment needs are similar at home and in the hospital, pumps with readouts that can be read in the dark minimize sleep disturbances. Poles that can be pushed easily over carpet also allow greater mobility for the patient.

Patients should be taught to check their weight and temperature regularly. The patient or caregiver should be instructed how to read accurately both the scale and the thermometer. They should be provided with a record to document weights and temperature readings.

Patients and families need assistance with organizing and storing supplies. Optimally, a home visit is made by the home health nurse before the patient's dismissal to prepare for the patient's homecoming. If the home health referral agency is in an outreach area, copies of all protocols help diminish confusion and disparities between services.

Geriatric Considerations

Peripheral parenteral nutrition (PPN) may be prescribed as an adjunct therapy when an elderly patient is hospitalized, particularly if the patient has a surgical procedure that interferes with gastrointestinal nutrient absorption.

Chapter Resources

CALCULATIONS FREQUENTLY USED IN NUTRITIONAL ASSESSMENT
Harris-Benedict Equation

Female: BEE = 655 + (9.6 × Wt) + (1.7 × Ht) − (4.7 × Age)

Male: BEE = 66 + (13.7 × Wt) + (5 × Ht) − (6.8 × Age)

Base Solutions	Bottle # _____ Infuse Over _____ Hours	
Aminosyn 3.5% M	ml	
Nephramine	ml	
Dextrose 70% & water	ml	
Freamine 11 8.5%	ml	
Dextrose 50% & water	ml	
Dextrose 20% & water	ml	
Dextrose 10% & water	ml	
Electrolytes & Vitamins		
Regular insulin	Units	
Heparin	Units	
Potassium acetate	mEq	
Potassium chloride	mEq	
Potassium phosphate	mM	
Sodium acetate	mEq	
Sodium chloride	mEq	
Sodium phosphate	mM	
Calcium gluconate	mEq	
Magnesium sulfate	mEq	
Hyperlyte	ml	
Multiple vitamin infusion	ml	
Folic acid	mg	
Vitamin K	mg	
Vitamin B-12	mcg	
Totals		

Date _____ Time ___ Dr. _____

Physician's Signature

where *BEE* stands for basal energy expenditure, *Wt* stands for patient weight in kilograms, and *Ht* is for patient height in centimeters.

Weight should be calculated according to the ideal body weight when the patient is in a state of starvation so that protein stores can be replenished.

Often an additional calculation is added to estimate activity, severity of illness, and other related disease states that may increase energy requirements. This requires a subjective evaluation of patient stress. This correction factor is listed below:

Bottle #_____ Infuse Over _____ Hours		Pharmacy Use
ml		
ml		
ml		
ml		
ml		
ml		
ml		
Units		
Units		
mEq		
mEq		
mM		
mEq		
mEq		
mM		
mEq		
mEq		
ml		
ml		
mg		
mg		
mcg		

Low stress: $1.3 \times \text{BEE}$

Moderate stress: $1.5 \times \text{BEE}$

Severe stress: $2.0 \times \text{BEE}$

Percentage of weight loss = number of kilograms lost/usual weight

Total lymphocyte count = WBC $\times$ percentage of lymphocytes/100

Creatinine/height index = actual urinary creatinine/ideal urinary creatinine $\times$ 100

Nitrogen balance = nitrogen intake − nitrogen excretion = protein intake in grams/6.25 = (UUN + 4) where UUN is the urine urea nitrogen.

Home Care Parenteral Nutrition Weekly Log

Dates:	M	T	W	T	F	S	S	Remarks
TPN completed								
Daily heparin flush								
Daily dressing change								
Daily catheter cap change								
Weight as ordered								
Temperature as ordered								
Blood Glucose AM								
Blood glucose PM								
Urine glucose (if applicable)								
Daily tubing change								
TPN started								
Meal(s) eaten daily (1) (2) (3)								
Bowel movements								

SKILL CHECKLIST

Total Parenteral Nutrition Administration

1. Checks solution against physician order.
2. Checks expiration date on the solution.
3. Ensures that TPN has reached room temperature before infusing the solution.
4. Checks solution for contamination.
5. Washes hands at least 10 seconds before spiking the solution with the tubing.
6. Spikes the solution while maintaining strict asepsis of the tubing spike.
7. Primes the tubing.
8. Labels tubing.
9. Places TPN on pump.
10. Sets flow rate.
11. Checks all connections.
12. Secures the tubing to prevent pull on the IV site.
13. Documents procedure according to policy.
14. Maintains constant rate.

Study Questions

1. Which of the following is included in the assessment of a patient's need for TPN?
   a. Medical history
   b. Serum albumin or prealbumin
   c. Weight history
   d. a and b only
   e. a, b, and c

2. Energy needs are met through TPN through the following components:
   a. Dextrose and lipids
   b. Vitamins and amino acids
   c. Trace elements
   d. All of the above

3. Fluid and electrolyte need of patients:
   a. Vary widely
   b. Are predictable across populations
   c. Increase when 10% dextrose is given
   d. b and c

4. Normal serum albumin levels range from:
   a. 2.5 to 3.5 g/dl
   b. 2.5 to 4 g/dl
   c. 3.5 to 5 g/dl
   d. 4 to 6.5 g/dl

5. Expect that many patients receiving TPN will express a desire to eat foods.
   a. True
   b. False

ANSWERS: 1. e   2. d   3. d   4. c   5. a

Vascular Access In Adult Critical Care

10

Objectives

1. Discuss nursing responsibilities related to the insertion and care of hemodynamic pressure lines.

2. Discuss nursing interventions for potential complications associated with hemodynamic monitoring, including pressure transducer systems, arterial line catheters, and pulmonary artery catheters.

3. List and discuss the clinical significance of each hemodynamic parameter monitored with the PA catheter.

4. State the nursing responsibilities related to fluid resuscitation and drug administration in the critical care setting.

5. Describe current controversies related to hemodynamic monitoring.

6. Develop nursing care plans for patients requiring hemodynamic monitoring.

Critically ill patients require IV therapy for resuscitation, fluid and electrolyte maintenance, medication administration, and nutritional support. These patients often suffer injuries or illnesses that require vascular access for advanced hemodynamic monitoring. Arterial line and pulmonary artery catheters provide continuous information regarding cardiovascular function as well as the effectiveness of fluid and medication therapy.

Pressure Transducer Systems

Pressure transducer systems provide a means to monitor and record pressures obtained through vascular access of the arterial and venous systems. These devices can be connected to hemodynamic monitoring catheters such as arterial line (A-line) and pulmonary artery (PA) catheters.

Various prepackaged sterile systems are available to meet the specific patient needs. Systems are available for monitoring single or multiple pressures.

These systems typically consist of the following elements:

- IV tubing: connects the flush solution to the transducer
- Transducer: converts the pressure into an electrical impulse
- Flush device: provides continuous delivery of flush solution at 2 to 5 ml/hr to maintain line patency; also has a fast-flush mechanism that allows intermittent rapid flush of the system
- Pressure tubing: connects the transducer to the catheter; is stiff and noncompliant specialized tubing that minimizes pressure fluctuation within the tubing
- Stopcocks: allow access to the system as appropriate; require sterile caps to cover all open ends of the stopcocks to prevent contamination of the system
- Additional equipment/supplies: include flush solution, a pressure infuser bag, and bedside monitor

The following steps are involved in setting up the pressure transducer system (Fig. 10-1):

1. Prepare the flush solution according to hospital policy.
   a. The flush solution is usually a 500 ml bag of heparinized D_5W or NS.
   b. Currently, there is much controversy and research regarding the flush solution used in hemodynamic pressure monitoring. Issues investigated include the type of IV fluid, the use of heparin, and the concentration of heparin in the IV fluid. Normal saline may be preferred for the flush solution because of the increased risk of infection with dextrose-based solutions. Heparin is often added to the IV fluid to maintain patency of the catheter and decrease the risk of thrombus

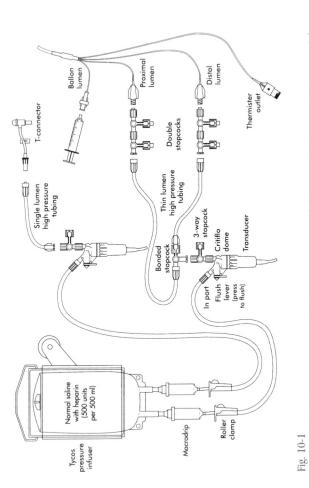

Fig. 10-1
Invasive blood pressure monitoring system used for monitoring systemic arterial pressure, right atrial pressure (CVP), and pulmonary artery pressure.
From Flynn J, Bruce N: *Introduction to critical care skills*, St. Louis, MO 1993, Mosby.

formation. However, it may be contraindicated for patients with bleeding disorders, patients with thrombocytopenia, or those receiving anticoagulants or thrombolytic agents.

2. Label the solution bag with the date and time. Indicate the addition of heparin (units/ml) on the IV label.

3. Assemble the pressure transducer system according to the instructions on the package insert and spike the flush solution bag. Label the tubing with the date and time.

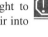

CLINICAL ALERT: Ensure that all connections are tight to prevent bacterial contamination, fluid leakage, or entry of air into the system.

4. Place the flush bag in the pressure infuser bag.

5. Prime the system with the flush solution by depressing the rapid flush device on the pressure transducer. Ensure that the transducer and all stopcocks are primed and that no air bubbles are in the system. "Vented" stopcocks must be replaced with "nonvented" stopcocks.

CLINICAL ALERT: Air bubbles in the system can cause inaccurate pressure readings and may introduce an air emboli into the arterial circulation.

6. Inflate the pressure infuser bag to 300 mmHg. Apply pressure uniformly on the IV fluid to prevent air from entering the system and to maintain line patency.

7. Connect the pressure tubing to the catheter.

8. Connect the transducer to the bedside monitor and set the appropriate scale and alarm limits.

   a. The monitor displays a graphic picture (waveform) and digital reading of the electrical impulses generated by the transducer.

   b. Monitor alarms alert the practitioner to changes in the patient's pressure being monitored or to complications with the equipment (e.g. catheter or tubing disconnection) that may lead to exsanguination.

CLINICAL ALERT: Never turn off the alarm system. Adjust the alarm limits to individual patient parameters.

9. Level the transducer, zero the pressure baseline, and calibrate the equipment.

   ▪ Leveling: Eliminates the influence of hydrostatic pressure. For monitoring pulmonary artery pressures (PAP), level the transducer to the phlebostatic axis (fourth intercostal space, midaxillary line). When monitoring arterial blood pressure,

level the transducer to the phlebostatic axis or secure it to the cannulated extremity, level with the insertion site.
- Zeroing: Eliminates the effects of atmospheric pressure. Turn the stopcock on the transducer "off to the patient" and "open to air," and then depress the zero key on the monitor.
- Calibrating: Ensures the accuracy of pressure readings by the monitor. Many monitors perform a self-calibration. Follow the instructions for individual monitors.

CLINICAL ALERT: Aseptic technique must always be maintained during preparation and manipulation of the equipment to minimize infectious complications.

Troubleshooting Pressure Transducer Systems

Many difficulties may occur with pressure monitoring systems. Table 10-1 lists some of these problems with possible causes and interventions.

Arterial Line Catheter

The A-line catheter is a rigid plastic catheter inserted by the physician into a peripheral artery. A-lines are useful for the management of patients requiring continuous arterial blood pressure monitoring. Continuous monitoring may be necessary for patients with unstable blood pressure, those with severe hypotension or hypertension, and those receiving medications affecting blood pressure (e.g., antihypertensives and vasoactive drugs). In critically ill patients with severe vasoconstriction, such as patients in shock, intraarterial monitoring provides a more accurate method of measuring blood pressure than does indirect blood pressure measurement using a cuff.

The A-line catheter is also used when frequent blood samples are necessary. Most laboratory specimens, including arterial blood gases (ABGs), can be drawn from the A-line catheter. Patients who may need frequent ABG sampling include those requiring mechanical ventilation and those with severe acid–base disturbance, such as patients in septic shock or with diabetic ketoacidosis.

Advantages of BP Monitoring with the A-line Catheter

- Provides accurate, direct blood pressure readings
- Provides continuous information regarding change in status and response to therapy
- Eliminates need for multiple sticks to obtain laboratory samples

Table 10-1 Pressure monitoring system problems and solutions

Problem	Causes	Interventions
Absence of waveform	Monitor turned off	Verify monitor on
	Disconnection	Tighten all connections
	Improper positioning of stopcocks	Check position of all stopcocks
	Inappropriate calibration or scale	Perform level-zero-calibrate process; select appropriate scale
	Faulty transducer	Replace transducer
Dampened waveform	Presence of air bubbles, blood, clot, or kink	Assess system and correct
	Catheter tip against vessel wall	Activate fast-flush, briefly
	Inadequate fluid or pressure in pressure infuser	Ensure adequate fluid and pressure at 300 mmHg
	Inappropriate calibration or scale	Perform level-zero-calibrate process
	Hypovolemia	Assess patient and report
Significant change in parameter unrelated to status change	Improper transducer level: too high causes low reading; too low causes high reading	Perform level-zero-calibrate process
Backup of blood in pressure line	Inadequate pressure or fluid in bag infuser	Ensure adequate fluid and pressure >300 mmHg
	Loose connections	Tighten all connections

Disadvantages as Compared with Manual Cuff Pressure

- Invasive
- Expensive
- Setup and maintenance require increased nursing time and knowledge
- Potential for infection, hemorrhage, vascular complications, and equipment-related complications

Preparation for A-line Insertion

- Assemble a single pressure transducer system and the flush solution as previously described.
- Label the tubing as the A-line to help prevent accidental disconnection or infusions into the site.
- Explain the procedure to the patient and family.
- Provide pain medication as appropriate.
- Prepare a sterile dressing to apply after insertion. The dressing should indicate the date and time of insertion and the last dressing change.

Sites for arterial cannulation

1. Radial artery (Fig. 10-2)
   a. Collateral circulation makes this the preferred site for cannulation.
   b. Before inserting the catheter, assess patency of the ulnar artery. The modified Allen's test is one method for assessing collateral circulation.
2. Femoral artery
   a. Advantages: It is easy to locate and access and can be used when the patient is severely vasoconstricted, hypotensive, or in cardiac failure.
   b. Disadvantages: The lack of collateral circulation increases the risk of limb ischemia and necrosis if the vessel becomes occluded. The site also makes immobilization and maintenance difficult.
3. Other arterial sites are used less frequently because of an increased risk of complications.
   - Axillary artery: greater rate of infection
   - Dorsalis pedis artery: increased risk of occlusion because of small vessel size
   - Brachial artery: increased risk of ischemia owing to the lack of adequate collateral circulation

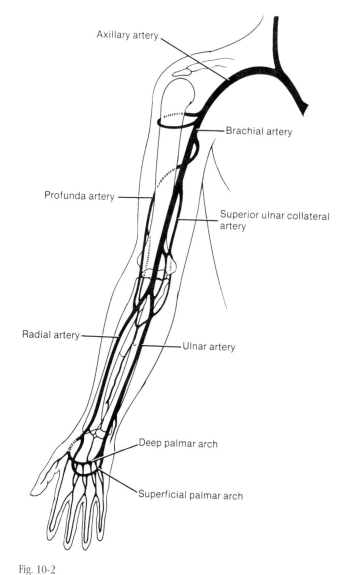

Fig. 10-2
Anatomic locations of the arteries of the arm.
From Daily EK, Schroeder JS: *Techniques in bedside hemodynamic monitoring,* ed 5, St. Louis, MO 1994, Mosby.

Maintenance

- Keep insertion site and tubing visible.
- Check connections frequently to prevent disconnection.
- Immobilize the cannulated extremity to prevent flexion, which may alter waveform and blood pressure readings.
- Level, zero, and calibrate every 8 hours or according to hospital policy, following significant changes in pressures, and after changes in the patient's position. Research demonstrates that this procedure may not be required as often as previously indicated.
- Perform noninvasive cuff pressure at least once each shift to compare pressure readings.
- Assess pulse, capillary refill, sensation, movement, color, and temperature distal to the insertion site a minimum of every two hours or as specified by hospital policy.

 CLINICAL ALERT: A decreased or absent pulse, cool or mottled skin, or changes in sensation or movement, may indicate occlusion of the artery.

- Change the flush solution every 24 hours or as directed by hospital policy.
- Change the pressure transducer system and dressing as directed by hospital policy. Much of the literature recommends changing gauze dressings every 24 hours and transparent dressings every 48 to 72 hours.
- Assess the insertion site for signs of infection as indicated by hospital policy. Some hospitals recommend changing the insertion site every 72 to 96 hours to reduce the risk of infection. Many clinicians believe that the benefits of routine replacement do not justify the risks of repeated cannulation and replace the A-line only if an infection or other complication is suspected.
- Maintain aseptic technique whenever manipulating the A-line setup.
- Monitor and assess the waveform continuously.
- Notify the physician of all abnormal pressure readings and any complications.

Complications

1. Hemorrhage
   - Hemorrhage is the most common complication associated with A-lines.
   - It may range from formation of a small hematoma, to oozing at the insertion site, to exsanguination.
   - Hematomas are usually the result of insufficient pressure

following removal of the A-line or laceration of the artery during insertion.

- Pressure must be applied a minimum of 5 to 10 minutes following removal.
- Oozing at the insertion site may occur in patients with bleeding disorders and those receiving anticoagulants or thrombolytics.
- Rapid exsanguination, which is potentially fatal, can occur if the tubing becomes disconnected.

2. Infection: Maintaining a closed system, ensuring use of aseptic technique, and limiting the number of blood samples may significantly reduce the risk of infection. "In-line" blood-sampling systems eliminate the need for opening stopcocks, which reduces the risk of bacterial contamination, clinician exposure, and blood loss. Recent advancement in the use of electrochemical and fiberoptic technology allows for continuous ABG monitoring in addition to BP monitoring. This technology decreases the frequency of blood sampling from the A-line.

CLINICAL ALERT: The immune system of critically ill patients is often suppressed by a multitude of factors, including trauma, disease processes, medications, and treatments. These patients frequently have multiple invasive lines, which increase their susceptibility to infection.

- Infection is associated with increased morbidity and mortality in patients with A-lines.
- Infection can be local or systemic. Signs and symptoms of a local infection include erythema, tenderness, swelling, and purulent drainage at the insertion site. The patient may also be febrile and have an elevated white blood cell count.
- Infection may be associated with catheter duration and site of cannulation.
- If line contamination is suspected, the catheter must be discontinued. The catheter tip may be sent to the laboratory for culture.

3. Vessel occlusion
- This may be caused by thrombosis or embolism.
- It may result in ischemia or necrosis of the cannulated extremity if untreated.
- Vessel occlusion is evidenced by diminished or absent distal pulse, pain, paresthesias, and pallor. If ischemia continues, the skin color can become mottled and eventually black as tissue death occurs.

- Factors that increase the risk of thrombosis include prolonged duration of catheter, large-gauge catheter in relation to vessel size, number of cannulation attempts, blood viscosity, and preexisting vascular disease.

4. Pain
   - Pain may be related to irritation from the catheter, immobilization, or site of cannulation.
   - It may be an indication of any of the previous complications.
   - Perform a complete pain assessment and physical exam, and notify the physician as indicated.
   - Provide pain medication as indicated, and evaluate effectiveness.

Pulmonary Artery Catheter

The pulmonary artery (PA) catheter is a multilumen, flow-directed, balloon-tipped catheter that is inserted into the PA and used for various functions:

- To evaluate cardiovascular function and tissue oxygenation
- To measure intracardiac pressures
- To measure cardiac output (CO) and calculate cardiac index (CI)
- To obtain mixed venous blood samples
- To administer fluids and medications
- To evaluate and guide patient therapy
- Recent advances in technology have produced PA catheters capable of cardiac pacing and continuous monitoring of CO and mixed venous oxygen saturation (SvO_2).

PA Catheter Lumens and Ports

1. Cordis - The cordis is not a part of the PA catheter (Fig. 10-3). It is a separate large-bore IV that attaches to an introducer, which is used to insert the PA catheter.
   - Inserted into a large peripheral or central vein (e.g., subclavian, internal jugular, femoral)
   - Terminates in the superior vena cava, slightly above the right atrium (RA)
   - Used to infuse IV fluid, and because of its large gauge, is often used to infuse blood and blood products
   - Can be connected to a pressure transducer and used to monitor central venous pressure (CVP)

2. PA (distal) lumen
   - Terminates in the PA; located at the distal tip of the catheter
   - Usually connected to a double pressure transducer system

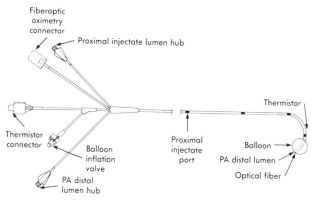

Fig. 10-3
Pulmonary artery catheter. The proximal injectate lumen hub
is attached to a pressure line to measure right atrial CVP. This
is also the hub where the solution will be injected to measure
CO. The injectate solution will exit at the proximal injectate
port, located in the right atrium.

- Provides continuous monitoring of the pulmonary artery
  systolic (PAS), diastolic (PAD), and mean (PAM) pressures
- Site for obtaining mixed venous gases

CLINICAL ALERT: The pulmonary artery pressure (PAP) must
be *continuously* monitored to allow immediate recognition of
catheter migration (see section on complications).

3. Right atrial (proximal) injectate lumen
   - Terminates in the RA
   - Usually connected to the same pressure transducer system as
     the PA lumen
   - Provides continuous or intermittent measurement of the right
     atrial pressure (RAP)
   - Injection port for boluses used to obtain CO measurements
   - Used for infusion of IV fluids or intermittent IV medications
     (antibiotics)

CLINICAL ALERT: Never infuse vasoactive or other continuous infusion drugs through the proximal injectate port. Interruption
of the drug would be required for CO measurement, and injection
would result in the patient receiving a bolus of the drug.

4. Proximal infusion (VIP) lumen
   - Additional lumen found on some PA catheters

- Terminates in the RA, approximately 1 cm distal to the right atrial injectate lumen
- Connected to a routine IV line or maintained with a heparin lock
- Provides infusion of IV fluid or total parenteral nutrition
- Provides infusion of IV medications, including continuous infusions

5. Balloon inflation port
   - Includes a volume-limited, 1.5 ml syringe
   - Balloon is located at the distal tip of the PA catheter
   - When inflated, cushions the catheter tip during insertion to prevent irritation of the right ventricle (RV)
   - Used to obtain the pulmonary artery wedge pressure (PWP) by "floating" the catheter into a small branch of the PA (done intermittently, lasting less than 15 seconds)

6. Thermistor port
   - Located approximately 3 cm from the catheter tip
   - Connected to the CO computer cable
   - Measures CO
   - Monitors continuous or intermittent core body temperature

Preparation for Insertion

The catheter is usually inserted by the physician with the RN's assistance. The RN is responsible for preparing the monitoring equipment, observing for complications during insertion, obtaining and interpreting data following insertion, and maintaining the catheter.

- Explain the procedure to the patient and family.
- Assemble a double pressure transducer system and flush solution for the PA distal and proximal injectate lumens.
- Connect the transducer to the bedside hemodynamic monitor, and perform the level-zero-calibrate function.
- Individualize pressure scale and alarms to patient.
- Prepare IV fluid and tubing for the cordis and VIP, per physician order.
- Prepare solution for priming the catheter according to hospital policy.
- Provide pain medication as appropriate.

Insertion of the PA Catheter

Before insertion, the physician will prime the PA, RA, and VIP ports. The PA distal and proximal injectate ports are then connected

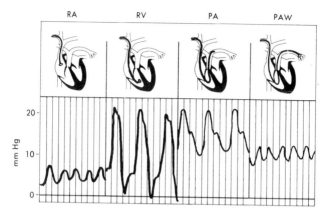

Fig. 10-4
Flow-directed, balloon-tipped catheter locations with corresponding pressure tracings.
From Schroeder JS, Daily EK: *Hemodynamic monitoring.* Tampa Tracings slide series, Tarpon Springs, FL, 1976, Tampa Tracings.

to the transducer tubings. The RA, RV, PA, and PWP waveforms will be displayed on the monitor as the catheter is advanced through the right heart and to the PA (Fig. 10-4). The physician and the nurse should observe these waveforms to monitor progression and position of the catheter.

The PA catheter is threaded into the RA through the subclavian or jugular vein via the cordis/introducer. The balloon is inflated in the RA, and the catheter floats through the tricuspid valve into the RV. The catheter should be advanced rapidly through the pulmonic valve into the PA to reduce right ventricular irritation. The balloon is deflated, and PAP measurements are recorded. The balloon is reinflated and slowly advanced until a "wedge" tracing is observed and a PWP is documented. Next, the balloon is allowed to passively deflate and the PAP waveform is displayed.

CLINICAL ALERT: The balloon must never remain inflated for more than 15 seconds. While inflated, the balloon occludes a branch of the pulmonary artery, and a pulmonary infarct or rupture can occur if inflation is prolonged.

CLINICAL ALERT: Ventricular arrhythmias may occur when the catheter reaches the RV. Monitor the ECG, and report ventricular irritability to the physician. Some hospitals recommend that lidocaine be immediately available during catheter insertion.

The catheter is secured to prevent migration and a portion is protected by a sterile sheath as it exits the skin. The sheath allows manipulation of the catheter, if necessary, without the risk of introducing contaminants into the vascular system. A chest x-ray is required following insertion to verify correct placement of the catheter.

Monitored Pressures

The PA catheter directly measures the RAP, PAS, PAD, and PWP. All pressures must be interpreted at the end of expiration because they are frequently altered by changes in intrapleural pressures during inspiration and expiration. The pressures can be read as digital values on the monitor, or paper strip recordings can be used to interpret waveforms and determine pressure values. Paper strip recordings provide the most accurate data but require greater skill and knowledge for interpretation.

Obtaining the PWP

The PWP is obtained when the PA balloon is inflated and the catheter advances and "wedges" in a small branch of the PA. The inflated balloon blocks the transmission of pressure from the right heart; however, because the catheter tip extends beyond the balloon, it continues to receive information from the left heart. The PWP is a left atrial tracing that is used as an indicator of left ventricular volume. Many clinical situations invalidate this pressure.

1. Verify the PAP tracing on the monitor.
2. Detach the volume-limited syringe from the balloon port and draw up 1.5 ml of air. Reconnect the syringe to the balloon port.
3. Slowly inflate the balloon until a PWP tracing is observed.

 CLINICAL ALERT: The waveform must be closely observed on the monitor throughout the procedure to prevent overinflation. Inflation is stopped as soon as the PWP tracing is observed and should not exceed 15 seconds. Inflation should require 1.25 to 1.5 ml of air.

4. Record the PWP.
5. Detach the syringe from the balloon port and allow the balloon to passively deflate. Never aspirate the air through the syringe; this may cause the balloon to rupture.
6. Verify return of the PAP waveform.

Maintenance

- Line and site care are similar to the care of other central line catheters and the A-line catheter.
- Follow-up chest X-rays to verify placement are done according to hospital policy.
- Continuously monitor the entire system for the presence of air.
- Monitor PAP waveforms *continuously* and PWP waveforms intermittently. (RAP can be monitored intermittently or continuously.)
- Maintain aseptic technique whenever manipulating system.

Complications

The complications that may be associated with hemodynamic monitoring using the PA catheter include those associated with central venous catheters and those discussed with A-line catheters. Additional complications include arrhythmias, spontaneous wedge, catheter migration, overwedge, knotting or kinking of the catheter, balloon rupture, pulmonary infarction, and pulmonary rupture (Table 10-2).

CLINICAL ALERT: Always deflate the balloon before with-drawing the catheter. Pulling the catheter back with the balloon inflated can cause severe valvular and myocardial damage. Hospital policy should be followed regarding manipulation of the PA catheter. Some hospitals allow only physicians to manipulate these catheters.

Cardiac Output

Cardiac output is the amount of blood ejected from the heart every minute, measured in liters per minute. The thermodilution method of CO measurement is most commonly used in critical care. A bolus of room temperature or iced fluid is injected into the proximal injectate port of the PA catheter. The thermistor located at the distal end of the PA catheter registers the change in blood temperature over time, and the CO is displayed on the monitor.

Thermodilution CO Monitoring (Fig. 10-5)

Equipment

1. CO computer and injectate temperature probe
2. Sterile, prepackaged, closed CO injectate system
3. IV solution for injectate, per hospital policy

Table 10-2 Cardiac complications and interventions

Complication	Causes and Indications	Interventions
Arrhythmias • Transient PVCs and short runs of VT • Persistent ectopy	• Irritation of myocardium	• Observe ECG • Notify the physician • Physician may reposition • May require antiarrhythmics
Spontaneous wedge • Risk of pulmonary infarction or rupture	• Kinking or looping in the RV • PA tip migrates forward into "wedge" position • PAP replaced by permanent PWP tracing	• Ensure balloon is deflated • Flex/extend arm • Reposition (side to side) • Encourage cough • Suction, if appropriate • Notify the physician • Pull the catheter back until PAP tracing observed*
Migration of the catheter tip backward into RV • May cause lethal dysrhythmias	• PAP replaced by RV tracing (RV should only be seen during insertion)	• Monitor ECG for lethal dysrhythmias • Inflate balloon and monitor for return of PAP

Migration of RA port forward into RV • Not serious	• Often seen with cardiomyopathies	• Notify the physician • Pull the catheter back until the RA tracing is observed*
Overwedge	• RA replaced by RV tracing • Overinflation of balloon • Catheter advanced too far (inflated requires <1 ml to obtain PWP tracing)	• Notify the physician to reposition catheter • Inflate slowly and stop when PWP tracing observed • Verify location with chest x-ray • Notify the physician to reposition catheter
Balloon rupture	• Duration/frequency of use • Manual deflation of balloon • Indicated by loss of resistance to inflation, inability to obtain PWP tracing, or lack of passive deflation	• Limit frequency of inflations • Tape end of syringe to prevent further attempts • Label as "broken balloon"

Continued.

Table 10-2 Cardiac complications and interventions—cont'd

Complication	Causes and Indications	Interventions
Pulmonary infarct	• Distal movement of catheter into "wedge" position • Embolization of thrombus	• Monitor waveform for spontaneous wedge • Maintain continuous flush of pressure lines • Verify placement with chest x-ray • Limit frequency of inflation • Stop inflation when PWP tracing observed
Pulmonary rupture • Death may occur owing to pulmonary hemorrhage	• Arterial wall punctured by catheter tip • Balloon overinflation in small branch of PA • Sudden hemoptysis with bright red blood	• If suspected, put in decubitus position (bleeding lung down) • Notify the physician • Discontinue anticoagulant therapy as ordered

*CLINICAL ALERT: Always deflate the balloon before withdrawing the catheter. Pulling the catheter back with the balloon inflated can cause severe valvular and myocardial damage. Hospital policy should be followed regarding manipulation of the PA catheter. Some hospitals allow only physicians to manipulate these catheters.

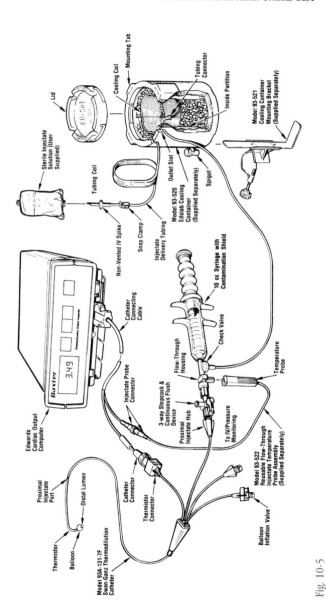

Fig. 10-5

CO-Set + Closed Injectate Delivery System, Cold Injectate.
(Courtesy Baxter Healthcare Corporation, Edwards Critical-Care Division, Irvine, CA.)

4. Labels for IV fluid and tubing
5. IV pole
6. Ice bucket and ice slush (if using iced injectate)

Procedure

- Explain the procedure to the patient/family.
- Assemble the injectate system according to the package insert.
- Label the IV bag with solution type, amount, date, and time.
- Spike the IV bag with the injectate system tubing, and hang it on the IV pole.
- Prime the tubing.
- If using iced injectate, attach the ice bucket to the IV pole, and place the coiled portion of the tubing into the bucket. Fill the bucket with ice slush.
- Attach the injectate syringe to the proximal injectate port of the PA catheter.
- Connect the thermistor port to the CO computer, and the in-line temperature probe to the system.
- The procedure for measuring CO will depend on the type of monitors being used. Follow the manufacturer's directions and hospital policy.

   CLINICAL ALERT: A computation constant must be entered into the monitor before performing the CO. The constant is a correction factor for variances in temperature change related to the size and type of PA catheter and the volume and temperature of injectate. Computation constants are generally listed in the package inserts of the PA catheter or are available from the manufacturer.

   Some disease processes (e.g., congestive heart failure (CHF), pulmonary edema) require fluid restriction; therefore, the volume of injectate, as well as the number of boluses, must be dictated by patient status as well as hospital policy.

   Generally, three CO measurements are done, and readings within 10% of one another are considered acceptable. Readings outside this range are eliminated, and additional measurements may be necessary. The acceptable CO readings are averaged for the recorded CO.

Complications

1. Infection
2. Poor technique, generating inaccurate data

3. Fluid overload
4. Arrhythmias owing to irritation from cold injectate
5. Inadvertent bolus of medications if injectate port is used for continuous infusions (This port should never be used for continuous infusions.)

A recent advancement in measuring CO is the introduction of continuous cardiac output (CCO) monitoring. CCO uses small pulses of heat as a thermal indicator. The thermistor at the distal tip of the PA catheter detects changes in the blood temperature and updates the information every 30 to 60 seconds. The monitor averages and records an updated CO every 3 to 6 minutes.

Advantages of CCO

- Continuous display of CO allows immediate response to a change in status.
- No manual bolus is required, which decreases the potential for human error, risk of infection, and fluid overload.
- Intermittent boluses can be administered as needed for comparison with the CCO readings.

Disadvantages of CCO

- The cost of equipment increases.
- Additional research is still needed. One area of investigation is determining which patient populations would benefit from this technology.

Clinical Significance of Hemodynamic Parameters (Table 10-3)

The pressures measured by the PA catheter and the CO provide information about cardiac function and fluid volume status. The body is always attempting to maintain a normal blood pressure (BP). The determinants of BP are CO and systemic vascular resistance (SVR). If CO falls, the sympathetic nervous system is stimulated, and SVR increases (vasoconstriction). The major determinants of CO are heart rate (HR) and stroke volume (SV).

HR is the primary compensatory mechanism of the body. If CO drops for any reason (e.g., hemorrhage, shock), the body attempts to maintain perfusion by increasing the HR to maintain tissue perfusion. If this mechanism is unsuccessful, the SV is affected.

SV is determined by preload, afterload, and contractility.

Table 10-3   Hemodynamic parameters

Hemodynamic Parameter	Normal Range*	Method of Obtaining or Calculation
Mean arterial pressure (MAP)	70–105 mmHg	$\dfrac{(2 \times \text{Diastole}) + \text{systole}}{3}$
Right atrial pressure (RAP)	2–6 mmHg	Measured by RA port of PA catheter as a mean pressure
Pulmonary artery systolic pressure (PAS)	15–30 mmHg	Measured by distal lumen of PA catheter
Pulmonary artery diastolic pressure (PAD)	8–15 mmHg	Measured by distal lumen of PA catheter
Pulmonary artery mean pressure (PAM)	10–20 mmHg	$\dfrac{(2 \times \text{PADS}) + \text{PAS}}{3}$
Pulmonary artery wedge pressure (PWP)	6–12 mmHg	Measured by distal lumen of PA catheter with balloon inflated
Cardiac output (CO)	4–8 l/min	$HR \times SV$ Measured with thermodilution method
Cardiac index (CI)	2.5–4.0 l/min/m^2	$\dfrac{CO}{BSA}$

Parameter	Normal range	Formula
Stroke volume (SV)	60–130 ml/beat	$\dfrac{CO}{HR} \times 1000$
Stroke volume index (SVI)	30–65 ml/beat/m²	$\dfrac{SV}{BSA}$
Systemic vascular resistance (SVR)	900–1400 dynes/sec/cm^{-5}	$\dfrac{MAP - RAP}{CO} \times 80$
Systemic vascular resistance index (SVRI)	1900–2390 dynes/sec/cm^{-5}/m²	$\dfrac{MAP - RAP}{CI} \times 80$
Pulmonary vascular resistance (PVR)	100–250 dynes/sec/cm^{-5}	$\dfrac{PAM - PWP}{CO} \times 80$
Pulmonary vascular resistance index (PVRI)	200–450 dynes/sec/cm^{-5}/m²	$\dfrac{PAM - PWP}{CI} \times 80$
Right ventricular stroke work index (RVSWI)	4–8 gram-meters/m²/beat	$SVI \times (PAM - RAP) \times 0.0136$
Left ventricular stroke work index (LVSWI)	45–75 gram-meters/m²/beat	$SVI \times (MAP - PWP) \times 0.0136$

*The normal range for hemodynamic parameters varies slightly between references. The values provided are meant only as a guide. Consult hospital policy for standard values.

Preload

- Preload is the filling pressure in the ventricles at the end of diastole.
- It is generated by the volume of blood in the ventricle.
- The Frank-Starling law holds that increased preload causes greater stretch of the myocardial fibers, which increases the strength of contraction and SV. If optimal preload is exceeded, the fibers become overstretched, and SV decreases.
- RV preload is obtained by monitoring the RAP.
- LV preload is obtained by monitoring the PWP and PAD (with limitations). Normally, the PAD is 1 to 4 mmHg greater than the PWP. A gradient greater than 4 represents factors other than preload (e.g., pulmonary emboli, hypoxia, chronic obstructive pulmonary disease, or COPD, or adult respiratory distress syndrome [ARDS]) causing elevation of the PAD. These conditions preclude the use of the PAD in determining LV preload. The PWP is not affected by these conditions.

Afterload

- Afterload is the resistance to ejection of blood from the ventricles.
- RV afterload is measured by a pulmonary vascular resistance (PVR) calculation.
- LV afterload is measured by a systemic vascular resistance (SVR) calculation.

Contractility

- Contractility is the force of myocardial contraction.
- It is generated by myocardial fiber shortening.
- RV contractility is derived from calculation of the right ventricular stroke work index (RVSWI).
- LV contractility is derived from calculation of the left ventricular stroke work index (LVSWI).

All hemodynamic parameters should be indexed to body surface area for the most accurate measurement. Indexed parameters are individualized to the patient's height and weight.

Documentation of Hemodynamic Monitoring

- Vital signs, hemodynamic parameters, and pertinent physiologic assessment should be recorded according to hospital policy and whenever there is a change in patient status.

- Paper strip recordings of hemodynamic pressures should be labeled with the date, time, waveform identification, and pressure values.
- Documentation should include all line and site care (e.g., change of flush solution, tubing, and dressing); condition of vascular access site; volume of flush solution received; the insertion, manipulation, or removal of all monitoring catheters; patient response to all therapies and procedures; and patient and family education.

Fluid and Drug Therapy in Critical Care

Patients who require fluid resuscitation in critical care include those with trauma, neurological respiratory, or cardiac illnesses. The type and amount of IV fluid is influenced by the injury or disease process. Many resuscitation regimes have been established based on an understanding of the pathophysiology of injury and disease processes.

A common goal for all patients is the prevention of end-organ damage. To prevent such damage, intravascular volume, venous return to the heart, CO, and tissue oxygenation may need to be restored and monitored. One complication of fluid resuscitation is the effect of large fluid volumes on individual organs (e.g., lungs, heart). ARDS, which impairs oxygen delivery, is one complication that may be associated with massive fluid resuscitation, yet it is often accompanied by decreased circulating blood volume requiring boluses of IV fluid. Patients with cardiac disease may require fluid resuscitation, although cardiac function may be compromised by the increased volume. The challenge is to meet the need for volume repletion while maintaining adequate cardiopulmonary function.

Hemodynamic parameters reflect both volume and cardiovascular status. Trending of these parameters, along with the patient's physical assessment, can help guide fluid and drug administration in the critically ill patient. The PA catheter is used to monitor the CO, PWP, and LV function during fluid challenges to determine the minimal volume (preload) needed to optimize cardiopulmonary function.

Vasoactive drugs are administered to control hypertension or hypotension, to increase or decrease preload, and to increase cardiac contractility. Vasoactive drugs commonly used in the critical care setting include the following:

- Dopamine
- Epinephrine
- Norepinephrine
- Dobutamine

- Phenylephrine
- Sodium nitroprusside
- Nitroglycerine
- Diltiazem

- Amrinone lactate
- Esmolol

Nurses have various responsibilities during the administration of each of these drugs:

- Knowledge and understanding of the actions, indications, dosage, method of administration, metabolism, possible side effects, and drug compatibility
- Knowledge of drug calculations
- Continuous monitoring of vital signs and hemodynamic parameters as appropriate
- Frequent assessment of venous access site, especially if infusing in peripheral site
- Evaluation of effectiveness and reporting of all negative outcomes of drug therapy
- Documentation of drug administration, including the name of the drug, concentration, rate, and dosage
- Use of a continuous infusion device to administer all vasoactive drugs

Syringe pumps or buretrol administration sets may be used to deliver intravenous medications when large volumes are contraindicated (e.g., myocardial infarction, congestive heart failure, and renal failure). Syringe pumps deliver concentrated medications in small volumes at a consistent flow rate. Disadvantages include an increased risk of infiltration, air emboli, and accidental bolus infusion. Newer infusion devices have the capability of performing drug calculations when dosing determinants (volume of diluent, amount of drug, dose, patient weight) are entered into the computer. This feature can increase the efficiency of drug titration.

 ## Nursing Diagnoses

- Infection, risk for, related to break in skin integrity, multiple invasive lines, and altered immune function
- Cardiac output, decreased, related to decreased volume, altered vascular tone, impaired contractility
- Pain, related to catheter insertion, immobilization
- Tissue perfusion, altered, related to presence of catheter in vascular bed

- Hemorrhage, risk for related to use of heparinized flush solution, coagulopathies, tubing disconnection
- Fluid volume excess, related to fluid resuscitation, excess fluid maintenance, impaired renal function
- Fluid volume deficit, risk for related to decreased fluid intake, gastrointestinal loss of fluid, pharmacological agents
- Injury, risk for, related to complications of hemodynamic monitoring

This chapter is intended to provide a brief introduction to hemodynamic monitoring in critical care. The reader is encouraged to refer to other sources for additional information, including waveform recognition, interpretation, and clinical management based on hemodynamic parameters.

The author of this chapter would like to acknowledge and thank Josette Etcheverry RN, MSN, CCRN and Robin Tyler RN, MSN, CCRN for their assistance in editing the content.

Study Questions

1. What nursing measures can reduce the risk of infection in patients receiving hemodynamic monitoring?

2. What are the advantages of direct arterial BP measurement? What are the disadvantages?

3. What are common causes of complications associated with A-line catheters? What are the nursing interventions for these complications?

4. What is the function of each lumen/port of the PA catheter?

5. Where is the PA catheter positioned within the vascular bed?

6. How is the pulmonary artery wedge pressure obtained?

7. What is the significance of hemodynamic parameters obtained or derived from the PA catheter?

8. What are the complications associated with PA catheter monitoring? What are the nursing interventions?

9. What are the nursing responsibilities in relation to fluid and drug administration in critical care?

ANSWERS: Answers to questions provided within chapter text.

Pediatric Intravenous Therapy

11

Objectives

1. Discuss the principles of metabolism and body surface area for fluid and electrolyte balance in the pediatric patient.

2. Describe principles of selecting an IV site and securing an IV device for the child up to 3 years of age.

3. Identify the nursing management interventions for pediatric IV medication administration.

4. List three primary blood products with indications for use in the pediatric patient.

5. Define the criteria used to determine if a child is a potential candidate for parenteral nutrition.

Providing care for pediatric patients can be a rewarding and challenging experience. Intravenous therapy for these patients presents its own unique challenges. Children require IV therapy for many of the same reasons as adults:

- Medication administration
- Fluid and electrolyte maintenance
- Parenteral nutrition
- Chemotherapy
- Blood transfusions
- Pain management

However, unlike most adults, pediatric patients have not yet developed the cognitive or coping skills necessary to prepare them for many aspects of IV therapy. A basic knowledge of the child's growth and developmental process is a crucial step for nurses to prepare themselves, the patient, and the child's family for all the IV therapy procedures. Table 11-1 lists guidelines for child and family preparation, correlated with the child's age, developmental level, and psychological characteristics.

The nurse should keep in mind that chronological age and the stage of psychosocial development in children may not always coincide. Children often temporarily regress to an earlier stage during an illness or hospitalization. It is important to remember that every child is unique, with different life experiences and different reactions to varied life events. In the provision of care, safety must prevail as the main concern through every age and stage of the developmental process.

Similarly, the nurse should establish a good rapport with the family and the child, using good communication techniques. Well-informed parents are more likely to remain calm, and the child will cue into this behavior and be less apprehensive about the therapy. Following are recommendations to use when initiating or maintaining pediatric intravenous therapy:

- Explain the procedure and its purpose.
- Encourage questions.
- Allow the parents to decide if they wish to be present for the procedure.
- Allow the child to remain in the parents' arms as long as possible, for those parents who chose to be present for the procedure.
- Encourage parents to remain close to the child throughout the procedure and to comfort the child by touching, caressing, talking, or singing to the child.
- Avoid doing procedures in the child's room, and opt for a procedure room or neutral room.

CLINICAL ALERT: Never ask the parent to assist with restrain-ing the child for the procedure. Enlist the assistance of a coworker to restrain the child.

The previous chapters in this text have discussed the theoretical and clinical components required for each topic. Fundamental guidelines presented in those chapters for all the varied therapies should be followed in providing IV therapy for the child. Additional practice guidelines related to the child's growth and developmental process with physiological rationale will be presented in this

Table 11-1 Developmental stages of childhood

Age	Developmental Level	Characteristics	Child/Family Preparation
Infants (birth–1 year)	Trust versus mistrust: Consistent response to needs allows infant to predict responses and develop trust	Fear of separation Fear of strangers Behavior is under reflexive control Uses cry to communicate	Attempt to provide consistent caregivers. Prepare equipment out of view. Avoid feeding child immediately before procedure. Decrease parental anxiety by keeping parents well informed. Minimize parental separation. Never use parents or family members to assist with restraining the child. If feasible, utilize a procedure room.

| Toddlers (1–3 years) | Autonomy versus shame and doubt: Desire to do things independently | Fear of injury
Fear of loss of control
Fear of the dark
Separation anxiety
Egocentricity
Ritualistic behavior helps to master skills and decrease anxiety
Magical thinking
Lack of concept of time | If parents choose to remain during procedure, encourage tactile and verbal soothing during and after procedure (i.e., cuddling the child).
Keep security objects close (i.e., teddy bear, blanket).
Minimize parenteral separation.
Explain only shortly before procedure.
Use a calm, quiet tone with simple and honest explanations.
If feasible, allow child to handle equipment.
Use immediate and concrete rewards (i.e., stickers). |

Continued.

Table 11-1 Developmental stages of childhood—cont'd

Age	Developmental Level	Characteristics	Child/Family Preparation
Preschool (4–6 years)	Initiative versus guilt	Short attention span Tend to mimic behavior Involved in parallel play Developing body image Fears concerning body integrity, loss of control, the dark, being alone	Use pictures, models, dolls, and actual equipment to demonstrate procedure. Emphasize that the procedure will help make the child healthy. Reinforce that the procedure is not punishment for bad behavior. Encourage choices (i.e., which arm) and assistance (i.e., opening alcohol wipes) when possible. Use simple terms and prepare only shortly before procedure. Praise cooperation and provide rewards (i.e., stickers).

Age Group	Developmental Stage	Characteristics	Interventions
School Age (6–12 years)	Industry versus inferiority: Using hands to make things, being helpful and mastering tasks	Fears loss of control, death, bodily injury, and failure to meet expectations of significant others Plays with peers Developing a sense of belonging, cooperation, and compromise Engages in fantasy play Enjoys learning Peer group becoming increasingly important	Prepare in advance so child has a greater sense of control. Use pictures, models, and videos. Allow time to handle equipment, if possible. Have child explain what he or she already knows of procedure. Include the child in decision-making (i.e., which arm) to increase sense of control.
Adolescents (13–19 years)	Identity versus identity diffusion: Defining self related to others, vacillating between dependence and independence	Fears loss of control, altered body image, and separation from peer group	Give immediate tactile and verbal praise for cooperation. Advance preparation is vital for adolescent's coping, cooperation, and compliance.

Continued.

Table 11-1 Developmental stages of childhood—cont'd

Age	Developmental Level	Characteristics	Child/Family Preparation
		Developing maturation and independence Strong need for privacy Peer acceptance is important May use noncompliance as a means of exerting independence and control	Explain the procedure using adult terms. Include adolescent in decision making. Models, diagrams, and videos are useful. Encourage participation in self-care (i.e., monitoring IV site). Coping/relaxation techniques may be useful.

chapter. Patient and family teaching for self-care management will be incorporated into all the topics, and a section at the end of the chapter will address the issues related to home care and the discharge process.

Fluid and Electrolyte Balance

Fluid and electrolyte balance in the child has a different physiological rationale than it does for the adult patient. The significant differences are described in the following list.

- Children have proportionally more body water than do adults. Water constitutes approximately 75% to 80% of the full-term infant's weight, compared with 60% to 70% of the adult's weight. The *proportion* of the body water to the body weight decreases with increasing age, development of body fat, and growth of the solid body structures. Table 11-2 shows body water in proportion to age and weight.
- The distribution of body water in the child also differs from that in the adult. Infants have more total body water in the extracellular compartment (42% to 45%) compared with adults (20%) (see Table 11-2). Because of the increased percentage of water in the extracellular fluid, the child's water turnover rate is two to three times greater than that of the adult. Fifty percent of the infant's extracellular fluid is

Table 11-2   Body water in proportion to age and weight

| | Percentage of Body Water | | |
Age/Weight	Total Body Water	Extracellular Fluid	Intracellular Fluid
Premature infant (1.2 kg)	81	59	22
Full-term infant (3.6 kg)	69	42	27
1-year-old child (10 kg)	60	32	28
Adult male (70 kg)	54	23	31
Adult female (60 kg)	49	23	26

Terry J and others: *Intravenous therapy: clinical principles and practice,* Philadelphia, 1995, WB Saunders. Reprinted with permission.

Table 11-3 Daily caloric requirements by age

Age	Daily Caloric Requirement
High-risk neonate	120–150 cal/kg
Normal neonate	100–120 cal/kg
Age 1–2 years	90–100 cal/kg
Age 3–6 years	80–90 cal/kg
Age 7–9 years	70–80 cal/kg
Age 10–12 years	50–60 cal/kg

Hazinski MF: *Nursing care of the critically ill child,* ed 2, St Louis, 1992, Mosby. Reprinted with permission.

exchanged every day, compared with only 20% of the adult's. Additionally, the smaller the child, the less fluid volume there is in each compartment, specifically in the intracellular fluid. Lower fluid volume results in less fluid reserve.

- The child's metabolism is two to three times greater than an adult's. A higher pulse and higher respiratory and peristaltic rates result in a greater proportion of insensible water loss and more metabolic waste. Therefore, a child requires more water per kg of body weight than an adult.
- Children have more body surface area (BSA) in proportion to body mass. This increased BSA ratio results in greater fluid loss through the skin by evaporation.
- An infant's kidneys do not concentrate urine at an adult level until after age 2; as a result, they are less able to conserve water in the event of excessive fluid loss or diminished fluid intake.
- Children have a greater daily fluid requirement (per kg of body weight) than do adults. Following are the three common methods used to determine the child's fluid requirements:
  - Meter-squared method: A nomogram is used to calculate the child's BSA; then 1500 ml to 1800 ml of fluid per square meter is calculated for the fluid replacement.
  - Calorie method: The usual fluid expenditure is approximately 150 ml for every 100 calories metabolized. Table 11-3 lists the daily caloric requirements by age.
  - Weight method: The child's weight in kg is used to estimate

Table 11-4   Maintenance fluid requirements in children

Weight	Formula
Body Weight Daily Maintenance Formula	
Neonate (<72 hours)	60–100 ml/kg
0–10 kg	100 ml/kg
11–20 kg	1000 ml for the first 10 kg + 50 ml/kg for kg 11–20
21–30 kg	1500 ml for the first 20 kg + 25 ml/kg for kg 21–30
Body Weight Hourly Maintenance Formula	
0–10 kg	4 ml/kg/hr
11–20 kg	40 ml/hr for first 10 kg + 2 ml/kg/hr for kg 11–20
21–30 kg	60 ml/hr for first 20 kg + 1 ml/kg/hr for kg 21–30

Hazinski, MF: *Nursing care of the critically ill child,* ed 2, St Louis, 1992, Mosby. Reprinted with permission.

the fluid requirements. Table 11-4 provides maintenance fluid requirements in children.

The weight method is used most frequently, but it tends to be less accurate than other methods when the child weighs more than 10 kg. The most accurate method is based on the child's BSA using the meter-squared formula.

Monitoring Fluid Replacement

Although the fluid requirement per kg of body weight is greater for a child than an adult, the actual fluid volume amount required by the child is minimal. Following are recommendations to avoid fluid volume overload in the child:

- Regulate all pediatric infusions with volumetric chambers (e.g., Buretrol sets).
- Use volume-controlled infusion pumps to ensure accurate fluid delivery.
- Use microdrop tubing (60 drops/ml) to administer small-volume infusions and help prevent bolus infusions.
- Measure and evaluate intake and output with fluid balance every 4 to 8 hours.

Table 11-5   Grades of pediatric dehydration

	Mild	Moderate	Severe
Weight Loss	3%–5%	6%–10%	9%–15%
BP	Normal	Normal–low	Low
Pulse	Rapid	Rapid	Rapid/weak
Eyeball	Normal	Sunken	Sunken
Fontanelle	Flat	Sunken	Sunken
Tears	Normal	Absent	Absent
Mucous membranes	Dry	Dry	Dry
Skin turgor	Mild decrease	Tenting	Severe decrease

- Monitor IV site, infusion, and equipment at least hourly.

Dehydration

The younger the child, the more rapid fluid and electrolyte imbalances develop. Children become dehydrated more quickly than adults and require more urgent replacement for those losses. Common dehydration symptoms for children and adults include dry mucous membranes, weight loss, poor skin turgor, and decreased urine volume with increased urine concentration. Specific dehydration characteristics found in the dehydrated infant include a sunken anterior fontanelle, lethargy, irritability, high-pitched weak cries, creases on the soles of the feet, and an increased basal body temperature.

Oral intake is often compromised during a child's illness and can expedite the dehydration process, requiring intravenous fluids to maintain the fluid and electrolyte balance. It is a common practice to grade the severity of dehydration and prescribe fluid replacement accordingly. Tables 11-5 and 11-6 list grades of pediatric dehydration and treatment by grade respectively.

Depending on the type of fluid and electrolyte imbalance, a hypertonic, hypotonic, or isotonic IV solution will be indicated in the intravenous management of the dehydration. Dextrose water is an isotonic solution and may be administered to children, but it should be used with extreme caution. If dextrose water is administered in large amounts it can alter the child's extracellular osmolarity, resulting in cerebral edema.

Table 11-6   Treatment of dehydration according to grade

Grade	Treatment
Mild	Maintenance fluid + (maintenance × 0.5)
Moderate	Maintenance + (maintenance × 1.0)
Severe	Maintenance + (maintenance × 1.5)

Intravenous Site Selection and Maintenance

The following principles are used for IV site selection:

- Always select a site at the most distal point on an extremity.
- Avoid previously used sites.
- Avoid joints and areas that may restrict extremity movement (potential increased risk for infiltration).
- Consider age, hand dominance, and mobility when selecting an IV site (Table 11-7, Fig. 11-1, Fig. 11-2).

Venipuncture Procedure Recommendations:

- Apply topical anesthetic cream 1 to 4 hours before the IV access procedure.
- Wrap the extremity in a warm compress for 10 minutes before IV access to assist in vein dilation.
- Use a cannula gauge (20 gauge to 24 gauge), depending on infusion solution.
- Apply a Penrose drain or rubber band for a tourniquet in a small child.
- Consider placing a flashlight or transilluminator device beneath the extremity to outline the vein and improve vein visualization.
- Insert the cannula with the bevel pointed downward, to prevent puncturing the far wall of the vessel and minimize occurrence of fluid extravasation in small veins.
- Never attempt to start an IV access on an infant or young child alone or without a passive restraining device.
- Consider using appropriate-sized arm and foot boards to secure the IV site.
- Never tape all the way around an extremity, because of the potential for blood flow obstruction.
- Ensure that the ID band is *not* placed on the same extremity with the IV access.

Table 11-7   Pediatric intravenous site access

Age	Site	Example
Neonates and premature infants	Upper arms Inner thighs Scalp	Upper arms: axilla Scalp: superficial temporal, frontal, occipital, postauricular, supraorbital, posterior facial areas Inner thighs: popliteal
Infants and toddlers	Scalp Antecubital area Foot Hand	Antecubital area: cephalic, basilic, median areas Foot: saphenous, median, marginal areas; dorsal arch Hand: metacarpal, dorsal venous arch, tributaries of cephalic and basilic
Preschool through adolescents	Hand Forearm	Forearm: cephalic, basilic, median, antebrachial areas

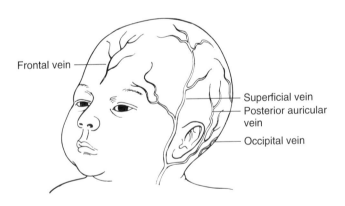

Fig. 11-1
Scalp veins of an infant.
Wheeler C, Frey AM: *Intravenous therapy in children.* In Terry J and others, editors: *Intravenous Therapy: Clinical Principles and Practice,* Philadelphia, 1995, WB Saunders.

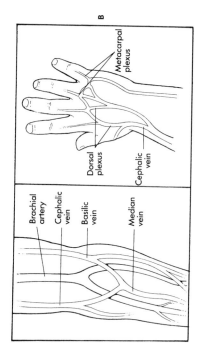

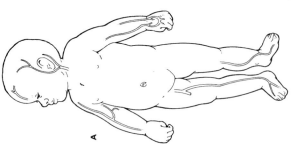

Fig. 11-2

A, Preferred sites for venous access infants. *B,* Preferred sites for venous access in toddlers, older children, and adolescents. Summerfield AL: *Inserting intravenous (IV) catheters.* In Smith DP and others, editors: *Comprehensive Child and Family Nursing Skills,* St. Louis, 1991, Mosby.

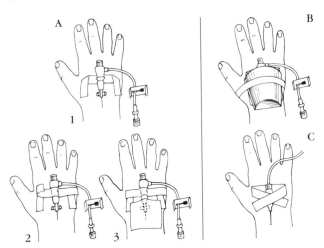

Fig. 11-3
Taping techniques for keeping IV devices in place. *A,* Catheter.
B, Butterfly needle.
Wheeler C, Frey AM: *Intravenous therapy in children.* In Terry J and others, editors: *Intravenous Therapy: Clinical Principles and Practice,* Philadelphia, 1995, WB Saunders.

- Use plastic medication cups to cover and protect the IV site in young, active children (Fig. 11-3).
- Protect the IV site from accidental dislodgment with stretch netting in older children.

CLINICAL ALERT: Monitor the IV site for pain, redness, edema, phlebitis, and infiltration every 30 to 60 minutes.

Central Venous Catheters

Intravenous access is often achieved through the peripheral veins in the pediatric patient's hand, forearm, foot, leg, or scalp. When inadequate peripheral access is present or long-term or aggressive IV therapy is required, central venous access becomes a viable option. Central venous access provides options for drug and fluid delivery and blood sampling for diagnostic testing. Needlesticks are a source of fear and pain in the child, and the central venous access offers a less traumatic approach to IV therapy. Using CVCs also eliminates the invasive procedure of peripheral IV site rotation every 48 to 72 hours.

Central venous access devices commonly used in pediatric patients include umbilical, percutaneous, tunneled, and peripherally inserted central catheters and implantable ports. The appropriate device depends on vein access, prescribed type and duration of therapy, disease process, and patient/family preference. Additionally, the device selection should include the child's age and size, cognitive ability, body image considerations, and self-care management requirements. The anatomical placement and potential advantages and disadvantages of each device follows.

Umbilical Catheter

Use of the umbilical catheter is common practice in neonatal and intensive care units for the acutely ill infant. The umbilical vein is the anatomical placement.

- Advantages: Easy route for IV fluid or drug administration; can be used for central venous pressure measurements, venous blood sampling, and exchange blood transfusions; catheter can be removed as soon as an alternate IV access is established
- Disadvantages: Site not accessible after the fourth day of life; potential complication for thrombosis, embolism, vasospasm, vascular perforation, infection, and hemorrhage

Percutaneous Central Venous Catheter

Catheter placement for the neonate and infant is the jugular vein. The site of choice for older children is the subclavian vein. The femoral vein with catheter tip placement in the vena cava can be used; however, use this site with caution if the child is in diapers, because of potential increased infection risk

- Advantages: Venous access is obtained without needlestick to child; can be used for short-term intermittent or continuous infusion therapy
- Disadvantages: Requires prudent daily aseptic site care, dressing change, and heparinization; alteration in body image

Tunneled Catheters

Device options include single- or double-lumen Broviac and Groshong catheters. Catheter placement for infants and children under age 5 is access through the facial vein threaded into the superior vena cava (Fig. 11-4); for older children the catheter is inserted percutaneously into the subclavian vein. When the chest is not a viable access site, the catheter can be inserted into the inferior

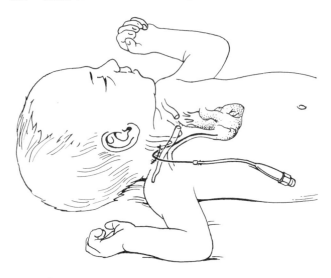

Fig. 11-4
Example of infant-sized Broviac catheter.
Weinstein SM: *Pediatric Intravenous Therapy.* In *Plumer's Principles and Practice of Intravenous Therapy*, Philadelphia, 1993, JB Lippincott.

vena cava through the femoral vein with the catheter exit site on the abdomen, thigh, or back. To avoid catheter dislodgment, loop the external "tail" of the catheter under the dressing and secure it with tape to the chest. T-shirts and binders are also recommended to secure the catheter.

CLINICAL ALERT: **Never** use a tie or string around the child's neck to secure the catheter because of the potential risk of strangulation.

- Advantages: Catheter longevity (months/years); easy access by patient or caregiver, catheter repair options; clean dressing technique can be used after tissue healing; IV access possible without needlestick; child may swim in chlorinated water after tissue site healing, based on immune status and physician order
- Disadvantages: Daily to weekly catheter heparinization and site care; alteration in body image; risk of accidental catheter dislodgment or puncture (e.g., infant may bite catheter during teething, or toddler may pull out catheter)

Peripherally Inserted Central Catheter

Catheter placement is through the basilic, cephalic, or median cubital veins in older children. The saphenous, superficial temporal, external jugular, popliteal, or axillary veins are used most often in newborns, infants, and toddlers.

- Advantages: Catheter can be inserted by specially trained nurses; allows repeated venous access without needlestick; a safe and less-expensive option than tunneled catheters; catheter size is French 2, 3, or 4, depending on child size and type or duration of therapy
- Disadvantages: Requires daily catheter heparinization and site care; PICC site should not be submerged in water; should avoid blood pressures and venipuncture in affected extremity; small-gauge PICCs are not recommended for blood sampling; repetitive movements in the affected extremity should be avoided; alteration in body image

Implantable Port

Device placement is the anterior chest under the skin via the subclavian vein, with the catheter tip in the superior vena cava.

Alternate site placement is the anterior fossa of the arm, with the catheter threaded via the basilic/cephalic vein into the superior vena cava.

- Advantages: Ideal for the child who requires intermittent therapy or long-term therapy for a child aged 3 and older (before age 3 the lack of sufficient subcutaneous tissue may allow the port to erode through the skin); requires minimal site care and maintenance; intact body image; device longevity (2–3 years); child may bathe or swim when port is not accessed; no external components to break or malfunction
- Disadvantages: Needlestick is required for IV access; potential pain associated with needle aspiration; vigorous contact sports may be restricted because of the potential risk for port displacement; requires monthly heparinization with needle access

Clinical Guidelines for Pediatric Central Venous Devices

- Heparin concentration, volume of flush per lumen, and frequency of catheter maintenance need to be correlated with the child's body requirements, fluid balance, and medical diagnosis.

- Three-way stopcocks may be used during blood sampling procedure, and the discarded blood sample is returned to the patient. Follow the institution or agency guidelines for this procedure.
- Blood sampling discard volume should be limited in volume (e.g., 5 ml or less).
- Normal saline flush volume is 5 ml or less; *calculate* the total volume of these flushes in the child's daily intake.
- Consult the manufacturer's recommendations for device flush protocols and site/dressing requirements.
- Assess the child, parent, or caregiver's ability and compliance for catheter/device management.
- Teaching strategies for catheter/device management should include the child's growth, developmental, and psychosocial status.

Intraosseous Route

The intraosseous route (into the bone) is an emergency measure used in infant and child resuscitation when immediate vascular access is required. This route is used only when conventional IV access is unobtainable. A needle is inserted into the bone marrow of a long bone, and blood, fluid, or drugs are then infused.

The fluid injected into the bone marrow cavity is rapidly drained into the central venous channel into the systemic circulation. The intraosseous route is as effective as the central venous route for delivering IV solutions. The optimal sites for intraosseous needle placement in infants and children include the distal tibia and distal femur (Fig. 11-5). Other sites include the iliac crest and the humerus. The sternum is never used in children. Complications are rare but can include osteomyelitis, sepsis, cellulitis, abscess, local necrosis, and fat embolism.

CLINICAL ALERT: The intraosseous route is intended for short-term use only, and once the child is stabilized, an alternate IV access route must be obtained.

Intravenous Medication Administration

The pediatric patient is susceptible to drug and fluid overload with varied IV therapy infusions. To diminish this occurrence, minimal fluid amounts should be used for drug dilution and flushing the IV access. Additional precautions follow:

- Use preservative-free solutions for the neonate.

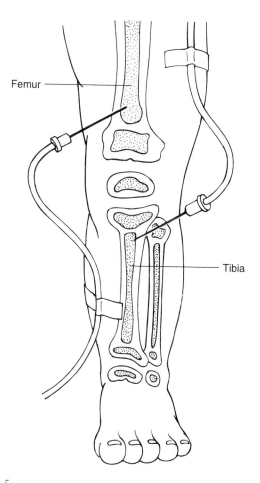

Fig. 11-5
Intraosseous access sites for IV infusion.
Wheeler C, Frey AM: *Intravenous therapy in children.* In Terry J and others, editors: *Intravenous Therapy: Clinical Principles and Practice,* Philadelphia, 1995, WB Saunders.

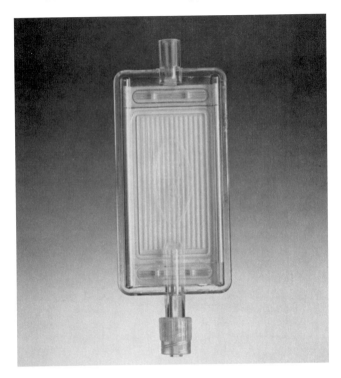

Fig. 11-6
Pall ELD 96 NT Set Saver Filter.
Courtesy Pall Biomedical Product Co., Port Washington, NY.

- Use small-volume infusion tubing with pumps and controllers to infuse drugs and solutions (Fig. 11-6).
- Pumps and controllers should have alarms and tamper-proof or locking features.
- Microinfusion pumps that can infuse fluids in increments of 0.1 ml/hr are the preferred choice for medication delivery in the neonate and infant.
- Knowledge of the child's body weight (kg/BSA/m^2) is essential for accurate drug dose calculations.
- Adhere to the prescribed or recommended infusion rates.

Table 11-8 lists common intravenous medications by drug, with indications and dosing guidelines with nursing considerations.

Table 11-8 Common IV medications

Drug	Indications	Dose	Nursing Considerations
Antibiotics			
Ampicillin			
Amcil	Systemic infections	100–300 mg/kg IV daily,	Drug should be discontinued if
Ampicin	Acute and chronic urinary	divided into 6-hour doses	immediate hypersensitivity
	tract infections caused by		reaction occurs.
	susceptible organisms		Use cautiously in patient with
	Meningitis		other drug allergies.
	Uncomplicated gonorrhea		Dosage should be altered in
			patients with impaired renal
			functions.
			Follow the manufacturer's
			directions for stability data.
			IV dose should be mixed in
			D5W or saline solution.
Sulfamethoxazole			
Bactrim	Urinary tract infections	8 mg/kg TMP per 40 mg/kg	Not recommended in children
Septra	Shigellosis	SMZ to 20 mg/kg TMP per	<2 months.
sulfamethoxazole-	Otitis media	100 mg/kg SMZ for serious	Infuse slowly over 60–90
trimethoprin	pneumocystis carinil	infections daily, divided into	minutes.
(SMZ-TMP)	pneumonia (PCP)	12-hour doses	

Continued.

Table 11-8　Common IV medications—cont'd

Drug	Indications	Dose	Nursing Considerations
			Use solution within 2 hours after preparation.
			Check solution carefully for precipitate.
			Monitor renal functioning.
			IV infusion must be diluted in D5W.
			Dose may be reduced for patients with impaired hepatic or renal function.
Cefazolin Ancef Kefzol	Serious respiratory, genitourinary, skin and soft tissue, bone, and joint infections Septicemis endocarditis	8–16 mg/kg IV every 8 hours of 6–12 mg/kg every 6 hours	Patients with altered renal functioning should be monitored closely.
Ceftazidime Fortaz Tazicef	Bacteremia Septicemia Serious respiratory, urinary, gynecological, intraabdominal, CNS, and skin infections	30–50 mg/kg IV every 8 hours	Monitor carefully for superinfections.

Drug	Uses	Dosage	Nursing Considerations
Cefuroxime Kefurox Zinacef	Serious lower respiratory tract, skin, and skin structure infections; Septicemia; Meningitis	50–100 mg/kg IV per day, divided into 6- or 8-hour doses	
Clindamycin Cleocin	Infections caused by Streptococci, Pneumococci, Bacteroides species, Fuso-bacterium species, and *Clostridium perfringens*	15–40 mg/kg IV divided into 6-hour doses	Culture and Sensitivity (C & S) testing should be done prior to starting IV. Administer no faster than 30 mg/min or 1.2 g/hr. Monitor renal, hepatic, and hematopoietic functions during prolonged therapy. Monitor closely for diarrhea.
Gentamicin Garamycin	Serious infections caused by susceptible organisms	2.0–2.5 mg/kg IV every 8 hours	Use cautiously in patients with impaired renal function.

Continued.

Table 11-8 Common IV medications—cont'd

Drug	Indications	Dose	Nursing Considerations
	Meningitis		Monitor renal function (output, specific gravity urinalysis, BUN, and creatine levels). Keep patient well hydrated. Monitor drug levels as ordered.
	Endocarditis prophylaxis		
	External ocular infections caused by susceptible organisms		
	Primary and secondary bacterial infections		
	Superficial burns		
	Skin ulcers and infected lacerations		
	Abrasions, insect bites, or minor surgical wounds		
Oxacillin Bactocill Prostaphlin	Systemic infections caused by susceptible organisms	100–200 mg/kg IV per day, divided into every 4- to 6-hour doses	Monitor renal and hepatic function. Watch for elevated serum glutamic-oxaloacetic transaminase (SGOT) and serum glutamate pyruvate transaminase (SGPT). IV infusion should be mixed with D5W saline solution. Monitor for superinfection.

Drug	Use	Dose	Comments
Tobramycin Nebcin	Serious infections caused by susceptible organisms	3 mg/kg–5 mg/kg, divided into 8-hour doses	Infuse over 20–60 minutes. Impaired renal function will require adjusted doses. Serum levels should be monitored.
Vancomycin Vancocin	Severe staph infections Enterocolitis Endocarditis prophylaxis	20–40 mg/kg IV daily, divided into 6-hour doses	Obtain C & S tests before starting therapy. Infuse over at least 60 minutes. Monitor BUN, creatine, and serum drug levels. If patient develops maculopapular rash on face, neck, trunk, and upper extremities, slow infusion rate. Monitor patient for ringing in the ears. Monitor renal function.

Continued.

Table 11-8 Common IV medications—cont'd

Drug	Indications	Dose	Nursing Considerations
Antivirals			
Acyclovir Zovirax	Initial and recurrent mucocutaneous herpes simplex virus Severe initial genital herpes in immunocompromised patients	For children > 12 years, 5 mg/kg over 1 hour every 8 hours For children < 12 years, 250 mg/m² over 1 hour IV every 8 hours	Infuse slowly over at least 1 hour to prevent renal tubular damage. Patients must be adequately hydrated.
Ganciclovir Cytovene	Treatment of CMV infections in immunocompromised patients	7.5 mg–10 mg/kg IV divided in 2 to 3 doses for induction, then 2.5–5 mg/kg/day	Monitor blood counts.
Antifungals			
Amphotericin B Fungizone	Systemic fungal infections caused by susceptible or ganisms Meningitis Coccidioidal arthritis	0.25 mg/kg daily by slow infusion over 6 hours to start; increase as tolerated to 1/mg/kg daily to a maximum of 1.5 mg/kg	If drug has been discontinued for > 1 week, then initial dose must be given and increased gradually. C & S testing must be completed.

Mix with D5W.

Use an in-line filter membrane with a mean pore diameter larger than 1 micron.

Do not mix or piggyback with other antibiotics.

Monitor hepatic and renal function studies.

Patients often premedicated with aspirin, antihistamines, antiemetics, or corticosteroids.

Monitor vital signs every 30 minutes for at least 4 hours after starting IV infusion.

Fever may appear within 1–2 hours of starting infusion but should subside in 4 hours of discharging drug.

Continued.

Table 11-8 Common IV medications—cont'd

Drug	Indications	Dose	Nursing Considerations
			Monitor I & Os closely and report changes. Monitor K+, Ca+, and Mg+ levels closely.
Antiemetic *Ondansetron* Zofran	Nausea and vomiting induced by chemotherapy	For > 4 years of age, 0.15 mg/kg over 15 minutes, 30 minutes before emetogenic chemotherapy. Repeated at 4 hours and 8 hours following the first dose.	

Blood and Blood Component Administration

Blood product administration for children requires precautions and monitoring guidelines similar to those used with adult patients. However, there are differences related to circulating blood volume, infused blood volume, red cell life span, hemoglobulin level, and maturation of the hematopoietic system. Children have a much greater circulating blood volume per unit of body weight than adults do, yet their absolute blood volume is very small (Table 11-9).

Indications for transfusion therapy in children include acute hemorrhage, anemia, abnormal blood component function or deficiency, and removal of harmful elements such as bilirubin during an exchange transfusion. Blood replacement should be considered when the blood loss is greater than 5% to 7% of the total circulating volume. Reduction in the child's blood volume by 30% to 40% produces evidence of clinical shock (Table 11-10).

Consider the following factors in transfusion therapy for children:

- Blood from the newborn is usually cross-matched against the mother's serum, which contains equal or greater quantities of antibodies present in the infant at birth.
- Neonates with severe hyperbilirubinemia or ABO incompatibility receive exchange transfusions by withdrawing small amounts of the infant's blood and infusing the same amount of plasma and red cells from one or more donors via an umbilical catheter. The neonate is typed and cross-matched before the transfusion process, and the blood transfusion is cleared of the offending antigen.
- Intrauterine blood exchange transfusion is considered when an amniocentesis test indicates increasing bilirubin in the

Table 11-9   Calculation of circulating blood volume in children

Age	Blood Volume Ml/kg
Neonates	85–90
Infants	75–80
Children	70–75
Adolescents	65–70

Hazinski MF: *Nursing care of the critically ill child,* ed 2, St Louis, 1992, Mosby. Reprinted with permission.

Table 11-10 Blood component therapy for pediatric patients

Blood Product	Indication	Dosage/Rate
Red blood cells (packed)	Treatment of anemia without volume expansion	10 ml/kg, not to exceed 15 ml/kg at 2.5 ml/kg/hr
Platelets	To control bleeding associated with deficiency in platelet number or function	1 u (50–70 ml)/7–10 kg body weight run over 30 minutes to a maximum of 4 hours; IV push or drip
Fresh frozen plasma	To increase levels of clotting factors in children with demonstrated deficiency	Acute hemorrhage: 15–30 ml/kg as indicated
	Occasionally volume expansion in acute blood loss	Clotting deficiency: 10–15 ml/kg at 1–2 ml/min

National Blood Education Program, Public Health Service, National Institutes of Health, US Department of Health and Human Services, *Transfusion therapy guidelines for nurses*, 1990, US Government Printing Office.

amniotic fluid of a fetus with Rh incompatibility or if the maternal indirect Coomb's test is strongly positive, to prevent kernicterus, severe anemia, brain damage, and death.

- *Only* qualified personnel (physicians and nurses) with advanced skills should perform newborn exchange transfusions or intrauterine transfusions. These transfusions should take place only in an appropriate clinical environment.
- Blood transfusion volume in children varies according to age and weight. The volume is calculated in ml/kg of body weight.
- Pediatric blood units are prepared in special units (e.g., Pedipacks) and usually equal half the volume of a conventional adult unit.
- Red cell transfusions require strict infusion times (e.g., calculate 5% of the total blood product to be transfused, and infuse this amount over the initial 15 minutes). This method facilitates early detection of a potential hemolytic reaction.
- Microaggregate filters are not routinely required in neonatal transfusions, because the blood neonates receive is usually less than 7 days old and rarely contains the microaggregate component; when microaggregate filters are used, they must be changed every 2 to 4 hours according to the manufacturer's recommendations.
- Blood warmers prevent hypothermia, which could result in potential cardiac dysrhythmia. The blood temperature should be maintained between 32° and 37°C.
- Infusion pumps capable of infusing blood are recommended for all transfusion therapies in children. The blood may be prefiltered and infused via a syringe pump for the neonate and infant.
- Blood and blood products may be administered via 27-, 26-, or 24-gauge peripheral IV access in the neonate and via 24- or 22-gauge peripheral IV access in older children.
- Straight line IV tubing should be used to minimize the volume of saline infused. Small amounts of normal saline (1 ml) should be used for flushing the IV line to prevent fluid overload.
- Explain the transfusion procedure to the parents, obtain their consent, and review the transfusion history of the child. Include the child in all the instructional preparations.

- Consider the child's and family's perspective of the transfusion process, their prior experiences, and their cultural and religious views related to transfusion therapy.

Chemotherapy Administration

Childhood cancers are treated with a combination of surgery, radiation therapy, chemotherapy, and biological response modifiers. Pediatric oncology diseases such as leukemia, lymphoma, neuroblastoma, Hodgkin's disease, Wilms' tumors, and brain tumors usually require intermittent chemotherapy to treat the disease. Aggressive chemotherapy used in many of these disease protocols frequently requires long-term venous access to deliver the prescribed drugs. The venous access devices used to deliver the varied chemotherapy drugs are tunneled catheters, PICCs, and implantable ports.

The chemotherapy drug side effects, duration of therapy, and maintenance of long-term venous access devices result in many physical and psychosocial changes for the child. Maintaining a child's developmental status to enable achievement of normal milestones throughout the course of chemotherapy can be a challenge. A change in body image (e.g., hair loss, weight changes) can have a significant impact on the child's self-concept, especially in the adolescent years. Focusing on the child's strengths and providing the child with as much autonomy as possible will promote a positive self-concept. Allowing children who are cognitively able to participate in decisions regarding their course of therapy will also enhance a positive outlook. Consider age-related diversionary activities selected by the child or parent to minimize distress associated with invasive procedures in the treatment regimens.

Clinical practice interventions recommended for pediatric chemotherapy administration include the following points:

- Consider the child's cognitive level, developmental level, and chronological age in preparation of instructional and recreational materials and resources. Chronically ill children often have developmental delays, and the child's response to the treatment may not be age-appropriate; interventions need to be based on the child's developmental level, not chronological age.
- Include caregiver education in all components of the chemotherapy (e.g., drug side effects and toxicities, administration route, and schedule). Encourage caregivers to actively participate in the child's care.

- Instruct the caregiver regarding safe handling precautions (e.g., wearing latex gloves when changing diapers; handling chemotherapy-contaminated linen; disposing of vomit, urine, or stool; disposing of chemotherapy drug and infusion supplies; managing a chemotherapy drug spill).
- Anticipate potential drug side effects such as nausea and vomiting; include age-appropriate assessments and interventions. Small children have an increased risk for aspiration; position children appropriately and monitor them according to a scheduled frequency.
- Calculate the prescribed drug dose with each course of chemotherapy. The child's height and weight will change throughout the treatment process.
- Keep an accurate, up-to-date, cumulative drug dose record on all children receiving drugs that have maximum dose limits.
- Intrathecal drug dosages may be based on age as an estimate of cerebral spinal fluid volume rather than on the BSA or weight.
- Never apply heat to suspected or actual drug infiltration, because tissue necrosis and sloughing may occur.

Parenteral Nutrition

Parenteral nutrition in the pediatric population is highly specialized. This therapy needs to sustain the child's life and weight and allow for the child's normal growth and developmental needs. Total parenteral nutrition (TPN) and partial parenteral nutrition (PPN) are most often used as supportive therapy for infants and children with complex illness and structural gastrointestinal anomalies.

Pediatric Indications for TPN and PPN

Gastrointestinal obstruction	Inflammatory bowel disease
Cystic fibrosis	Hirschsprung's disease
Crohn's disease	Congenital heart disease
Short bowel syndrome	Necrotizing enterocolitis
Pancreatitis	Cancer
Renal failure	AIDS

Gastroschisis (a congenital fissure in the wall of the abdomen that remains open)

Criteria used to determine if a child is a potential candidate for TPN or PPN include the following:

- Greater than 5% weight loss
- Height/weight ratio below the fifth percentile when plotted on a growth chart
- Serum albumin level below 3 g/dl
- Total lymphocyte count less than 1000/mm^3 (excluding granulocytopenia)

In the past several years it has been common practice to discharge the child to home care on TPN or PPN. Home parenteral nutrition allows the child a greater degree of normalcy in the growth and development process. Portable infusion pumps allow relative freedom, do not require an IV pole, and can be contained in an unobtrusive carrying case. Many children receive the TPN or PPN over 8 to 12 hours during the night, which allows the child a normal lifestyle of school and activities. TPN or PPN in the home setting requires individually tailored education and instruction for the child and parent or other caregiver. All educational components should be tailored according to the child's growth and developmental process and the prescribed TPN or PPN therapy.

Clinical Guidelines for TPN or PPN in Children

- The initial rate of infusion and glucose concentration must be low and increased gradually, to allow the child's insulin production to accommodate the continuous glucose load. Similarly, the glucose concentration and rate of infusion must be decreased gradually to wean the child from TPN or PPN. *Hypoglycemia* and *hyperglycemia* occur more rapidly in children than in adults.
- Dextrose provides the main calorie source and should be concentrated to provide enough energy requirements. However, the fluid volume required to dilute very concentrated dextrose is prohibitive to the *fluid balance* for infants and small children. The higher concentrations of dextrose (≥25%) can be administered via a central venous access device using less diluent.
- Fats are essential for the neurological development in the infant. The fatty acids in the TPN solution may displace the bilirubin from the albumin, causing a rise in the bilirubin level and an increased risk of kernicterus. Bilirubin levels should be obtained 4 hours after the fat emulsion has been infused.
- Children have higher metabolic rates than adults and required more calories per kilogram of body weight (Table 11-11). The

Table 11-11   Nutritional requirements for the pediatric patient

Age	Calories/kg/24 hours
Up to 6 months	120
6–12 months	100
12–36 months	90–95
4–10 years	80
>10 years—male	45
>10 years—female	38

Nutrient	Percent of Total Calories
Carbohydrates	40–45% carbohydrates and fats 85%–88%
Fat	40%
Protein	20%

Hazinski MF: *Nursing care of the critically ill child,* ed 2, St Louis, 1992, Mosby. Reprinted with permission.

active child will need maintenance caloric intake to provide the necessary energy requirements for basal metabolism, growth and development, and tissue healing. Children receiving long-term therapy (months or years) need to be continuously monitored to ensure that these nutritional requirements are met to allow a normal growth pattern.

- Infants receiving TPN are usually acutely ill and are deprived of maternal contact. It is important to hold and cuddle the child to help meet the emotional needs. If no oral intake is provided to the infant, ensure that the infant's sucking need is met.
- Children may develop adverse reactions to lipid infusions (e.g., dyspnea, flushing, nausea, headache, dizziness, chest pain, back pain). Therefore, lipids should be administered only 3 to 4 times a week, over a portion of the day, such as 8 hours. The maximum lipid infusion is 4 g/kg per 24-hour period and *should not exceed* 3 ml/kg/hr.
- Adjust the TPN or PPN rate by 10% increments, and never adjust the lipid infusion rate.
- Weigh children daily and infants every shift while they are receiving TPN or PPN.
- Maintain strict intake and output records. Obtain glucose level every 4 to 8 hours when initiating TPN or PPN, then every 4 hours for infants and every 8 hours for children. Obtain vital signs at least every 4 hours.

- Monitor liver function studies and serum liver enzymes on a scheduled frequency; abnormalities and elevations in these tests occur often in children.

Home Care Considerations

As the cost of health care continues to rise, the push to care for patients in the home setting increases. Pediatric home infusion therapy is a positive alternative to the traditional hospitalization process for the payer, physician, parent, and patient. Home infusion therapy allows the child to participate in normal activities related to school, family, and friends that the hospital setting often hinders.

Common pediatric infusion therapies administered at home include antibiotics, chemotherapy, parenteral nutrition, blood sampling for laboratory tests, and therapeutic drug monitoring. Maintaining therapeutic drug levels requires prudent monitoring. The prescribed drug should be administered at the scheduled time. Peak drug levels should be obtained 30 to 60 minutes after the drug has been infused, and trough drug levels should be obtained just before the next scheduled drug dose. The physician's order may vary the prescribed times for obtaining the peak- and trough-level blood sample. It is crucial to document the medication infusion dose and time with the time that the peak and trough levels were obtained. (See the box Therapeutic Drug Levels and box Normal Term Newborn Blood Values and Urinalysis Values for the levels that are frequently monitored in children.)

Therapeutic Drug Levels

Carbamazepine (Tegretol)	4–12 µg/ml
Clonazepam (Klonopin)	15–70 µg/ml
Digoxin (Lanoxin)	0.8–2.0 µg/ml
Gentamicin/Tobramycin	Peak 4–10 µg/ml trough 2 mcg/ml
Phenobarbital	15–30 µg/ml
Phenytoin (Dilantin)	10–20 µg/ml
Theophylline (Marax)	10–20 µg/ml
Valproic Acid (Depakene)	50–150 µg/ml
Vancomycin (Vancocin)	Peak 25–40 µg/ml; trough 10 µg/ml

Normal Term Newborn Blood Values and Urinalysis Values

Blood Values

Hemoglobin	15–20 g/dl
Hematocrit	43%–61%
WBC	10,000–30,000/mm^3
Neutrophils	40%–80%
Immature WBC	3%–10%
Platelets	100,000–280,000/mm^3
Reticulocytes	3%–6%
Blood volume	82.3 ml/kg (third day after early cord clamping)
	92.6 ml/kg (third day after delayed cord clamping)
Sodium	124–156 mmol/l
Potassium	5.3–7.3 mmol/l
Chloride	90–111 mmol/l
Calcium	7.3–9.2 mg/dl
Glucose	40–97 mg/dl
IEM-PKU*	<4mg

Bilirubin (capillary heel stick)†	4–6 mg/dl	Bilirubin level peaks
Cord blood bilirubin	1.0–1.8 mg/dl	3–5 days and should not exceed 13 mg/dl

Urinalysis Values

Protein	<5–10 mg/dl
WBC	<2–3
RBC	Negative
Casts	Negative
Bacteria	Negative
Specific gravity	1.001–1.025
Color	Pale yellow

*IEM, Inborn errors of metabolism; PKU, Phenylketonia.

†Breast-milk jaundice: Bilirubin rises the fourth day *after mature breast milk comes in;* Bilirubin peak of 20–25 mg/dl is reached at 2–3 weeks of age.

Discharge Teaching Process

Once the discharge criteria are met, the nurse must educate the family and child on the specific home infusion therapy prescribed. The following are important aspects to consider in the discharge teaching plan:

- Psychosocial, growth, and developmental aspects of the child
- Therapy effects on the child's body image
- The child's participation in certain sports or desired activities
- The child's peers' reactions to home infusion therapy
- The type, complexity, and duration of home infusion therapy
- The ability of the child and parent or other caregiver to meet the care requirements
- Home environment factors (e.g., patient care in a multiple-level home; need for refrigeration for parenteral nutrition and phone availability)
- Self-care processes such as catheter site care and medication administration, with return demonstration of learned techniques to ensure prudent technique and accuracy in dosing
- Instructional materials tailored to age and comprehension
- Verbal and written instructions regarding who, when, where, and how to call for assistance in an emergency or with significant concerns about the home infusion therapy

 Nursing Diagnosis

Table 11-12 lists potential nursing diagnosis and results of proper treatment.

 Documentation Recommendations

- Document exact placement of all peripheral IV devices and gauges, IV site management, and IV access securing.
- Document type, placement, site care, and maintenance for all central venous access devices.
- Document all drugs, solution types, volume and tubing, dose, time, date, weight/drug/solution calculations, and type of IV filter used.
- Document all infusion devices, type, infusion rate, alarm function, tubing, and volume.
- Document all therapeutic drug and laboratory diagnostic monitoring levels and blood sampling volumes.

Table 11-12   Nursing diagnoses and desired patient outcomes in children receiving intravenous therapy

Nursing Diagnosis	Patient Outcome
Fluid volume deficit, risk for, because of vomiting, diarrhea, burns, hemorrhage, wound drainage, or diabetic ketoacidosis	The child's hydration status will demonstrate improvement by improved skin turgor, moist mucous membranes, stable weight, 1 ml/kg/hr of urine output, serum electrolyte values within normal limits. Oral fluids will be tolerated. Urine specific gravity will be between 1,000 and 1,010.
Fluid volume excess, because of fluid overload, cardiac or renal disease, inappropriate secretion, or fluid shift	The child's weight will return to pre-illness status, edema will decrease, vital signs will return to normal, and no audible rales will be present.
Sensory/perceptual alteration (visual, auditory, gustatory, tactile), because of electrolyte imbalance, cerebral edema, or fever	The child will respond appropriately for age (e.g., smile at parents, suck from bottle).
Skin integrity impaired, risk for, because of diarrhea, edema, or dry skin	The child's skin will be free of signs of breakdown, excoriation in diaper area will decrease, and skin turgor will return to normal.
Diversional activity deficit, because of environmental lack of activity; frequent, lengthy treatments; or long-term hospitalization	The child will participate in chosen activities and will express interest in surroundings and activity.
Fear, because of separation from parent, unfamiliar environment, treatment, IV equipment, or normal developmental phobias	The child will demonstrate reduced fear behaviors (e.g., crying, wide-eyed gaze, tension, or hiding).

Continued.

Table 11-12   Nursing diagnoses and desired patient outcomes in children receiving intravenous therapy—cont'd

Nursing Diagnosis	Patient Outcome
Knowledge deficit (self-care, central venous catheter site care), because of lack of exposure, information misinterpretation, cognitive limitation	The child and family will verbalize understanding of what was taught and will demonstrate ability to perform new skills.
Mobility, impaired physical, because of restraints and IV support boards and decreased endurance and strength	The child will achieve maximum mobility within age and medical restrictions, no skin breakdown, no contractures, and maximum joint range of motion.
Nutrition, altered; less than body requirements, because of nausea, vomiting, diarrhea, and inability to absorb nutrients	The child will tolerate feedings via oral route, feeding tube, or IV line without side effects; will gain a predetermined amount per day; will experience an increased energy level, and will participate in diet decisions, if age appropriate.
Self-esteem disturbance/body image disturbance, because of venous access device, illness, and effects of treatment (e.g., alcopecia)	The child will participate in decision-making process about self-care, will take initiative to do tasks, will make eye contact, will interact freely with peers.
Urinary elimination altered, because of fluid shift, diarrhea, inadequate intake, and chronic illness	The child will have adequate output that is in balance with intake and will have urine specific gravity between 1,000 and 1,010.

Terry J and others: *Intravenous therapy: clinical principles and practice,* Philadelphia, 1995, WB Saunders. Reprinted with permission.

- Document all chemotherapy, blood and blood product, and parenteral solutions (type, dose, volume, weight/dose calculations such as kg/wt; m^2) and the type and number of product filters used.
- Document all educational strategies related to the child and parent or other caregiver; note their understanding of the instructions, techniques in drug dosing, catheter maintenance, chemotherapy precautions, emergency procedures.
- Document all assessment parameters related to fluid volume deficit or overload; pain, vital signs, and weight/BSA calculations.

Study Questions

Select the **one** best answer.

1. The physiological principles for fluid and electrolyte balance in the child compared with the adult are related to which factor?
   a. Children have proportionally less body water than adults do.
   b. Children have less BSA in proportion to body mass.
   c. A child's metabolism is two to three times greater than an adult's.
   d. A child's daily fluid requirement (kilogram of body weight) is less than that of an adult.

2. Strategies to facilitate an *infant* IV procedure include all but one of these child/family preparations:
   a. Decrease parenteral anxiety by keeping parents well informed.
   b. Feed the child immediately before the procedure.
   c. Minimize parental separation from the child.
   d. Never use parents or family members to assist with restraining the child.

3. Nursing management for IV fluid administration in the child includes which steps?
   a. All pediatric infusions should be regulated with volumetric chambers or volume-controlled infusion pumps.
   b. Measured intake and output and evaluate fluid balance every 4 to 8 hours.
   c. Evaluate IV site, infusion, and equipment hourly.
   d. All the above

4. Principles for IV site selection in the child include which of the following?
   a. Consider age, hand dominance, and mobility in IV site selection.
   b. Always select a site at the most proximal point on the limb.
   c. Insert the cannula with the bevel tip up.
   d. Wrap the extremity in a cold compress to aid in IV insertion.

5. Practice guidelines for the child with a central venous catheter include which of the following?
   a. Heparin concentration, volume of flush per lumen, and frequency of catheter flushing should be correlated with child's body weight, fluid balance, and medical condition.
   b. Blood sampling discard practice recommendation: small-volume discard, small-volume normal saline flush, and potential use of three-way stopcock.
   c. Self-care management strategies should include consideration of child's growth and development status.
   d. All the above

6. IV therapy practices that diminish drug and fluid overload in the child include which statement?
   a. Preservative-free solutions are necessary for all pediatric patients 6 years old or younger.
   b. Macro infusion pumps are needed to infuse fluids in increments of 10 ml/hr.
   c. Large volume tubing is needed for infusion of drugs or solutions.
   d. Knowledge of kg/BSA/m^2 is essential for correct drug dose calculations.

7. *Differences* in blood transfusion therapy for the child compared with that for the adult include all the following except which factor?
   a. Differences in white blood count
   b. Differences in red cell life
   c. Differences in circulating blood volume
   d. Differences in volume to be transfused

8. Which common malignancies in children often require chemotherapy administration?
   a. Leukemia, neuroblastoma, multiple myeloma
   b. Wilms' and brain tumors, Hodgkin's disease

    c. Leukemia, lymphoma, lung cancer
    d. Leukemia, brain tumors, myelodysplastic syndrome

9. Parenteral nutrition administration criteria for the child may include which element?
    a. Weight loss >2%
    b. Serum albumin level <5 g/dl
    c. Height/weight ratio below the fifth percentile when plotted on a growth chart
    d. Total lymphocyte count <3000/mm^3

10. Which home care considerations are relevant for pediatric infusion therapy?
    a. Infusion therapies: antibiotics, chemotherapy, parenteral nutrition
    b. Therapeutic drug monitoring
    c. Blood sampling for varied laboratory tests
    d. All the above

ANSWERS: 1. c   2. b   3. d   4. a   5. d
6. d   7. a   8. b   9. c   10. d

Calculations for IV Therapy

12

Objectives

1. Calculate IV flow rates using 10-, 12-, 15-, and 60-drop infusion sets.

2. Calculate drug dosage requirements for microgram and kilogram for the child and the adult patient.

3. Calculate body surface area drug doses for the child and the adult patient.

4. Calculate the pediatric IVs infusion rate using the rule of six.

Flow Rate Calculations

Flow rate calculations are integral to the safe delivery of IV fluids and medications. Information necessary to calculate the flow rate includes the following:

1. Volume of fluid to be infused
2. Total infusion time
3. Calibration of the administration set used (number of drops per milliliter it delivers; this information is found on the IV tubing package)

Manufacturers of IV tubings use 10, 12, 15, 20, or 60 drops (gtt) to deliver a milliliter (ml) of fluid. To calculate an *hourly* IV rate, use the following formula:

$$\frac{\text{gtt/ml of set}}{60 \text{ min}} \times \text{total hourly volume} = \text{gtts/min} \qquad \text{Equation 1}$$

1000 ml over 8 hours = 125 ml/hr; 10 gtt/ml infusion set

$$\frac{10 \text{ gtt/ml}}{60 \text{ min}} \times 125 \text{ ml/hr} = \frac{1 \text{ gtt}}{6 \text{ min}} \times 125 \text{ ml/hr}$$

$$\frac{1}{6} \times \frac{125 \text{ ml/hr}}{1} = \frac{1}{6} \times \frac{125}{1} = 20 \text{ gtt/min}$$

Since $^{10}\!/_{60}$ reduces to $^{1}\!/_{6}$, any hourly volume may be divided by 6 to determine the drops per minute of an IV set that delivers 10 drops per milliliter.

1000 ml over 10 hours = 100 ml/hr; 15 gtt/ml infusion set   Equation 2

$$\frac{15 \text{ gtt/ml}}{60 \text{ min}} \times 100 \text{ ml/hr} = \frac{1 \text{ gtt}}{4 \text{ min}} \times 100 \text{ ml/hr}$$

$$\frac{1}{4} \times \frac{100 \text{ ml/hr}}{1} = \frac{1}{4} \times \frac{100}{1} = 25 \text{ gtt/min}$$

CLINICAL ALERT: Calculations for other IV tubing sets include: gtt/ml/infusion set

$$\frac{12 \text{ gtt}}{60 \text{ min}} = \frac{1}{5} \text{ or divide by } 5 \qquad \text{Equation 3}$$

$$\frac{15 \text{ gtt}}{60 \text{ min}} = \frac{1}{4} \text{ or divide by } 4$$

$$\frac{20 \text{ gtt}}{60 \text{ min}} = \frac{1}{3} \text{ or divide by } 3$$

$$\frac{60 \text{ gtt}}{60 \text{ min}} = 1 \text{ or divide by } 1$$

Often a 24-hour volume is prescribed by a physician. Divide the desired volume by 24 before using the preceding formula.

3000 ml/24 hr   Equation 4

$3000 \div 24$

$$\frac{3000}{1} \times \frac{1}{24} = 125 \text{ ml/hr}$$

To calculate drops per minute for fluid volume that is prescribed in milliliters per hour, proceed to the step of

$$\frac{\text{gtt/ml of set}}{60 \text{ min}} = \text{total hourly volume} = \text{gtt/min} \qquad \text{Equation 5}$$

When small-volume IV piggyback medications are administered through the same IV line as a continuous infusion, the IV infusion will *not* stay on time unless the *time* needed to infuse the piggyback medications is included in the total calculations. Subtract the time required for the piggyback infusion from the 24-hour period before calculating the drops per minute for the continuous IV.

IV fluid 3000 ml 24 hr   Equation 6

Piggyback medication

50 ml over 20 min × 3 in 24 hr = 1 hour

24 hr − 1 hr = 23 hrs

3000 ml ÷ 23

$$\frac{3000}{1} \times \frac{1}{23} = 130 \text{ ml/hr}$$

This consideration is important for very ill patients receiving triple antibiotic therapy, especially if each drug dose is diluted in 50 to 100 ml of IV fluid.

Monitoring IV flow rate is facilitated by recording the milliliter per hour by hourly increments on each IV container. This information may be recorded on the IV time-tape affixed to the outside of the container.

Flow Rate	Time
0 ml	8 AM start
125	9
250	10
375	11
500	12 PM
625	1
750	2
875	3
1000 ml	4 PM end

Subsequent rate adjustments can be made throughout the IV fluid delivery by observing the desired milliliters to be infused at the scheduled time and adjusting the flow rate.

Drug Dose Calculations—Adult

IV drug dosage may be prescribed in microgram/kilogram/minute (µg/kg/min), milligram/hour, units of drug per hour, or by BSA requirements. Calculations of µg/kg/min include conversion of pounds to kilograms and milligrams to micrograms. Drug units per hour and milligrams per hour are determined by the concentration of a drug in a volume of solution. BSA requirements are calculated via a nomogram. The following formulas and examples describe a step-by-step process for each method.

Microgram/Kilogram/Minute

Convert weight in pounds to kilograms (divide the weight by 2.2):

132 lb ÷ 2.2 = 60 kg

Convert total milligram medication dose to microgram (multiply the milligram by 1000 or move decimal three places to the right)

100 mg × 1000 = 100,000 µg

In most instances a microdrop IV tubing will be used, and 60 microdrops per minute equal 1 milliliter.

Patient—176 pounds   Equation 7

Medication—dopamine 200 mg in 250 ml dilute strength (DS)/0.45 normal saline

Dose—dopamine 5 µg/kg/min

1. Convert 176 pounds to kg

    176 ÷ 2.2 = 80 kg

    Dopamine 200 mg to micrograms

    200 mg × 1000 = 200,000 µg

2. Determine µg/min dose based on kg weight

    5 µg/kg/min × 80 kg = 400 µg/min

3. Determine µg/ml dosage

    200,000 µg : 250 ml = x µg : 1 ml

    $$\frac{200,000}{250} = \frac{x}{1}$$

$$x = \frac{200,000}{250}$$

$x = 800$ μg/ml

4. Determine microdrops per minute

   microdrop tubing 60 mgtt/ml

   800 μg: 60 microdrops = 400 μg/min

   $$\frac{800}{60} = \frac{400}{x} : 800 \; x = 24,000$$

   $$x = \frac{24,000}{800}$$

   $x = 30$ microdrops/min

Milligram/Hour

Drug concentration in milligrams per milliliter will vary according to the dilution factor. Note the concentration milligrams per milliliter of each drug before calculation of flow rate.

Morphine—50 mg in 1000 ml = 1 mg/20 ml   Equation 8

Dose—morphine 4 mg/hr

Infusion set—60 gtt/min

1 mg = 20 ml

4 mg = x ml/hr

$4 \times 20 = 80$

80 ml/hr

$$\frac{60 \text{ microdrops}}{60 \text{ minutes}} \times 80 \text{ ml/hr} = \text{microdrops/min}$$

$$\frac{60}{60} \times 80$$

$1 \times 80 =$

80 microdrops/min

Units of Drug per Hour

Heparin—20,000 units in 500 ml dextrose in water (D/W) Equation 9

Dose—heparin 1000 units/hr

Infusion set—60 gtt/ml

20,000 units heparin ÷ 500 ml infusion

20,000 ÷ = 500 = x units/ml

$$x = \frac{20,000}{500}$$

$x = 40$ units/ml

$$\frac{1000 \text{ units/hour}}{40 \text{ units/ml/solution}}$$

$$\frac{1000}{40} : 1 \times \frac{1000}{40} = x \text{ ml/min}$$

$$\frac{1000}{40} = 25 \text{ ml/hour}$$

$$\frac{60 \text{ microdrops}}{60 \text{ minutes}} \times 25 \text{ ml/hour} = \text{microdrops/min}$$

$$\frac{60}{60} \times \frac{25}{1} = 1 \times 25 = 25 \text{ microdrops/min}$$

BSA Requirements

The dosages of some drugs are calculated proportionally to the BSA of the patient. BSA is calculated in square meters (m^2). A nomogram is used to correlate height (cm/in) with weight (kg/lb) to determine BSA in square meters (m^2). The drug dose is then ordered mg/m^2.

Height—68 inches   Equation 10

Weight—150 pounds

$m^2 = 1.80$ BSA

Dose 75 mg/m^2

$1.80 \times 75 = x$ dose

$x = 135$ mg dose

Drug Dose Calculations—Pediatric

There are several methods for calculating pediatric dosage based on age, weight, or BSA. The usual means of calculating pediatric dosage is the milligrams per kilogram or micrograms per kilogram methods. These methods require conversion of pounds to kilograms before determining the desired dose. Drug literature giving the recommended dose per kilogram or pound of body weight should be consulted before measuring the desired dose.

Milligram/Kilogram Body Weight

Convert weight in pounds to kilograms (divide the weight by 2.2).

Child—22 pounds   Equation 11

Medication—phenytoin 5 mg = 1 kg (child's body weight)

Required dose—mg

1. Convert 22 pounds to kg:

   $22 \div 2.2 = 10$ kg

2. Determine dose based on 1 kg = 5 mg phenytoin (Dilantin)

   1 kg (child) = 5 mg (drug)

   10 kg (child) = x mg (drug)

   10 kg × 5 = 50 mg

   50 mg = drug dose

Microgram/Kilogram Body Weight

Convert weight in pounds to kilograms (divide the weight by 2.2).

Child—33 pounds   Equation 12

Medication—Actinomycin 15 µg = 1 kg (child's body weight)

Required dose————µg

1. Convert 33 pounds to kg:

   $33 \div 2.2 = 15$ kg

2. Determine dose based on 1 kg = 15 µg Actinomycin:

   1 kg (child) = 15 µg (drug)

   15 kg (child = × µg (drug)

   15 kg × 15 µg = 225 µg

   225 µg = drug dose

Other Methods

If the dosage is not given in terms of milligrams per kilogram, then the pediatric dose is calculated from the standard adult dose. These methods are referred to as rules, and the dosage is calculated by weight in pounds, age in months, age in years, or surface area in square meters compared with an adult dose.

Clark's rule (child of 2 years or more)

This method is based on weight in pounds. The adult dose is multiplied by $\dfrac{\text{wt (lb)}}{150\ \text{lb}}$

$$\frac{\text{weight (in pounds)}}{150\ \text{lb}} \times \text{adult dose} = \text{approximate child dose} \quad \text{Equation 13}$$

$$\frac{50\ \text{lb}}{150\ \text{lb}} \times 150\ \text{mg adult dose} = \text{approximate child dose}$$

$$\frac{50}{1} \times \frac{1}{1} = 50\ \text{mg child dose}$$

Fried's rule (infant under 1 year)

This method is based on the age in months. The adult dose is multiplied by the following fraction:

$$\frac{\text{age (in months)}}{150\ \text{months}} \qquad\qquad \text{Equation 14}$$

(150 months is the age of a 12½-year-old child)

$$\frac{\text{age (in months)}}{150\ \text{months}} \times \text{adult dose} = \text{approximate infant dose}$$

$$\frac{9\ \text{months}}{150\ \text{months}} \times 200\ \text{mg} = \text{infant dose}$$

$$\frac{9}{150} \times \frac{200}{1} = \frac{9}{15} \times \frac{20}{1} = \frac{9}{3} \times \frac{4}{1} = \text{infant dose}$$

$$\frac{9}{3} \times \frac{4}{1} = \frac{36}{3} = 12\ \text{mg infant dose}$$

Young's rule (child of 2 years and older)

This method is based on the age in years of the child. The adult dose is multiplied by the following fraction:

$$\frac{\text{age of child in years}}{\text{age in years} + 12} \times \text{adult dose} = \text{approximate child dose}$$

Adult dose of penicillin 500 mg   Equation 15

Child age—8 years

Child dose $= x$ mg

$$\frac{8 \text{ yrs}}{8 \text{ yrs} + 12 \text{ yrs}} \times 500 \text{ mg} = \text{approximate child dose}$$

$$\frac{8}{8 + 12} = \frac{8}{20} = \frac{2}{5}$$

$$\frac{2}{5} \times \frac{500}{1} = \frac{2}{1} \times \frac{100}{1}$$

$$\frac{2}{1} \times \frac{100}{1} = \frac{200}{1} = 200 \text{ mg} = \text{child dose}$$

BSA method

A nomogram is used to correlate the height (cm/in) with the weight (kg/lb) to determine BSA in square meters (m^2). The drug dose is then ordered mg/m^2.

Height—23 inches   Equation 16

Weight—44 pounds

$m^2 = 0.50$ (BSA)

Dose—1 mg/m^2

0.50×1 mg = x dose

$x = 0.50$ mg drug

Other methods using surface area include the following:

$$\frac{\text{Surface area in square meters}}{1.75} \times \text{adult dose} = \text{approximate child dose}$$

$$\frac{\text{Surface area of child}}{\text{Surface area of adult}} \times \text{adult dose} = \text{approximate child dose}$$

Rule of 6 Calculating Intravenous Infusion in a Pediatric Crisis Situation*

The rule of 6 is a simplification of a complicated mathematical equation used to calculate the amount of drug needed to make an infusion. The rule of 6 is as follows:

---

*Consult with a pharmacist or physician regarding calculations, drug concentrations, and compatible IV fluids and solutions. McLeroy PA: Hosp Pharm 29(10): 939, 1994. Reprinted with permission.

6 × weight (wt) in kilograms (kg) = milligrams (mg) of drug to add to 100 ml of IV fluid (IVF). When the fluid is infused at 1 ml/hr, it will deliver drug at the rate of 1 µg/kg/minute.

Desired dose = µg/kg/min   Equation 17

$$= \mu g \times \frac{1\ mg}{1000 \mu g} \times kg \times min \times \frac{1\ hr}{60\ min}$$

$$= 0.06\ mg \times kg \times hr$$

$$\frac{Desired\ dose}{Desired\ rate} = \frac{0.06\ mg \times kg \times hr}{ml/hr}$$ Equation 18

$$\frac{Desired\ dose}{Desired\ rate} = \frac{kg \times 0.06\ mg}{ml} = \frac{mg\ drug}{100\ ml}$$ Equation 19

$$Amount\ of\ drug\ (mg) = \frac{kg \times 0.06\ mg \times 100\ ml}{ml}$$ Equation 20

$$Amount\ of\ drug\ (mg/100\ ml) = kg \times 6$$ Equation 21

The rule of 6 can be used with the following drugs: amrinone, dobutamine, dopamine, nitroglycerin, and nitroprusside. These drugs are dosed in terms of 1 µg/kg per minute or multiples thereof.

When using epinephrine, isoproterenol, norepinephrine, or prostaglandin E_1 multiply by 0.6 instead of 6, because these drugs are dosed in terms of 0.1 µg/kg per minute, because of their potency.

For lidocaine, multiply by 60 instead of 6, because doses are usually started at 20 to 50 µg/kg/min.

Example: A 7 kg infant is in heart failure and requires continuous dobutamine infusion to run at 5 ml/hr to deliver 5 µg/kg per minute. How many milligrams of dobutamine must be added to a 100 ml IVF bag?

Rule of 6: 6 × 7 kg = 42 mg

Therefore, 42 mg of dobutamine is added to 100 ml IVF and 1 ml/hour = 1 µg/kg per minute. Label the bag *dobutamine 42 mg/100 ml/D5W 1 ml/hour = 1 mcg/kg per minute.*

Study Questions

Refer to flow rate and drug dose calculation examples provided earlier in this chapter.

1. Calculate an infusion rate for 1000 ml every 10 hours using a 10 drop/ml infusion set.

   $$\frac{\text{gtt/ml of set}}{60 \text{ min}} \times \text{total hourly volume} = \text{gtts/min}$$

   _____ ml over _____ hours = _____ ml/hr

2. Calculate an infusion rate for 500 ml every 12 hours using a 12 drop/ml infusion set.

   gtt/ml _of set_ $\times$ total hourly volume = gtts/min

   _____ ml over _____ hours = _____ /hr

3. If a medication is to be added to 50 ml normal saline and administered over a 30-minute period, what should the flow rate be set at if a 60 gtt/ml calibration is used?

   $$\frac{50 \text{ ml} \times 60 \text{ gtt}}{30 \text{ minutes}} = \text{flow rate}$$

4. Calculate the flow rate for 250 ml D5W given over 2 hours with a 15 gtt/ml infusion set.

   $$\frac{250 \text{ ml} \times 15 \text{ gtt}}{120 \text{ minutes}} = \text{flow rate}$$

5. You are to administer Ancef 500 mg IV piggyback using a 15 gtt/ml secondary infusion set. If the medication is diluted in 100 ml of D5W, how fast should the drop/minute rate be to administer the medication in 30 minutes?

   _____ ml × _____ gtt = flow rate of _____ minutes

6. Agency standard solution for heparin is 25,000 units in D5W 500 ml. The order is to administer 1000 units per hour. Calculate the infusion rate using a 60 gtt/ml set.

   First calculate the volume of D5W that contains 1000 u using the proportion formula.

   $$\frac{25,000}{500 \text{ ml}} = \frac{1000 \text{ u}}{x}$$

   You must then calculate the flow rate per hour and the drops per minute using the gtt/ml infusion set.

7. The order is to infuse dopamine 200 mg diluted in 250 ml D5W at 5 µg/kg/min. The patient's weight is 132 lb. The infusion set = 60 gtt/ml.
   a. Convert 132 lb to _____ kg.
   b. How many mg of dopamine will each ml contain?
   c. What dose is the patient to receive per minute?
   d. How many gtt/min _____ ? How many ml/hr _____ ?

8. Calculate the body surface area (m²) for an adult 66 inches tall and weighing 200 lb. Then calculate the drug dosage mg/m² (order: cyclophosphamide 650 mg/m²; doxorubicin 50 mg/m²; and 5-fluorouracil 300 mg/m².

   Body Surface Area (BSA): = 2.00 via nomogram

9. Rule of 6: A child weighing 10 kg requires a continuous lidocaine infusion to deliver at the rate of 20 µg/kg per minute. (Rule of six for lidocaine: Multiply by 60 instead of 6, because doses are usually started at 20 µg to 50 µg/kg/min).
   a. _____ kg × 60 = _____ mg/100 ml IV fluid
   b. _____ ml/hr = _____ µg/kg/min

10. Rule of 6: A 7 kg infant is in heart failure and requires a continuous dobutamine infusion to run at 5 ml/hour to deliver 5 µg/kg per minute. How many milligrams of dobutamine must be added to a 100 ml IV fluid bag?
    a. Rule of six: _____ × 7 kg = _____ mg
    b. Therefore, _____ of dobutamine is added to 100 ml IV fluid and _____ ml/hour = _____ µg/kg per minute.

ANSWERS:

1. 1000 ml divided by 10 hours = 100 ml/hr
$$\frac{10 \text{ gtt/ml}}{60 \text{ min}} = \frac{1}{6} \times \frac{100 \text{ ml/hr}}{1} = \frac{1}{6} \times \frac{100}{1} = 16.6 = 17 \text{ gtt/min}$$

2. 500 ml divided by 12 hours = 41.6 = 42 ml/hr
$$\frac{12 \text{ gtt/min}}{60 \text{ min}} = \frac{1}{5} \times \frac{42 \text{ ml/hr}}{1} = \frac{1}{5} \times \frac{42}{1} = 8.3 = 9 \text{ gtts/min}$$

3. $\dfrac{50 \times 60}{30} = \dfrac{3000}{30} = 100$ gtts/min over 30 minutes

4. $\dfrac{250 \times 15}{120} = \dfrac{3750}{120} = 31.25 = 32$ gtt/min over 120 minutes

5. $\dfrac{100 \times 15}{30} = \dfrac{1500}{30} = 50$ gtt/min

6. $\dfrac{25,000 \text{ U}}{500 \text{ ml}} = \dfrac{1000 \text{ U}}{x \text{ ml}}$

   $= 500,000 = 25,000\, x$

   $x = 20$ ml/hr

   $\dfrac{60 \text{ gtt set}}{60 \text{ mins}} = \dfrac{1}{1} \times 20$ ml/hr $= 20$ gtts/min

7. a. $132 \div 2.2 = 60$ kg

   b. $\dfrac{200 \text{ mg}}{250 \text{ ml}} = 0.8$ mg/ml concentration

   0.8 mg $= x$ μg
   $0.8 \times 1000 = 800$ μg/ ml concentration

   c. 5 μg $\times 60$ kg/min
      $= 300$ μg/min

   d. $\dfrac{800 \text{ μg}}{1 \text{ ml}} = \dfrac{300 \text{ μg}}{x \text{ ml}} = \dfrac{0.375 \text{ ml} \times 60 \text{ gtt/ml set}}{1 \text{ minute}}$
   $= 23$ gtt/min $= 23$ ml/hr

8. BSA $= 2.0$
   Cyclophosphamide 650 mg $\times 2 = 1300$ mg
   Doxorubicin   50 mg $\times 2 = 100$ mg
   5-Fluorouracil   300 mg $\times 2 = 600$ mg

9. a. 10 kg $\times 60 = 600$ mg/100 ml IV fluid
   b. 1 ml/hr $= 10$ μg/kg/minute (Therefore, 2 ml/hr would deliver 20 μg/kg/min.)

10. a. 6×7 kg $= 42$ mg
    b. Therefore, 42 mg of dobutamine is added to 100 ml IV fluid and 1 ml/hour $= 1$ μg/kg per minute.

Appendix A
Adult
Infusion
Therapies

Biotherapy Drugs

Anticoagulants

Antifungals

Antimicrobials

Antivirals

Bronchodilators

Hypoglycemic drugs

Immunosuppressants

Cardiovascular drugs

These drug categories have been compiled to enable the nurse to more effectively and efficiently administer specific drug therapies. The drug category is described by action, therapy option, and broad administration guidelines. Refer to Tables A-1 and A-2 for drug, dose, infusion, dilution/concentration, therapeutic monitoring, comments and pertinent side effects and toxicities.

Therapeutic Drug Monitoring: Selected drugs are monitored by serum and urine for the purpose of achieving and maintaining therapeutic drug effect and for preventing drug toxicity. Drug levels are obtained at peak time and trough time after a steady state of the drug has occurred. Selected drug groups listed in Table A-2 include: anticoagulants, antimicrobials, bronchodilators, cardiovascular drugs, hypoglycemic drugs, and immunosuppressants. To effectively conduct therapeutic drug monitoring, the laboratory needs the following information:

Drug name	Daily or intermittent dose
Time and amount of last dose	Time blood sample was drawn

Text continued on p. 411.

Table A-1 Biotherapy drugs

Drug Class	Disease	Route*	Dose (mg/m²)	Major Side Effects Toxicities	Nursing Action
Bacillus Calmette-Guérin (BCG)	Acute leukemia and melanoma (scarification); bladder papillomas	IV Intravesical	Varies	Local pain, swelling, fever, chills	May require self-administration; teach patient/caregiver drug administration techniques.
Epoetin Alfa Epogen (Amgen) Procrit (Ortho Biotech)	Anemia in patients with dialysis-dependent end-stage renal disease; anemia in patients with corticotropin releasing factor (CRF); HIV-zidovudine treated patients; anemia in patients receiving chemotherapy	SQ IV Reconstitute with accompanying diluent; refrigerate	Anemia/CRF/dialysis = 50–100 u/kg 3× weekly; Chemotherapy 15 u/kg 3× weekly	Mild flulike symptoms with arthralgias and myalgias; irritation at the injection (SQ) site; transient rash and urticaria; a rise in BP associated with a rise in hematocrit	May require self-administration; teach patient/caregiver drug administration techniques. *Do not shake* when drug is reconstituted. Dose titration is based on hematocrit levels (i.e., drug dose may be increased/

| | | | | | decreased/ maintained or discontinued). Monitor hematocrit values weekly with initial therapy and on a scheduled frequency thereafter |
| Granulocyte Colony Stimulating Factor (G-CSF) Filgrastim Neupogen (Amgen) | Accelerated recovery from chemotherapy-induced neutropenia (granulocytes); mobilization of stem cells (preautologous BMT); post-allogenic bone marrow transplantation (BMT) | SQ IV over 30 minutes | 5 µg/kg daily until neutrophil counts > 10,000/m³ > 10 µg/kg varied | Myalgias, arthralgias, chills, fever, fatigue, anorexia, headache, rash, fluid retention, bone pain in areas of high bone marrow reserve | Follow recommended reconstitution guidelines (e.g., 5 µg/ml); Do not mix with normal saline or flush IV lines with N/S; use nonfiltered tubing. Refrigerate. *Do not freeze;* avoid shaking vial. Administer drug> 24 hours after last dose of chemotherapy. |

Continued.

*IV, intravenous; IM, intramuscular; SQ, subcutaneous.

Table A-1   Cont'd

Drug Class	Disease	Route*	Dose (mg/m²)	Major Side Effects Toxicities	Nursing Action
Granulocyte Macrophage Colony Stimulating Factor (GM-CSF) Sargramostim Leukine (Immunex)	Accelerated recovery from chemotherapy-induced neutropenia (granulocytes, eosinophils, monocytes); induction chemotherapy (AML); post–autologous transplantation in NHL, ALL, Hodgkin's;	IV Administer over 2 hours; infuse daily for 2–3 weeks; protocol varies	250 µg/m² daily; varies with protocol	Fever, malaise, dose-related fluid retention, myalgias, joint and bone pain, rash. *First-dose phenomenon* in 15%–30% of patients characterized by flushing, tachycardia, hypotension,	Follow reconstitution guidelines. Use only normal saline; final concentration 10 µg/ml. Do not shake after mixing; use nonfiltered tubing. Designate a specific IV line to avoid drug incompatibility. Administer drug

		mobilization of stem cells (preautologous BMT); BMT engraftment failure	dyspnea, vomiting, and syncope	> 24 hours after last dose of chemotherapy and >12 hours after radiotherapy; discontinue if ANC > 20,000 mm^3.
Immunoglobulin (IgG)	IV	Idiopathic thrombocytopenia purpura, aplastic anemia, agammaglobulinemia,	Dose and administration protocols vary with manufacturer	Chills, fever, nausea, myalgias, rash, headache, hypotension, dyspnea, and a	Compatible with D5W only; incompatible with any other drug in syringe

Continued.

Table A-1　Cont'd

Drug Class	Disease	Route*	Dose (mg/m²)	Major Side Effects Toxicities	Nursing Action
	CLL-B cell, allogenic BMT, prophylactic to prevent CMV infections in patients post BMT; pediatric AIDS			sensation of tightness in chest (incidence is related to volume and rate of IVIG infusion). Individuals with IgA deficiency can develop anaphylactic reactions: hypotension, tachycardia, urticaria, edema of eyelids, lips, and tongue; respiratory and gastrointestinal distress.	or solution. Stable for a very short period after reconstitution. Monitor vital signs every 15 minutes for an hour, then every 1–2 hours for the duration of the infusion. Recommended infusion rates: *Gamimune* (Miles): 0.01–0.02 ml/kg initial 30 minutes; increase to maximum of 0.08 ml/kg/min.

Gammagard
(Baxter): 0.5 ml/
kg; increase to
maximum of 4
mg/kg/hr.
Gammar (Armour):
0.01 ml/kg/hr;
increase to 0.2
ml/kg/min after
15 to 30 minutes.
Iveegam (Immuno-
US): 1 ml/min.
up to 2 ml/min.
Sandoglobulin
(Sandoz): 0.5–1
ml/min (10–15
drops); increase
after 15 to 30
minutes to
1.5–2.5 ml/min
(30–50 drops)
Venoglobulin (Al-
pha Thera-
peutic): 0.01–
0.02 ml/kg/min
for first 30
minutes.

Continued.

Table A-1   Cont'd

Drug Class	Disease	Route*	Dose (mg/m²)	Major Side Effects Toxicities	Nursing Action
Interferon Alfa-2A, Interferon Alfa-2B Roferon-A (Roche) Intron A (Schering)	Antiviral and anti-tumor activity; hair cell leukemia, renal cell cancer, Kaposi's sarcoma, venereal warts; hepatitis C and B	IM SQ IV	1–3 million IU varies with disease protocol	Flulike syndrome, myalgias, arthralgias, headache, fatigue, chills, taste changes, rash, alopecia, hypersensitivity, hypotension, tachycardia, chest pain, dizziness, temporary impotence.	Follow reconstitution guidelines; store in refrigerator. Symptoms of infection may be masked by side effects of drug; teach patient/caregiver to report sore throat, fever, diarrhea, vomiting.
Interleukin-2 (IL-2) Proleukin (Chiron)	Metastatic renal cell carcinoma; melanoma; produces "killer" lymphocytes	IV	600,000 IU/kg every 8 hours; 14 total doses	Dose dependent: fever, chills, anemia, skin changes, fatigue, diarrhea, nausea and vomit-	*Monitor side effects:* Follow guidelines for reconstitution, filtration and

Drug	Action/Use	Route	Dose	Side Effects	Nursing Considerations
				ing, anorexia, pulmonary dyspnea/congestion, hypotension, tachycardia, oliguria/anuria, lethargy, hallucinations, restlessness, headache, blurred vision, myalgia, stomatitis, myelosuppression.	evaluation of compatability with concomitant medications such as steroids, vasopressors, colloid and crystalloid solutions (5% plasma protein), diuretics, antiemetics, sedatives, and antidiarrhea drugs.
Interleukin-3 (Sandoz, Immunex, Hoechst, Behringwerke)†	Bone marrow suppression associated with chemotherapy, tumor infiltration, myelodysplasia, or aplastic anemia; stimulates the	IV SQ	Varies; µg/kg	Dose and route dependent: Flu-like syndrome, headache, fever, fatigue, lethargy, dyspnea, myalgias, erythema at the injection site,	Follow reconstitution guidelines. Teach patient/caregiver drug administration techniques and side effects to monitor.

Continued.

†Investigational Agents.

Table A-1   Cont'd

Drug Class	Disease	Route*	Dose (mg/m²)	Major Side Effects Toxicities	Nursing Action
	leukocyte count with variable effects on platelets and reticulocytes		rash, urticaria, nausea, and vomiting.		
Interleukin-6 (Sandoz, Serono)†	Myelosuppressive chemotherapy regimens; regulates the immune response by stimulating both B and T lymphocytes	IV SQ	Varies; µg/kg	Flu-like syndrome, fever, chills, headache, nausea & vomiting, anorexia, transient mild increases in alkaline phosphatase, transaminases, creatinine, and fasting glucose.	Follow reconstitution guidelines. Drug may be administered in combination with other colony-stimulating-factors. Monitor side effects.

Drug	Action	Route	Dose	Side Effects	Nursing Considerations
Interleukin-11 (Genetics Institute)†	Promotes production of platelets	SQ	75 µg/kg	Mild fatigue, myalgias and arthralgias, fluid retention	Follow reconstitution guidelines and dose escalation titrations.
PIXY-321 (GM-CSF + Interleukin-3) (Immunex)†	Myelosuppressive chemotherapy regimens; promotes recovery of granulocytes and platelets	SQ IV	500–750 µg/m2	Headache, myalgia, malaise, bone pain, fever, nausea, fatigue, local skin reactions at the injection site	Follow reconstitution guidelines; monitor side effects.

†Investigational Agents.

Table A-2 Adult Intravenous Infusion Therapies

Drug	Dose:	Infusion	Dilution/ Concentration	Therapeutic Monitoring	Comments
Anticoagulant Heparin	IV bolus dose is based on u/kg (e.g., DVT/PE 85 u/kg; others 70 u/kg rounded to nearest 100 u) Increase by infusion aPTT= ≤47/200u/h	Continuous infusion regulated by a aPTT, PT, (e.g., 20 u/kg; round to nearest 50 u/hr); (aPTT = >47/200 u/hr;	Dilute in 0.9% N/S, D5W, Ringer's solution; heparin units/ml/hr; titrate to aPTT, PT; via IV pump.	CBC, aPTT, PT initial; aPTT at 8 hours after infusion; then frequency based on aPTT and heparin infusion	Incompatible with amikacin, ampicillin, atropine, codeine, dacarbazine, daunorubicin, diazapam, dobutamine, and multiple antimicrobials. Monitor aPTT, PT with heparin infusion, BP, P; do not administer concomitantly with IV nitroglycerine. Avoid IM injection.

Antifungal Drugs				
Amphotericin B	0.1 mg/ml, over 2–4 hours and/or 0.25 mg/kg/day; may increase up to 1 mg/kg/day; not to exceed 1.5 mg/kg	Test dose 1 mg/20 ml D5W given over 10 to 30 minutes; continuous infusion; titrate infusion reside effects	Use 1 mg/250 mg D5W (0.1 mg/ml)/ may dilute 50 mg/10 ml N/S then dilute with 500 ml of solution to conc. 0.1 mg/ml.	Peaks 1–2 hours	Incompatible with multiple medications. Avoid concurrent blood administration. Use in-line filter; monitor BP, P, R, T Q15 min × 2, then Q2–4hr. Premedicate with antipyretics. Obtain accurate intake and output and daily/weekly weights. Monitor for fever/chills.
Fluconazole	50–400 mg initially, then 200 mg daily for 4 weeks	Infuse at 200 mg/hr or less; do not use plastic containers in connections	Follow manufacturer's guidelines.	Administer drug only after C & S confirms organism	Monitor BP, P, R, T Q15 min × 2 then Q4hr. Assess intake and output and weigh daily to weekly. *Incompatible with other drugs in solution or*

Continued.

Table A-2   Cont'd

Drug	Dose	Infusion	Dilution/ Concentration	Therapeutic Monitoring	Comments
					syringe. Potentiates anticoagulation (warfarin); increases renal dysfunction-cyclosporine.
Antimicrobial Drugs Amikacin	15 mg/kg/day in 2–3 divided doses	Over 30–60 minutes; not to exceed 1.5 g	Use 100–200 ml D5W.	Peak 20–30 µg/ml after 30 minute infusion; trough 4–8 µg/ml immediately before the next dose	Monitor side effects: GU—oliguria, hematuria, azotemia, nephrotoxicity; EENT—Ototoxicity; leukopenia; nausea and vomiting, neurotoxicity.

Drug	Dose	Infusion	Reconstitution	Peak	Notes
Aztreonam	1–2 g in 2–3 divided doses	Intermittent infusion, 30–60 mins	Follow manufacturer's reconstitution guidelines.	IV peak immediate; trough 8 hours later	Incompatible with nafcillin, metronidazole, cephradine. Continue Aztreonam treatment for 48 hours after negative culture or until patient is asymptomatic. Monitor myelosuppression, neurotoxicity, liver enzymes.
Ceftazidime (Fortaz)	1 g Q8–12 hr for 5–10 days	1 g/10 ml sterile water, then into 50–100 N/S over 30–60 mins via y-site	Use 1 g/10 ml sterile water, then 50/100 ml N/S.	Peaks 1 hour	Incompatible with aminoglycosides. Monitor nephrotoxicity, intake and output, myelosuppression; lab studies: BUN, ALT, AST, CBC, LDH, Bilirubin; Irritant: phlebitis or extravasation.

Continued.

Table A-2   Cont'd

Drug	Dose	Infusion	Dilution/ Concentration	Therapeutic Monitoring	Comments
Gentamicin	3–5 mg/kg per day, in 3 doses	Intermittent over 30 minutes to 120 minutes	Dilute in 50–200 ml N/S or D5W.	Peak 4–10 μg/ml after 30 minute infusion; trough 4–8 μg/ml immediately before the next dose	Increased ototoxicity, neurotoxicity, nephrotoxicity with other aminoglycosides, amphotericin, chemotherapy. Incompatible with many medications; monitor nephrotoxicity, ototoxicity, myelosuppression.
Imipenem-Cylastatin	250–500 mg Q8 hr; 1 g for severe infection	Intermittent 30 to 60 minutes	Dilute into 100 ml N/S or D5W.	Peak 30–60 minutes	Potential for anaphylaxis; *incompatible* with aminoglycosides in solution or syringe.

Drug	Dosage	Administration	IV/Diluent	Peak	Nursing considerations
Piperacillin	100–300 mg/kg day in divided doses Q4–6hr	Intermittent 1 g/5 ml over 3–5 minutes; 50 to 100 ml over 30 minutes	Use 1 g/3–5 ml IVP 3–5 min N/S or D5W 50–100 ml.	Peaks 30 minutes	Monitor GI (diarrhea), CNS (somnolence), neutropenia, elevated AST, ALT, LDH, and BUN laboratory tests. Incompatible with aminoglycosides, amphotericin B. Monitor nephrotoxicity, myelosuppression, nausea, vomiting, diarrhea.
Tobramycin	3–5 mg/kg/day in divided doses Q6–8 hr	Intermittent 30–60 minutes	Use 50–100 ml N/S or D5W.	Peak 4–10 µg/ml after 30 minute infusion; trough 0.5–2.0 µg/ml, immediately before next dose	Weigh before treatment: calculation of dosage is based on ideal body weight. Monitor intake and output, BP, P, T, R on a scheduled frequency. Increased ototoxicity, neu-

Continued.

Table A-2   Cont'd

Drug	Dose	Infusion	Dilution/ Concentration	Therapeutic Monitoring	Comments
					rotoxicity, and nephrotoxicity with other aminoglycosides; *incompatible* with heparin.
Vancomycin	500 mg Q6hr to 1 g Q12hr	Intermittent over 60 minutes	Use 500 mg/100 ml N/S or D5W.	Peak 20–40 μg/ml after 1–2 hr infusion; trough 5–10 μg/ml immediately before next dose	Anaphylaxis, nephrotoxicity, ototoxicity, myelosuppression; side effects are increased with aminoglycosides and cephalosporins, amphotericin B. *Incompatible* with multiple medications; Monitor intake and output, BP, P, T, R; Redman's syndrome.

Antivirals			
Acyclovir	5 mg/kg over 1 hr, Q8hr	Intermittent; infuse via IV pump; increase fluids to 3 l/day	Reconstitute with 10 ml compatible solution/500 mg of drug; concentration 50 mg/ml. Use within 12 hours; store at room temperature.	Peak 1 hour; half-life 20–180 minutes	*Incompatible* with dobutamine, dopamine, all protein and blood products. Monitor myelosuppression, nephrotoxicity, lab studies (CBC, AST, ALT, BUN, CrCL). Increased neuro-nephrotoxicity with aminoglycosides, amphotericin, methotrexate; ensure IV hydration.
Foscarnet	Initial: 60 mg/kg over 1 hour Q8hr × 2–3 weeks, then 90–120 mg/kg/day over 2 hours	Intermittent Q8hr over 1–2 hour infusion times. Use infusion device; no more than 1 mg/kg/min via central	Use concentration 12 mg/ml with N/S or D5W if using peripheral vein; 24 mg/ml if using central venous access.	Half-life 2–8 hours	Increased nephrotoxicity with aminoglycosides, amphotericin B, IV petamidine. Monitor neurotoxicity,

Continued.

Table A-2   Cont'd

Drug	Dose	Infusion	Dilution/ Concentration	Therapeutic Monitoring	Comments
		venous access; *do not give IV bolus*			myelosuppression, esophageal ulceration, nephrotoxicity, bronchospasm. Increase IV fluids before and during drug administration. Assess BUN, AST.
Ganciclovir	5 mg/kg over 1 hour daily × 7 days	Intermittent over 1 hour; *do not give IV bolus*	Reconstitute 500 mg in 10 ml; further dilute in 100 ml D5W, N/S, LR. Use solution within 24 hours.	Half-life 3–4 hours	Incompatible with other drugs in syringe or solution. Drug is mutagenic; use chemotherapy precautions. Severe granulocytopenia with zidovudine.

					Monitor neurotoxicity, GI and GU hemorrhage, myelosuppression.
Bronchodilators Aminophylline	0.3–0.9 mg/kg/hr maintenance dosing	Continuous infusion; titrate dose (CI)	Dilute in compatible solution; D5W mg/ml.	10–20 µg/ml; obtain serum level 24 hrs after starting CI and immediately before next dose CI	Hypersensitivity to xanthines; incompatible with multiple medications; Monitor CNS side effects; ensure precautions with elderly population. May increase effects of anticoagulants; monitor respiratory status for duration of drug infusion.

Continued.

Table A-2   Cont'd

Drug	Dose	Infusion	Dilution/ Concentration	Therapeutic Monitoring	Comments
Hypoglycemic Drugs Insulin—regular	2–12 u IV (50–100 ml/NS) IDDM, KETOACIDOSIS	Continuous infusion via IV pump; decrease rate when serum glucose is 250 mg/ml	Dilute in 0.9% N/S or 0.45 saline for IV infusion.	Serum glucose levels monitored at least Q1hr for the duration of IV insulin therapy	Ensure accurate monitoring of insulin IV dose hourly correlated with serum glucose levels; incompatible with aminophilline, heparin, dopamine. Monitor CNS, anaphylaxis, GI side effects.
Immunosuppressant Antithymocyte Globulin (Atgam) (ATG)	10–15 mg/kg daily for 14 days; then QOD for 7–14 days	Intradermal skin test before drug administration; infuse over > 4 hours	Reconstitute with N/S; refrigerate after reconstitution. Use in-line filtered tubing.	Not applicable	Incompatible with all drugs in solution or syringe. Monitor skin test dose

site: if a local reaction (wheal, erythema, itching, edema), notify physician. Monitor for anaphylaxis, myelosuppression, fever, chills, phlebitis at IV site.

Drug	Dose	Administration	Special Considerations
Cyclosporine (CyA)	5–15 mg/kg/day	BMT: continuous infusion Q12hr daily; other protocols: 2–6 hour infusions daily	Dilute 50 mg/20–100 ml N/S. Use a glass bottle and compatible tubing.	Obtain CYA level from a separate IV access than drug administration; obtain trough 12 hrs after CYA is infused daily.

Do not mix with other drugs in same bottle. May be infused through TPN/lipid line. Monitor nephrotoxicity, hepatotoxicity, neurotoxicity, hypertension. Vital signs Q15 min ×4; then Q2–4 hr. Ensure accurate serum trough levels, accurate intake and output, weight.

Continued.

Table A-2 Cont'd

Drug	Dose	Infusion	Dilution/ Concentration	Therapeutic Monitoring	Comments
Azathioprine (Imuran)	3–5 mg/kg/day	Intermittent over 30 mins	Dilute with N/S or D5W in 50–100 ml solution	Not applicable	Do not mix with other drugs in same solution container; monitor for hepatotoxicity, myelosuppression.
Muromonab CD3 (Orthoclone OKT3)	5 mg IV bolus Qd × 10–14 days	Use a 0.22 micron filter needle to withdraw medication into the syringe; administer drug IV bolus over 1 min without the filter	Follow the manufacturer's guidelines for drug reconstitution.	Serum values are obtained on a scheduled basis for the duration of therapy.	Cyclosporine is discontinued the day OKT3 is initiated. Monitor pulmonary edema; patient must have a clear chest x-ray within 24 hours of drug therapy. Weight gain is limited to <3%; premedicate prior to drug administration.

Select Cardiovascular Drugs

Antiarrhythmia drugs, antihypertensives, diuretics, beta blockers, and channel blockers

Drug	Dosage	Preparation	Pharmacokinetics	Nursing Considerations
Adenosine (antiarrhythmia)	IV bolus 6 mg; may give 12 mg IV bolus × 2	Follow manufacturer's guidelines.	Half-life 30 seconds	*Contraindications:* second or third degree heart block, AV block, atrial flutter/ventricular tachycardia, atrial fibrillation, ventricular tachycardia. Monitor BP continuously for fluctuations or EKG changes.
Amrinone (Inocor) (cardiac inotropic)	IV bolus 0.75 mg/kg given over 2–3 min; then infusion 5–10 μg/kg/min	Follow manufacturer's guidelines; do not mix with glucose directly.	Onset 2–5 minutes; peak 10 minutes; half-life 4–6 hours	IV bolus then IV infusion via IV pump. Incompatible with furosemide and dextrose solution for direct dilution; monitor BP, P, Q5min during

Continued.

Table A-2   Cont'd

Drug	Dose	Infusion	Dilution/ Concentration	Therapeutic Monitoring	Comments
					the drug infusion. Monitor cardiac glycosides, ALT, AST, bilirubin daily.
Atropine (antiarrhythmia and bradycardia)	IV bolus 0.5–1 mg every 3–5 minutes. Dose not to exceed 2 mg.	IV bolus	May administer undiluted in urgent need; may dilute in 10 ml N/S at rate of 0.5 mg/min.	IV peak 2–4 minutes; half-life 2–3 hours	Incompatible with multiple medications. Evaluate therapeutic effects; monitor vital signs, cardiac status, and rhythm continuously during IV dosing.
Bretylium Tosylate (antiarrhythmia agent for ventricular fibrillation, ventricular tachycardia)	Initial dose 5–10 mg/kg up to 30 mg/kg; continuous IV infusion 1–4 mg/min (1 g/250 ml)	IV bolus over 10 minutes; repeat as needed 15–30 min up to 30 mg/kg. If continuous infusion use IV pump.	Dilute 500 mg in 50 ml N/S or D5W. Infuse over 10–30 minutes. Continuous infusion: dilute 1 g/250 ml; infuse 1–4 mg/min.	Onset 5 minutes	Monitor cardiac status/rhythm and vital signs continuously during drug dosing. Drug may cause severe nausea and vomiting,

Drug	Dose	Route	Dilution	Onset/Peak	Considerations
Digoxin (antiarrhythmia)	IV bolus 0.5 mg over 5 minutes	IV bolus	Use in IV undiluted or 1 mg of drug in 4 ml N/S or D5W.	Onset 5–30 minutes 0.8–2.0 ng/ml immediately before next dose every 7 days	respiratory depression, rebound hypertension after 1–2 hours. Assess apical pulse for 1 minute before drug administration. Monitor CNS (headache); GI (nausea and vomiting, anorexia, diarrhea); EENT (blurred vision, diplopia, and muscle weakness); intake and output, daily weights, and therapeutic drug level.
Dobutamine HCL (vasopressor)	Infusion 2.5–10 µg/kg/min up to 40 µg/kg/min	Continuous infusion via IV pump	Dilute 250 mg/10 ml of D5W or N/S, then further dilute in 50 ml or more. Titrate dose.	Onset 1–5 minutes; peak 10 minutes.	Incompatible with acyclovir, amphotericin B, cephalothin, gentamicin, sodium bicarbonate.

Continued.

Table A-2   Cont'd

Drug	Dose	Infusion	Dilution/ Concentration	Therapeutic Monitoring	Comments
					Monitor vital signs, cardiac status/rhythm continuously during drug infusion. Evaluate therapeutic response.
Dopamine HCL (vasopressor)	Begin infusion at 10 μg/kg/min for severe hypotension or 0.5–2 μg for renal perfusion	Continuous infusion via IV pump	Use N/S, D5W, LR2 g in 500 ml solution for 4 mg/ml.	Onset 5 minutes; duration < 10 minutes	Incompatible with acyclovir, amphotericin, cephalothin, gentamicin, sodium bicarbonate. Monitor vital, cardiac status/rhythm Q5min during initial infusion; thereafter, on a scheduled fre-

Drug	Dose	Administration	Onset/Duration	Dilution	Nursing Considerations
Esmolol HCL Brevibloc (beta adrenergic blocker)	IV loading dose 500 μg/kg/min for 1 min; maintenance 50 μg/kg for 4 minutes. Increase maintenance infusion by 50 μg/kg/min.; maximum 200 μg/kg/min; titrate to patient response	Continuous infusion via IV pump	Onset—rapid; duration—short; half-life 9 minutes	Dilute 5 g/20 ml, then dilute in the remaining 480 ml of N/S, D5W, D5R; D5NS, 0.45% NaCL.	quency. Evaluate therapeutic response. Monitor CVP initial infusion. Incompatible with furosemide, sodium bicarbonate. Do not mix with any drug before full dilution. Monitor vital signs, continuously on initial dosing then on a scheduled frequency. Monitor respiratory status, hypotension, intake and output. Evaluate therapeutic outcome.
Isoproterenol HCL (Isuprel) (antiarrhythmia)	IV 0.02–0.06 or 5 μg/min	5–10 μg continuous infusion via IV pump	Onset rapid; duration ~ 10 minutes	Infuse 1 mg/250 ml D5W.	Incompatible with aminophylline, barbiturates,

Continued.

Table A-2   Cont'd

406   Pocket Guide to Intravenous Therapy

Drug	Dose	Infusion	Dilution/Concentration	Therapeutic Monitoring	Comments
					carbenicillin, epinephrine, lidocaine, and sodium bicarbonate. Monitor BP, P, R continuously; monitor for cardiac arrest, bronchospasms.
Lidocaine (antiarrhythmia)	Initial dose 1–1.5 mg/kg; then 0.5 mg/kg to maximum 3 mg/kg	Continuous infusion 2–4 mg/min via IV pump	2 g/500 ml D5W = 4 mg/ml 1 g 500 ml D5W = 2 mg/ml 2 g/250 ml D5W = 8 mg/ml concentration	Onset 2 minutes; duration 20 minutes 6–12 hours after starting continuous IV infusion; 1.5–5 μg/ml	Monitor ECG and BP continuously for fluctuations. Incompatible with ampicillin, cefazolin, phenytoin, and blood. Evaluate therapeutic response; monitor intake and output, respiratory depression and cardiovascular response

Drug	Dosage	Administration	Dilution	Onset	Nursing considerations
Mannitol (osmotic diuretic)	IV 300–400 mg/kg of 20%–25% solution up to 100 g of a 15%–20% solution for oliguria; IV 1.5–2 g/kg of 15%–25% solution over 30–60 min for intracranial pressure; 50–200 g/24 hr for renal failure to maintain output 30–50 ml/hr	IV 15%–25% solution with filter over 30–90 minutes; *test dose in severe oliguria;* 0.2 g/kg over 3–5 min; may repeat ×2; if no urine response, reassess patient	Follow manufacturer's guidelines.	Onset 30–60 minutes for diuresis; 30–90 minutes for intraocular pressure	Incompatible with whole blood, potassium, and sodium chloride. Monitor CNS status, vital signs, intake and output. Evaluate therapeutic response.
Nitroglycerin (vasodilator)	IV 5 µg/min; then increase by 5 µg/min Q3–5 min; if no response after 20 µg/min, increase by 10/20 µg/min until desired response	Continuous infusion via IV pump; use glass bottle and non-PVC tubing; no filters	50 mg/250 ml D5W = 0.2 mg/ml concentration; 50 mg/500 ml D5W = 0.1 mg/ml concentration; 100 mg/250 ml = 0.4 mg/ml.	Onset—immediate	Incompatible with any drug in solution or syringe; monitor vital signs continuously during initial dosing, then as scheduled. Assess cardiovascular and CNS status.

Continued.

Table A-2 Cont'd

Drug	Dose	Infusion	Dilution/ Concentration	Therapeutic Monitoring	Comments
Nitroprusside (antihypertensive)	5–8 µg/kg min IV continuously	Continuous IV via IV pump	Dissolve 50 mg in 2–3 ml of D5W; then dilute in 250–1000 ml D5W.	Onset 1–2 minutes; duration 1–10 minutes; half-life 4 days	Incompatible with any drug in solution or syringe. Monitor vital signs, BP, P Q5–15min. Assess intake and output, daily weight, electrolytes. Evaluate therapeutic response.
Procainamide (Pronestyl) (antiarrhythmia)	IV bolus 100 mg Q5min given 20–50 mg/min; not to exceed 500 mg; then IV infusion	Continuous IV infusion via IV pump 2–6 mg/min	Dilute 100 mg/ml D5W; give 20 mg or less for 1 minute; Dilute 1 g in 250–500 ml D5W, run at 2–6 mg/minute; Half-life 3 hours 16–24 hours after starting continuous IV infusion, at 4–8 µg/ml		Monitor vital signs, BP, P continuously for fluctuations; monitor ECG to determine increased PR or QRS segments. If these develop, discontinue drug

Propranolol HCL (Inderal) (antihypertensive)	IV bolus 0.5–3 mg over 1 mg/min; may repeat in 2 minutes for dysrhythmia	Bolus and/or short term (10–15 minutes) only	Dilute drug in 50 ml N/S and infuse 1 mg over 10–15 minutes.	Onset 2 minutes; peak 15 minutes; duration 3–6 hours; half-life 3–5 hours	immediately. Monitor intake and output and electrolytes; potential for heart block, cardiac arrest. Incompatible with any drug in solution or syringe. Monitor vital signs, BP, P continuously during IV dosing. Assess intake and output, ECG, daily weight; watch for hypotension and bronchospasm. Evaluate therapeutic response.
Quinidine (antiarrhythmia)	IV infusion 800 mg in 40 ml D5W run at 16 mg/min	Continuous infusion via IV pump	Dilute 800 mg into 40 ml or more D5W; give 16 mg or less over 1 minute as infusion.	Immediately before next dose, 2–5 μg/ml	Considered incompatible with any drug in solution or syringe. Monitor vital signs, BP, P continu-

Continued.

Table A-2 Cont'd

Drug	Dose	Infusion	Dilution/ Concentration	Therapeutic Monitoring	Comments
					ously for fluctuations; watch ECG to determine increased PR or QRS complex. If these develop, discontinue or reduce drug dose. Evaluate therapeutic response.
Verapamil HCL (calcium channel blocker)	IV bolus 5–10 mg over 2 minutes; repeat if necessary in 30 minutes	IV bolus only	Follow manufacturer's guidelines.	Onset 3–5 minutes; peak 3–5 minutes; duration 10–20 minutes	Incompatible with albumin, amphotericin, ampicillin, dobutamine, hydralazine, mezlocillin, nafcillin, oxacillin, and sodium bicarbonate. Monitor cardiac status BP, P, ECG; evaluate therapeutic response.

Drug name	Daily or intermittent dose
Route of drug administration	Patient age

Patient diagnosis—pertinent to multiple drug therapies (e.g., anticoagulants).

Biotherapy Drugs

These drugs augment, modulate, or restore the host's immunologic defense mechanism. Their antitumor activity (cytotoxic and antiproliferative) affects differentiation or maturation of cells and interferes with the ability of the tumor to metastasize. Biotherapy drugs may be given in combination with surgery, chemotherapy, radiation therapy, or bone marrow and solid organ transplantation or may be given as a single agent. They are being used extensively in bone marrow and organ transplant protocols to decrease the intensity and duration of the nadir and thereby enhance the patient's recovery process. Additional pertinent uses of the colony-stimulating factors is to stimulate stem cells to appear in the peripheral blood. These stem cells are then harvested via apheresis and used in peripheral blood stem cell transplantation.

Anticoagulant Drugs

Anticoagulants alter the patient's coagulation status by preventing conversion of fibrinogen to fibrin and prothrombin to thrombin and by enhancing inhibitory effects of antithrombin III. These drugs are given for varied medical conditions—deep vein thrombosis, pulmonary emboli, and disseminated intravascular clotting syndrome—and as an anticoagulant in open heart surgery, transfusion, and dialysis procedures.

Antifungals

Antifungal drugs increase cell membrane permeability in susceptible organisms by binding sterols. Fungal infections such as candidiasis, cryptococcosis, histoplasmosis, and aspergillosis are treated with antifungal agents.

Antimicrobials

Antimicrobial drugs interfere with or inhibit microbial cell wall synthesis, which renders the cell osmotically unstable. Multiple drug therapies may be selected for the varied medical diagnoses. Safe antimicrobial administration includes following the manufacturer's reconstitution guidelines, knowing specific drug incompatibilities, observing and reporting side effects, following therapeutic drug monitoring techniques, and administering the drug in a timely and cost-effective manner.

Antivirals

Antiviral drugs interfere with DNA synthesis needed for viral replication. These drugs are used most often for the immunocompromised person for treatment of herpes simplex and cytomegalovirus. These drugs have significant toxicities, dosing guidelines, and hydration requirements.

Bronchodilators

These drugs relax the smooth muscles of the respiratory system by blocking phosphodiesterase, which increased cyclic AMP. These drugs are used to treat respiratory diseases such as bronchial asthma and bronchospasm. Ensure therapeutic drug infusion, monitoring, and observe the patient for potential CNS side effects.

Hypoglycemic Drugs

Hypoglycemic drugs decrease blood sugar and should be adjusted by monitoring blood glucose levels on a scheduled frequency. Ensure that patient assessment includes blood glucose levels, vital signs, level of consciousness, and intake and output with intravenous insulin dosing.

Immunosuppressants

Pharmacological immunosuppressants inhibit the T-lymphocytes (responsible for tissue or organ graft rejection and graft-versus-host-disease) and are used in multiple immunosuppression regimens. Patients receiving solid organ transplantation or donor bone marrow transplantation receive these drugs over extended periods of time. Follow drug dose preparation and administration guidelines, and monitor the side effects and toxicities.

Cardiovascular Drugs

- *Antiarrhythmias:* slow conduction through the AV node, can interrupt reentry pathways through the AV node; decrease rise of depolarization phase of action potential
- *Antihypertensives:* directly relax arteriolar and venous smooth muscle, resulting in reduction in cardiac preload and afterload
- *Beta blockers:* block stimulation of beta adrenergic receptors in the myocardium (which decreases the rate of SA node discharge, slows conduction of the AV node, and decreases O_2 consumption in the myocardium); reduce cerebral flow and cerebral perfusion
- *Calcium channel blockers:* inhibit calcium ion influx across cell membrane during cardiac depolarization, produce relaxation of coronary vascular smooth muscle, dilate coronary arteries

- *Osmotic diuretics:* act by increasing osmolarity of glomerular filtrate, which raises osmotic pressure of fluid in renal tubules; decrease reabsorption of water electrolytes; increase urinary output and sodium and chloride excretion
- *Vasodilators:* decrease preload and afterload, which is responsible for decreasing left ventricular end-diastolic pressure, systemic vascular resistance
- *Vasopressors:* cause increased contractility and increased coronary blood flow and heart rate by acting on beta receptors in the heart

Adult Intravenous Infusion Therapies Guidelines

Consult with the physician, pharmacist, or agency or institution guidelines for drug administration protocols (infusion, solution, dilution/concentration, dosing amounts and frequency, and patient monitoring requirements). The patients' medical diagnosis may require staff competency in advanced drug administration requirements (including staff ACLS certification), intensive care patient status, and continual ECG monitoring of the patient during drug dosing/infusion.

Appendix B
Use of Nursing Diagnoses with Sample Charting

P-Problem   I-Intervention   E-Evaluation of outcome

Topics			Notes
Infusion guidelines			

Date 10/96	Time 0900	P	Fluid volume deficit, related to nothing by mouth, postoperative day (3) following right colectomy, manifested by thirst and dry mucous membranes.
		I	1000 ml D5 0.45 N/S with 40 mEq KCL at 125 ml/hr using macrodrop tubing initiated. Insertion site right cephalic vein without redness or discomfort; sterile dressing in place.
	1100	E	Urine volume from 0700 to 1100 is 250 ml. Thirst diminished, mucous membranes pink and sticky. IV fluids continue at 125 ml/hr.
	1500	E	Urine volume from 1100 to 1500 is 1050 ml. Physician notified of increased urinary output. Mucous membranes pink and moist, skin warm and dry to touch.

Topics			Notes

Venipuncture

Dates 10/96	Time 0830	P	Anxiety, related to invasive procedure, as manifested by, "This is the first time I've had an IV and I'm nervous."
		I	Explained the procedure to the patient. Coached in deep breathing exercise and instructed to focus attention on the picture on center wall during venipuncture.
			Peripheral IV site established in right cephalic vein using 20-gauge 1½ inch angiocath. Sterile technique used and catheter secured according to policy. 1000 ml D5 0.45 N/S with 40 mEq KCL infusion at 125 ml/hr.
		E	IV infusing at desired rate. Appears calm and at ease postprocedure. "The IV start was not as bad as I thought it would be."

(Nurse's name)

Central venous catheters

Dates 10/96	Time 1000	P	Skin integrity, impaired; infection, risk for, access of Port-A-Cath.
		I	Access of Port-A-Cath, sterile technique used. Huber needle 19-gauge, 1½-inch, 90-degree inserted, good blood return, flushed with 10 ml N/S, then connected to 1000 ml D5 N/S at 125 ml/hr.
		E	Transparent dressing intact over needle site. Placement site without redness and tenderness. IV fluids infusing at 125 mg/hr.
		P	Injury, risk for, related to catheter potential occlusion, after IV infusion.

Topics			Notes
		I	IV fluids discontinued. Port-A-Cath system flushed with 10 ml N/S, then heparin 5 ml (100 u/ml) as needle was removed from the portal septum leaving a heparin lock.
		E	Port-A-Cath access site intact. Skin without redness or oozing.
			(Nurse's name)

IV fluids

Date 10/96	Time 1530	P	Fluid volume deficit, risk for, related to excessive fluid loss from surgical procedure (right colectomy) and previous NPO status.
		I	IV fluids 1000 ml D5 0.45 N/S with 40 mEq increased to 120 ml/hr. Clear oral fluids provided.
		E	Insertion site without redness. No complaints of discomfort at IV site or right arm. States is less thirsty this afternoon. Breath sounds clear in both lung bases.
			(Nurse's name)

IV medication administration

Date 10/96	Time 1300	P	Injury, risk for, related to positive venogram of right leg.
		I	Discontinued D5 0.45 N/S IV solution, 600 ml infused. Initiated heparin infusion (25,000 U/500 ml) at rate of 750 U/hr. Placed on infusion pump at rate of 15 ml/hr.
		E	IV site 12 hours old and no erythema or edema noted. Right leg warm and dry to touch, red area 4 cm in diameter noted in midcalf area.
			(Nurse's name)

Topics			Notes

Blood administration

Date 10/96	Time 1000	P	Injury, risk for, related to altered clotting mechanism, manifested by nose bleed; platelet count 50,000 mm^3. BP 112/72, P 108, R 20, T 98.4 as baseline vital signs.
		E	10 units pooled random platelets initiated. (ID #02G54496, O positive) via Y-set IV tubing with 100 ml normal saline bag for flushing of multilumen subclavian catheter. ID numbers on donor unit and patient bracelet verified by Nurse, RN and Nurse, RN.
		E	No active bleeding at this time from central line exit site: nose bleed diminished; 2 cm diameter pinkish red fluid on tissue. BP 114/76, P 112, R 18, T 98. No complaints of discomfort, e.g., shortness of breath, chills, or urticaria. Urine clear.
	1100	E	Bleeding from nose has ceased; BP 116/80, P 116, R 20, T 98.2 Platelet transfusion is completed. Time, date, ID number, and signature completed on transfusion record and record returned to blood bank. Postplatelet count ordered for 1200.
		P	Injury, risk for, related to catheter occlusion, following transfusion.
		I	Subclavian catheter flushed 2 ml normal saline, then tubing disconnected from catheter. Sterile injection cap attached. Catheter lumen heparin locked with 2 ml heparin (100 u/ml).
		E	Catheter flushes with ease during normal saline and heparin infusion.

(Nurse's name)

Topics			Notes

Chemotherapy

Date 10/96	Time 1030	P	Knowledge deficit, related to chemo-therapy side effects.
		I	Discussion of potential side effects (nausea, hair loss, and tingling of fingers and toes) reviewed with patient. Written materials regarding drugs, potential side effects, and self-management interventions given to patient and spouse. Patient or spouse to notify physician after discharge if temperature is over 38°C, or persistent nausea. Appointment for lab work next Fri. Granisetron 1 mg and dexamethasone 20 mg diluted in 60 ml D5W administered over 15 minutes prior to chemotherapy drug infusions.
			Doxorubicin 37.5 mg given IV push over 10 minutes; bleomycin 15 mg infused over 20 minutes (fourth cycle receiving Bleomycin and no reactions thus far); vinblastine 9 mg given IV push over 5 minutes, and dacarbazine 562.5 mg given IV push over 10 minutes excellent blood returned obtained before, during, and after all chemotherapy drug infusions. Chemotherapy drugs given through a free-flowing IV of normal saline into peripheral site (20-gauge 1½ inch angiocath) in right hand dorsal vein.
		E	No complaints of burning or pain before, during, or after drug administration. States understanding of side effects (as above), self-management interventions (rest, drink fluids, empty bladder every 4 hours), and pertinent instructions for next 48 hours.

(Nurse's name)

Topics			Notes

Parenteral nutrition

Date 10/96	Time 2100	P	Self-esteem disturbance, body image, related to placement of vascular device. Manifestated by: "I'm very concerned about summertime clothing and have ceased activities I normally pursue. I feel embarassed when disrobing in locker room because of the catheter."
		I	Discussed feelings at length about these issues. Discussed coiling and taping catheter inside bra to secure placement; suggestions given for clothing styles.
		I	Appeared more at ease at the end of the discussion. "I will try suggestions and share at the next clinic appointment."
10/96	1400	P	Infection, risk for, related to break in technique when managing catheter and initiating parenteral nutrition, during return demonstration technique.
		I	Reviewed steps for catheter preparation and initiation of parenteral nutrition.
		I	Observed patient in return demonstration of above procedure. Maintained sterile technique while cleansing catheter, setting up and connecting parenteral nutrition solution. Patient and caregiver can state signs and symptoms of infection: fever >38°C, chills, nausea and vomiting, pain or redness at catheter exit site; know when and where to seek follow-up care.

(Nurse's name)

Critical care

| Date 10/96 | Time 1000 | P | Pain, recurrent anginal
Alteration in tissue perfusion |

Topics			Notes
		I	Nitroglycerin infusion 50 mg/250 ml D5W [0.2 mg/ml]; titrate for relief of anginal pain, maintain systolic BP < 130. Infusion at 6 gtts/min (20 μg/min) via infusion pump. Oxygen per nasal cannula/6 LPM. States pain is 5 out of 10.
	1010	E	BP 142/70, P 88, R 24, ECG rhythm NSR with 6 ectopic BPM. States pain is 3 out of 10. Nitroglycerin infusion 9 gtts/min (30 μg/min). Oxygen/cannula 4 LPM.
	1020	E	BP 138/68, P 84, R 20, ECG rhythm NSR with occasional ectopic BPM. States pain is 1 out of 10. Nitroglycerin infusion 12 gtts/min (40 μg/min). Oxygen/cannula 4 LPM.
Pediatrics			
Date 10/96	Time 2200	P	Fluid volume deficit, related to emesis in past 48 hours; mild dehydration Fear, related to unfamiliar environment, IV equipment (18 mo child/12 kg wt.)
	2215	I	Procedure (IV access) explained to parent. Parent holding child on lap. Child with parent transferred to IV procedure room, 2 nurses restrained child with mummy wrap, allowing left arm extended, parent talking to child at head of table and stroking face. (Topical anesthetic cream applied at 2100 to left hand.) IV prep to left hand; IV access to dorsal metacarpal vein via 24-gauge angiocath; good blood return. IV site secured with tape; transparent dressing and plastic med cup secured with tape and IV netting.

Topics			Notes
			Child can move all fingers well; no discoloration. IV D5W/Lactated Ringer's 500 ml via microbore tubing with Buretrol set and infusion pump. [Calculated 1100 ml/for maintenance fluid +550 ml for mild dehydration = 1650 ml/24 hours.] (IV rate = 69 ml/hr) Infusion initiated at 69 gtts/min. IV pump alarm set. Child/parent returned to patient room.
	2300	E	IV site intact; no evidence of edema or discoloration in hand/arm. Child sleeping on parent's lap. Parent stated child went to sleep about 5 minutes ago. Infusion at 69 gtts/min.

Appendix C
Risk Management Considerations in IV Therapy

Increasingly, nurses are involved in malpractice suits, either by being called as witnesses or by being named in malpractice claims. To minimize personal exposure, assume accountability for all your actions. Provide reasonable and prudent care in all circumstances, and never provide a treatment or perform a procedure or skill that is not thoroughly understood and where competence has not been demonstrated. Some proactive risk management strategies for IV nurses to use to prevent or limit liability include the following:

- Know and follow standards of care. Nurses are responsible for upholding both professional organization standards and community standards. Follow agency policies. Be aware of the trends of incidents in your setting.
- Educate patients so they can form realistic expectations for their IV treatment or procedure. Gear education to the patient's level of understanding. Do not use words such as "routine" or "simple" when explaining a procedure.
- Be knowledgable about patient rights: the right to privacy, the right to refuse treatment, the right to obtain treatment, the right to know the caregiver. Attempt to resolve conflicts immediately.
- Document all procedures, treatments, and education carefully and completely. Include actions taken to minimize patient complications, such as replacement of a malfunctioning IV pump.
- Keep an open line of communication between all health care providers. Some situations where failure to communicate may

lead to adverse patient outcomes include failing to notify a physician of a patient status change, failing to chart vital signs, and failing to give a receiving nursing area a report of patient condition during a transfer.

- Communicate a sense of caring to each patient. Be especially aware of nonverbal communication.

- These patients require support and encouragement as they adjust to a worsening health status.

- Do not render an opinion in areas of care that are outside of nursing practice and where nurses are not generally recognized as experts on the basis of education or practice. Nurses have a responsibility as patient advocates to use the designated chain of command to resolve concerns related to patient care.

- Generate incident reports when unusual occurrences happen. This will alert agency risk management personnel of potential liability exposures. Some situations in IV therapy where incident reports should be generated include medication extravasation into surrounding tissue, medication errors, flow rate errors, equipment or product failures, infection control issues, patient care procedure breakdowns, laboratory processing delays that adversely affect patient outcome, and the patient/family statement that a lawsuit is intended.

Appendix D
Basic IV Therapy
Course Objectives

A. Be knowledgable of the state Nurse Practice Act as it relates to IV therapy.

B. Understand anatomy and physiology as applied to IV therapy.
   1. Identify protective functions of the skin.
   2. Differentiate between arteries and veins.
   3. Identify venous anatomical structures.
   4. Demonstrate appropriate vein selection for prescribed IV treatment.
   5. Know measures that reduce the vasovagal response.
   6. List IV therapy–related factors that can cause alterations of the cardiopulmonary system.
   7. Identify factors that can alter normal blood clotting.
   8. List the functions of blood.

C. Understand fundamental concepts of fluid and electrolyte balance and relate these to prescribed treatment modalities. Understand the relationship between IV fluids and the body's homeostatic and regulatory functions.
   1. Identify the major homeostatic mechanisms that regulate fluid and electrolyte balance.
   2. Describe the influence of age on maintenance of fluid and electrolyte balance.
   3. Name the function of the following laboratory parameters: sodium, potassium, creatinine, BUN, and glucose.
   4. Recognize the importance of abnormal parameters for the following laboratory panels: complete blood count, electrolyte profile, renal function profile.
   5. List nursing responsibilities in monitoring a patient's fluid and electrolyte status.
   6. List types of fluid and electrolyte imbalances.
   7. List types of acid–base imbalances.
   8. Identify specific IV fluids and indications for use.

      9. Recognize major adverse patient outcomes related to fluid and electrolyte IV therapy.

D. Demonstrate competency in venipuncture techniques.
    1. Prepare the patient for IV therapy by providing patient education.
    2. Select the correct-size IV catheter for therapy prescribed.
    3. Assemble all equipment.
    4. Select the appropriate vein for the prescribed therapy.
    5. Insert the catheter following agency policy.
    6. Secure the catheter according to policy.
    7. Document the procedure according to policy.

E. Recognize measures that prevent IV therapy–related infections.
    1. List ways in which the system may become contaminated.
    2. Demonstrate aseptic assembly of IV infusion.
    3. Identify CDC guidelines for prevention of intravascular infections and transmission of blood-borne infections.
    4. Rotate the IV site every 72 hours or in the presence of redness or inflammation.
    5. Identify indications for changing the entire IV administration set.

F. Demonstrate knowledge and competency in the administration of intravenous fluids.
    1. List nursing responsibilities when monitoring fluid administration.
    2. Assemble needed equipment.
    3. Identify principles and equipment used to maintain an accurate flow rate.
    4. Change tubing and bags using aseptic technique.
    5. Maintain and monitor heparin lock patency.
    6. Calculate flow rates correctly.
    7. Discontinue infusion.

G. Demonstrate knowledge and competency in the administration of IV medications.
    1. State objectives of IV drug administration.
    2. Name factors that affect patient response to drugs.
    3. List factors that influence drug compatibility and stability.
    4. State five rights of medication administration.
    5. Demonstrate IV piggyback drug administration.
    6. Demonstrate IV push administration.
    7. Set up a medication infusion using a pump.
    8. Calculate the rate required to administer the prescribed dose.
    9. Assess the patient for adverse effects.

H. Demonstrate knowledge of blood administration.
   1. Report the clinical objective for the patient's blood transfusion.
   2. State the indications for administration of the various blood products.
   3. State the IV solution used for the initiation of blood or component therapy.
   4. Identify signs and symptoms of blood transfusion reactions.
   5. Describe the identification and verification procedure that must be followed before transfusing a blood product.

I. Demonstrate knowledge of TPN.
   1. Define TPN.
   2. Recognize terms used to describe TPN.
   3. Identify indications for TPN administration.
   4. List potential complications of TPN.
   5. Identify principles of TPN administration.

BIBLIOGRAPHY

Central venous catheters

Andris DA and others: Pinch-off syndrome: a rare etiology for central venous catheter occlusion, *JPEN J Parenter Enteral Nutr* 18(6):531, 1994.

Bagnall-Reeb H, Ryder M, Anglim MA: *Venous access device occlusions,* Abbott Park, IL, 1993, Abbott Laboratories.

Baranowski L: Central venous access devices, current technologies, uses, and management strategies, *J Intravenous Nurs* 16(3):167, 1993.

Barone CP: Drawing blood from central lines—concern about infection control, *Crit Care Nurse* 14(3):150, 1994.

Brant JM: The use of access devices in cancer pain control, *Semin Oncol Nurs* 11(3):203, 1995.

Buchman AL and others: Catheter-related infections associated with home parenteral nutrition and predictive factors for the need for catheter removal in their treatment, *JPEN J Parenter Enteral Nutr* 18(4): 297, 1994.

Cunningham RS, Bonam-Crawford: The role of fibrinolytic agents in the management of thrombotic complications associated with vascular access devices, *Nurs Clin North Am* 28(4):899, 1993.

Doane LS: Administering intraperitoneal chemotherapy using a peritoneal port, *Nurs Clin North Am* 28(4):885, 1993.

Dool J, Rodehaver CB, Fulton JS: Central venous access devices: issues for staff education and clinical competence, *Nurs Clin North Am* 28(4):973, 1993.

Erdman SH and others: Central line occlusion with three-in-one nutrition admixtures administered at home, *JPEN J Parenter Enteral Nutr* 18(2):177, 1994.

Freedman SE, Bosserman G: Tunneled catheters: technologic advances and nursing care issues, *Nurs Clin North Am* 28(4):851, 1993.

Gullo SM: Implanted ports: technologic advances and nursing care issues, *Nurs Clin North Am* 28(4):859, 1993.

Hadaway LC: Comparison of vascular devices, *Semin Oncol Nurs* 11(3):154, 1995.

Ingle RJ: Rare complications of vascular access devices, *Semin Oncol Nurs* 11(3):184, 1995.

Johnson GB: Nursing care of patients with implanted pumps, *Nurs Clin North Am* 28(4):873, 1993.

Johnson JC: Complications of vascular devices, *Emerg Med Clin North Am* 12(3):691, 1994.

Keller CA: Methods of drawing blood samples through central venous catheters in pediatric patients undergoing bone marrow transplant: results of a national survey, *Oncol Nurs Forum* 21(5):879, 1994.

Kelly C and others: A change in flushing protocols of central venous catheters, *Oncol Nurs Forum* 19(4):599, 1992.

Kupensky DT: Use of hydrochloric acid to restore patency in an occluded implantable port: a case report, *J Intravenous Nurs* 18(4):198, 1995.

Lapka DMV, Wild LD, Barbour LA: Heparin-induced thrombocytopenia and thrombosis: a case study and clinical overview, *Oncol Nurs Forum* 21(5):871, 1994.

Lawson M, Vertenstein MJ: Methods for determining the internal volume of central venous catheters, *J Intravenous Nurs* 16(3):148, 1993.

Lilienberg A, Bengtsson M, Starkhammar H: Implantable devices for venous access: nurses' and patients' evaluation of three different port systems, *J Adv Nurs* 19(1):21, 1994.

McDermott MK: Patient education and compliance issues associated with access devices, *Semin Oncol Nurs* 11(3):221, 1995.

Nace CS, Ingle RJ: Central venous catheter "pinch-off" and fracture: a review of two under-recognized complications, *Oncol Nurs Forum* 20(8):1227, 1993.

Northsea C: Using urokinase to restore patency in double lumen catheters, *J Amer Nephrology Nurses Assoc* 21(5):261, 1994.

Oncology Nursing Society, *Access device guidelines, module I catheters,* 1989, The Society.

Passaro ME and others: Long-term silastic catheters and chest pain, *JPEN J Parenter Enteral Nutr* 18(3):240, 1994.

Pinherio JM, Fisher MA: Use of a triple-lumen catheter for umbilical access in the neonate, *J Pediatr* 120(4:1):624, 1992.

Pinto KM: Accuracy of coagulation values obtained from a heparinized central venous catheter, *Concol Nurs Forum* 21(3):573, 1994.

Rapsilber LM, Camp-Sorrell D: Ambulatory infusion pumps, *Semin Oncol Nurs* 11(2):213, 1995.

Rumsey KA, Richardson DK: Management of infection and occlusion associated with vascular access devices, *Semin Oncol Nurs* 11(3):174, 1995.

Ruschman KL, Fulton JS: Effectiveness of disinfectant techniques on intravenous tubing latex injection ports, *J Intravenous Nurs* 16(5):304, 1993.

Sansivero GE: Why pick a PICC? *Nursing* 25(7):35, 1995.

Scharping S, Hirschman L: Venous access device study: identification of number of patients with venous access device lines, *J Intravenous Nurs* 17(6):277, 1994.

Smith RM: A nurse's guide to implanted ports, *RN* 56(4):48, 1993.

Stephens LC, Haire WD, Kotulak GD: Are clinical signs accurate indicators of the cause of central venous catheter occlusion? *JPEN J Parenter Enteral Nutr* 19(1):75, 1995.

Welker DL: *Troubleshooting vascular access devices,* St Paul, MN, 1993, Pharmacia Deltec.

Winslow MN, Trammell L, Camp-Sorrell D: Selection of vascular access devices and nursing care, *Semin Oncol Nurs* 11(3):167, 1995.

Peripherally inserted central catheters

Abi-Nader JA: Peripherally inserted central venous catheters in critical care patients, *Heart Lung* 22(5):428, 1993.

Cardella JF, Fox PS, Lawler JB: Interventional radiologic placement of peripherally inserted central catheters, *J Vasc Intervent Radiol* 4(5): 653, 1993.

Cardella JF, Lukens ML, Fox PS: Fibrin sheath entrapment of peripherally inserted central catheters, *J Vasc Interven Radiol* 5(3):439, 1994.

Dotan KS: Development of PICC criteria leads to increased patient satisfaction, *Oncol Nurs Forum* 20(4):699, 1993.

Frederick DG: Tongue blade stabilizes PICC to prevent flow occlusion, *Oncol Nurs Forum* 20(4):699, 1993.

Goodwin ML, Carlson I: The peripherally inserted central catheter: a retrospective look at three years of insertions, *J Intravenous Nurs* 16(2):92, 1993.

Greene LM, Gerlach CJ: Central lines have moved out, *RN* 57(5):26, 1994.

Greenspoon JS, Rosen DJ, Ault M: Use of the peripherally inserted central catheter for parenteral nutrition during pregnancy, *Obstet Gynecol* 81 (5:2):831, 1993.

Hedges C, Karas BS: Peripherally-inserted central catheters: challenges for hospital management, *Medsurg Nurs* 2(6):443, 1993.

Hovsepian DM, Bonn J, Eschelman DJ: Technique for peripheral insertion of central venous catheters, *J Vasc Intervent Radiol* 4(6):795, 1993.

James L, Bledsoe L, Hadaway LC: A retrospective look at tip location and complications of peripherally inserted central catheters lines, *J Intravenous Nurs* 16(2):104, 1993.

LaFortune S: The use of confirming x-rays to verify tip position for peripherally inserted catheters, *J Intravenous Nurs* 16(4):246, 1993.

Lam S and others: Peripherally inserted central catheters in an acute-care hospital, *Arch Intern Med* 154(16):1833, 1994.

Linz DN, Bisset GS III, Warner BW: Fracture and embolization of a peripherally inserted central venous catheter, *JPEN J Parenter Enteral Nutr* 18(1):79, 1994.

Loughran SC, Borzatta M: Peripherally inserted central catheters: a report of 2506 catheter days, *JPEN J Parenter Enteral Nutr* 19(2):133, 1995.

Meares C: PICC and MLC lines: options worth exploring, *Nursing* 22 (10):52, 1992.

Merrell SW and others: Peripherally inserted central venous catheters. Low-risk alternatives for ongoing venous access, *West J Med* 160(1): 25, 1994.

Orr ME: Issues in the management of percutaneous central venous catheters: single and multiple lumens, *Nurs Clin North Am* 28(4): 911, 1993.

Pauley SY and others: Catheter-related colonization associated with percutaneous inserted central catheters, *J Intravenous Nurs* 16(1):50, 1993.

Ryder MA: Peripherally inserted central venous catheters, *Nurs Clin North Am* 28(4):937, 1993.

Sansivero GE: Why pick a PICC? What you need to know, *Nursing* 25 (7):34, 1995.

Valk WJC, Liem KD, Geven WB: Seldinger technique as an alternative approach for percutaneous insertion of hydrophilic polyurethane central venous catheters in newborns, *JPEN J Parenter Enteral Nutr* 19 (2):151, 1995.

Blood and blood component administration

American Association of Blood Banks: *Accreditation requirements manual,* ed 6, Arlington, VA, 1996, The Association.

American Association of Blood Banks: *Blood bank operations manual,* Arlington, VA, 1995, The Association.

American Association of Blood Banks: *Blood transfusion therapy: a physician's handbook,* ed 5, Arlington, VA, 1995, The Association.

American Association of Blood Banks: *Standards for blood banks and transfusion services,* ed 17, Arlington, VA, 1996, The Association.

Benson K and others: The platelet-refractory bone marrow transplant patient: prophylaxis and treatment of bleeding, *Semin Oncol* 20(5 suppl 6):102, 1993.

Bordin JO, Blajchman MA: Immunosuppressive effects of allogenic blood transfusions: implications for the patient with a malignancy, *Hematol Oncol Clin North Am* 9(1):205, 1995.

Buschel PC, Kapustay PM: Peripheral stem cell transplantation, *Oncol Nurs* 2(2):1, 1995.

Coffland FL, Sheleton DM: Blood component replacement therapy, *Crit Care Nurs Clin North Am* 5(3):543, 1993.

College of American Pathologists: Practice parameter for the use of fresh-frozen plasma, cryoprecipitate, and platelets, *JAMA* 271(10): 777, 1994.

Cook LS: An overview of leukocyte depletion in blood transfusion, *J Intravenous Nurs* 18(1):11, 1995.

Cottler-Fox M, Klein HG: Transfusion support of hematology and oncology patients. The role of recombinant hematopoietic growth factors, *Arch Pathol Lab Med* 118(4):417, 1994.

Dodsworth H: Making sense of the use of blood and blood products, *Nurs Times* 91(1):25, 1995.

Fakhry SM, Sheldon GF: Blood administration, risks, and substitutes, *Adv Surg* 28:71, 1995.

Food and Drug Administration: *Code of federal regulations,* title 21, 600-799, Washington, DC, 1994, US Government Printing Office.

Friedberg RC: Issues in transfusion therapy in the patient with a malignancy, *Hematol Oncol Clin North Am* 8(6):1223, 1994.

Gerber L: Autologous blood transfusion: why and how, *J Intravenous Nurs* 17(2):65, 1994.

Gonterman R, Kiracofe S, Owens P: Administering, documenting, and tracking blood products and volume expanders, *Medsurg Nurs* 3(4): 269, 1994.

Goodnough LT, Bodner MS, Martin JW: Blood transfusion and blood conservation: cost and utilization issues. *Am J Med Qual* 9(4):172, 1994.

Hammond LC, Machemer SA: Myths and facts about blood and its components, *Nursing* 23(9):29, 1993.

Jassak PF, Riley MB: Autologous stem cell transplant, *Cancer Pract* 2 (2):141, 1994.

Lange EG and others: Hemolytic transfusion reaction, *Nursing* 25(7): 33, 1995.

Lawrence VA, Birch S, Gafni A: The impact of new clinical guidelines on the North American blood economy, *Transfus Med Rev* 8(4):232, 1994.

Lichtiger B: Monitoring the safety of transfusion practices in the United States, *Transfus Clin Biol* 1(3):247, 1994.

Mijovic A, Pagliuca A, Mufti GJ: Autologous blood stem cell transplantation in hematological malignancies, *Leuk Lymphoma* 13(1–2): 33, 1994.

Mintz PD: Quality assessment and improvement of transfusion practices, *Hematol Oncol Clin North Am* 9(1):219, 1995.

Mummert TB, Tourault MA: Transfusion-related fatality reports—a summary, *Nurs Manage* 25(10):801, 1994.

Norville R and others: The effects of infusion methods on platelet count, morphology, and corrected count increment in children with cancer: in vitro and in vivo studies, *Oncol Nurs Forum* 21(10):1669, 1994.

Oddi LF: Disclosure of human immunodeficiency virus status in healthcare settings, *J Intravenous Nurs* 17(2):93, 1994.

Roberts A: Systems of life: blood pt 6, *Nurs Times* 90(45):31, 1994.

Rosen NR, Bates LH, Herod G: Transfusion therapy: improved patient care and resource utilization, *Transfusion* 33(4):341, 1993.

Sciortino AD and others: The efficacy of administering blood transfusions at home to terminally ill cancer patients, *J Palliat Care* 9(3):14, 1993.

Shanberge JN: Guidelines for blood component therapy, *J Fla Med Assoc* 80(1):43, 1993.

Shanberge JN, Quattrociocchi-Longe T: Analysis of fresh frozen plasma administration with suggestions for ways to reduce usage, *Transfus Med* 2(3):189, 1992.

Shulman IA and others: Monitoring transfusionist practices: a strategy for improving transfusions safety, *Transfusion* 34(1):11, 1994.

Smith RN and others: Instilling the facts about autotransfusion, *Nursing* 25 (3):52, 1995.

Spector D: Transfusion-associated graft-versus-host disease: an overview and two case reports, *Oncol Nurs Forum* 22(1):97, 1995.

Stadtmauer EA, Schneider CJ, Silberson LE: Peripheral blood progenitor cell generation and harvesting, *Semin Oncol* 22(3):291, 1995.

Stehling L and others: Guidelines for blood utilization review, *Transfusion* 34(5):438, 1994.

Strauss RG and others: National acceptability of American Association of Blood Banks Pediatric Hemotherapy Committee guidelines for auditing pediatric transfusion practices, *Transfusion* 33(2):68, 1993.

Suez D: Intravenous immunoglobulin therapy: indications, potential side effects, and treatment guidelines, *J Intravenous Nurs* 4(18):178, 1995.

Sweeney JD, Holme S, Heaton A: Quality of platelet concentrates, *Immunol Invest* 24(1–2):353, 1995.

Tartter PI: Immunologic effects of blood transfusion, *Immunol Invest* 24 (1–2):277, 1995.

Walker FE and others: Guiding patients and their families through peripheral stem cell transplantation with the help of a teaching booklet, *Oncol Nurs Forum* 21(3):585, 1994.

Walker FE, Roethke SK, Martin G: An overview of the rationale, process, and nursing implications of peripheral blood stem cell transplantation, *Cancer Nurs* 17(2):141, 1994.

Winston DJ and others: Intravenous immunoglobulin and CMV-seronegative blood products for prevention of CMV infection and disease in bone marrow transplant recipients, *Bone Marrow Transplant* 12 (3):283, 1993.

Wright D: Peripheral stem cell transplantation, *Medsurg Nurs* 3(1): 40, 1994.

Chemotherapy administration

Aapro MS: Docetaxel (taxotere): a highly active taxoid with manageable toxicity, *Semin Oncol* 22(2, suppl 4):1, 1995.

ASHP Special Interest Group, ASHP technical assistance bulletin on handling cytotoxic and hazardous drugs, *Am J Hosp Pharm* 47 (5):1033–1049, 1990.

Bicher A and others: Infusion site soft tissue injury after paclitaxel administration, *Cancer* 76(1):116, 1995.

Brogden JM, Nevidjon B: Vinorelbine tartate (navelbine): drug profile and nursing implications of a new vinca alkaloid, *Oncol Nurs Forum* 22 (4):635, 1995.

Chisholm LG and others: Cancer chemotherapy: alternative administration routes, *Cancer Nurs* 16(3):237, 1993.

Cooke J and others: Use of cytotoxic methods to determine mutagenic changes in the blood of pharmacy personnel and nurses who handle cytotoxic agents, *Am J Hosp Pharm* 48(6):1199–1205, 1991.

Davis ME, DeSantis D, Klemm K: A flow sheet for follow-up after chemotherapy extravasation, *Oncol Nurs Forum* 22(6):979, 1995.

DeVita VT Jr: *Principles of chemotherapy.* In DeVita VT Jr, Hellman S, Rosenberg SA, editors: *Cancer: principles and practice of oncology,* ed 4, Philadelphia, 1993, JB Lippincott.

Dorr RT, Von Hoff DD: *Cancer chemotherapy handbook,* ed 2, Norwalk, 1994, Appleton and Lange.

Drugs of choice for cancer chemotherapy, *Med Lett* 37(945):25, 1995.

Ensminger WD: Regional chemotherapy, *Semin Oncol* 20(1):3, 1993.

Fossella FV and others: Summary of phase II data of docetaxel (taxotere), an active agent in the first- and second-line treatment of advanced non-small cell lung cancer, *Semin Oncol* 22(2, suppl 4): 22, 1995.

Gullo SM: Safe handling of cytotoxic agents, *Oncol Nurs Forum* 22(3): 517, 1995.

Kaye SB: Docetaxel (taxotere) in the treatment of solid tumors other than breast and lung cancer, *Semin Oncol* 22(2, suppl 4):30, 1995.

LePage E: Using a ventricular reservoir to instill amphotericin B, *J Neurosci Nurs* 25(4):212, 1993.

Lesser GJ, Grossman SA: The chemotherapy of adult primary brain tumors, *Cancer Treat Rev* 19(3):261, 1993.

Lynes AC: Percutaneous hepatic arterial chemotherapy and chemobolization, *Cancer Nurs* 19(4):283, 1993.

McCaffrey Boyle D, Engelking C: Vesicant extravasation: myths and realities, *Oncol Nurs Forum* 22(1):57, 1995.

McDevitt JJ and others: Exposure to hospital pharmacists and nurses to antineoplastics agents, *J Occup Med* 35(1):57, 1993.

Mahon SM and others: Safe handling practices of cytotoxic drugs: the results of a chapter survey, *Oncol Nurs Forum* 21(7):1157, 1994.

Mayer DK: Hazards of chemotherapy, implementing safe handling practices, *Cancer* 70(suppl 4):988–992, 1992.

Mayer RJ: Chemotherapy for metastatic colorectal cancer, *Cancer* 70 (suppl 5):1414, 1992.

Mayo DJ, Pearson DC: Chemotherapy extravasation: a consequence of fibrin sheath formation around venous access devices, *Oncol Nurs Forum* 22(4):675, 1995.

Meyer M and others: Pre- and perioperative perfusion chemotherapy for soft tissue sarcoma of the limbs, *Cancer Treat Research* 56:105, 1991.

Nieweg RMB and others: Safe handling of antineoplastic drugs, *Cancer Nurs* 17(6):501, 1994.

Noone MH, Fioravanti SG: Taxol: past, present, and future, *Oncol Nurs* 1 (4):1, 1994.

Oncology Nursing Society, Cancer Chemotherapy Guidelines and Recommendations for Practice, Pittsburgh, 1996, Oncology Medical Press Inc.

Otto SE: Advanced concepts in chemotherapy drug delivery: regional therapy, *J Intravenous Nurs* 18(4):170, 1995.

Parillo VL: Documentation forms for monitoring occupational surveillance of healthcare workers who handle cytotoxic drugs, *Oncol Nurs Forum* 21 (1):115–120, 1994.

Ravidin PM, Valero V: Review of docetaxel (taxotere), a highly active new agent for the treatment of metastatic breast cancer, *Semin Oncol* 22(2, suppl 4):17, 1995.

Rittenberg CN, Gralla RJ, Rehmeyer TA: Assessing and managing venous irritation associated with vinorelbine tartrate (navelbine). *Oncol Nurs Forum* 22(4):707, 1995.

St Germain B, Houlihan N, D'Amato S: Dimethyl sulfoxide therapy in the treatment of vesicant extravasant: two case presentations, *J Intravenous Nurs* 17(5):261, 1994.

San Angel F: Current controversies in chemotherapy administration, *J Intravenous Nur* 18(1):16, 1995.

Terry J and others, editors: *Intravenous therapy, clinical principles and practice,* Philadelphia, 1995, WB Saunders.

US Department of Labor, Office of Occupational Medicine, Occupational Safety and Health Administration: *Controlling occupational exposure to hazardous drugs,* CPL 2-2.20B CH-4, Washington, DC, 1995, US Government Printing Office.

Valanis BG and others: Acute symptoms associated with antineoplastic drug handling among nurses, *Cancer Nurs* 16(4):288, 1993.

Valanis BG and others: Association of antineoplastic drug handling with acute adverse effects in pharmacy personnel, *Am J Hosp Pharm* 50 (3):455–462, 1993.

Valanis BG and others: Staff members' compliance with their facility's antineoplastic drug handling policy, *Oncol Nurs Forum* 18(3):571–576, 1991.

Vokes EE and others: A phase II study of cisplatin, 5-fluorouracil, and leucovorin augmented by vinorelbine (navelbine) for advanced non-small cell lung cancer: rationale and study design, *Semin Oncol* 21(5, suppl 10):79, 1994.

Williams SA: Using oncology nursing society cancer chemotherapy guidelines as a basis for continuing education in rural hospitals, *Oncol Nurs Forum* 22(4):689, 1995.

Wood LS, Gullo SM: IV vesicants: how to avoid extravasation, *Am J Nurs* 93(4):42, 1993.

Workman ML: Occupational absorption of chemotherapeutic agents among health care professionals, *Oncol Nurs Forum* 18(2):346, 1991 (abstract).

Yucha CB and others: Effect of elevation on intravenous extravasations, *J Intravenous Nurs* 17(5):231, 1994.

Vascular access in adult critical care

Bearden EF: The costs and benefits of monitoring perfusion in the critically ill, *Crit Care Nurs Clin North Am* 7:239–248, 1995.

Chernow B: *Essentials of critical care pharmacology,* ed 3, Baltimore, 1994, Williams and Wilkins.

Daily EK, Schroeder JS: *Techniques in bedside hemodynamic monitoring,* ed 5, St Louis, 1994, Mosby.

Ditmyer CE and others: Comparison of continuous with intermittent bolus thermodilution cardiac output measurements, *Am J Crit Care* 4:460–465, 1995.

Ermakov S, Hoyt JW: Pulmonary artery catheterization, *Crit Care Clin* 8:773–806, 1992.

Flynn JB, Bruce NP: *Introduction to critical care skills,* St Louis, 1993, Mosby.

Franklin C: The technique of radial artery cannulation: tips for maximizing results while minimizing the risks of complications, *J Crit Illness* 10:424–432, 1995.

Haupt MT, Kaufman BS, Carlson RW: Fluid resuscitation in patients with increased vascular permeability, *Crit Care Clin* 8:341–353, 1992.

Johnson MK, Schumann L: Comparison of three methods of measurement of pulmonary artery catheter readings in critically ill patients, *Am J Crit Care* 4:300–307, 1995.

Kadota LT: *Hemodynamic monitoring.* In Clochesy JM and others, editors: *Critical care nursing,* Philadelphia, 1993, WB Saunders.

Kern LS: *Hemodynamic monitoring.* In Boggs RL, Wooldridge-King M, editors: *AACN procedure manual for critical care,* ed 3, Philadelphia, 1993, WB Saunders.

Parson R, Hotter A: *Invasive vascular techniques—arterial puncture.* In Boggs RL, Wooldridge-King M, editors: *AACN procedure manual for critical care,* ed 3, Philadelphia, 1993, WB Saunders.

Ramsey JD, Tisdale LA: Use of ventricular stroke work index and ventricular function curves in assessing myocardial contractility, *Crit Care Nurs* 15:16–67, 1995.

Pediatrics

Baranowski L: *Central venous access devices—current technologies, uses and management strategies,* J Intraven Nurs 16(3):167–194, 1993.

Drug information for the healthcare professional, 1994, The United States Pharmacopeial Convention.

Frederick V: *Pediatric IV therapy—soothing the patient,* RN 54(12):40–42, 1991.

Hazinski MF: *Nursing care of the critically ill child,* ed 2, St Louis, 1992, Mosby.

Hutchinson D: *Pediatric IV therapy—starting the line,* RN 54(12):43–48, 1991.

Jackson PL, Saunders SE: *Child health nursing—a comprehensive approach to the care of children and their families,* Philadelphia, 1993, JB Lippincott.

James SR, Mott SR: *Child health nursing—essential care of children and families,* Menlo Park, CA, 1988, Addison-Wesley.

LaRocca JC, Otto SE: *Pocket guide to intravenous therapy,* St Louis, 1993, Mosby.

Mahan LK, Arlin MT: *Krause's food, nutrition and diet therapy,* Philadelphia, 1992, WB Saunders.

Millam DA: *How to teach good venipuncture technique,* Am J Nurs 93(7):38, 1993.

Millam DA: *Starting IV's—how to develop your venipuncture skills,* Nursing 22(9):33, 1992.

Ringel M: *For pediatric infusion—there's no place like home,* Infusion 2(1), 1995.

Sansweri GE: *Why pick a PICC? Nursing* 25(7):35, 1995.

Selekman J: *Pediatric nursing—a study and learning tool,* Springhouse, PA, 1988, Springhouse.

Springhouse drug reference, Springhouse, PA, 1988, Springhouse.

Terry J and others, editors: *Intravenous therapy—clinical principles and practice,* Philadelphia, 1995, WB Saunders.

Transfusion therapy guidelines for nurses, 1990, National Blood Resource Education Program.

Weinstein SM: *Plumer's principles and practice of intravenous therapy,* Philadelphia, 1993, JB Lippincott.

Calculations for IV therapy

Brown M, Mulholland JL: *Drug calculations, process and problems for clinical practice,* ed 4, St Louis, 1992, Mosby.

Dison N: *Simplified drugs and solutions for nurses, including mathematics,* ed 10, St Louis, 1992, Mosby.

Hart LK: *The arithmetic of dosages and solutions: a programmed presentation,* ed 7, St Louis, 1989, Mosby.

McLeroy PA: The rule of six: calculating intravenous infusions in a pediatric crisis situation, *Hosp Pharm* 29(10):939, 1994.

Shannon MT, Wilson BA: In Givoni, Hayes, editors: *Drugs and nursing implications,* ed 7, Norwalk, 1992, Appleton and Lange.

Skidmore-Roth L: *Mosby's drug reference,* St Louis, 1995, Mosby.

Whisler BL, Whisler LL, Whisler DD: Mathematics for health professionals, ed 3, Boston, 1992, Jones and Bartlett.

Woodrow R: Essentials of pharmacology for health occupations, ed 2, Albany, NY, 1992, Delmar.

Adult infusion therapies

Abernathy E: Role of hematopoietic growth factors: nursing care issues in adult acute leukemia, *Pharmacia* 2:20, 1995.

Appelbaum FR: The application of hematopoietic colony stimulating factors (CSFs) in cancer management, *Curr Iss Cancer Nurs Prac Updates* 2(2):1, 1993.

Banks MA: Home infusion of intravenous immunoglobulin, *J Intravenous Nurs* 17(6):299, 1994.

Bender CM: Cognitive dysfunction associated with biological response modifier therapy, *Oncol Nurs Forum* 21(3):515, 1994.

Blanford NL: Renal transplantation: a case study of the ideal, *Crit Care Nurs* 13(2):46, 1993.

Caliendo G, Joyce D, Altmiller MC: Nursing guidelines and discharge planning for patients receiving recombinant interleukin-2, *Semin Oncol Nurs* 9(3, suppl 1):25, 1993.

Camp-Sorrel D, Wujcik D: Intravenous immunoglobulin administration: an evaluation of vital sign monitoring, *Oncol Nurs Forum* 21(3):531, 1994.

Gano JB, Kleinerman S: Liposomal MTP-PE: a promising new biologic response modifier, *Oncol Nurs Forum* 22(5):809, 1995.

Holmes W: Cyclosporine immunosuppression: clinical practice issues, *Curr Iss Cancer Nurs Prac Updates* 1(10):1, 1993.

King CR: Outpatient management of myelosuppression, *Clin Perspect Oncol Nurs* 1(4):1, 1995.

Rieger PT, Haeuber D: A new approach to managing chemotherapy-related anemia: nursing implications of Epoetin Alfa, *Oncol Nurs Forum* 22 (1):71, 1995.

Rowe JM and others: A randomized placebo-controlled phase II study of granulocyte-macrophage colony-stimulating factor in adult patients, *Blood* 86(2):457, 1995.

Sharp E and others: A teaching tool for patients receiving continuous IV infusion recombinant interleukin-2 therapy, *Oncol Nurs Forum* 21 (5):911, 1994.

Stone RM and others: Granulocyte-macrophage colony-stimulating factor and initial chemotherapy for elderly patients with primary acute myelogenous leukemia, *N Engl J Med* 332(25):1671, 1995.

Straw LJ, Conrad KJ: Patient education resources related to biotherapy and the immune system, *Oncol Nurs Forum* 21(7):1223, 1994.

Suez D: Intravenous immunoglobulin therapy: indications, potential side effects, and treatment guidelines, *J Intravenous Nurs* 18(4):178, 1995.

Trusler LA: OKT 3: nursing considerations for use in acute renal transplant rejection, *J Amer Nephrology Nurses Assoc* 17(4):299, 1990.

Vadham-Raj S and others: Effects of PIXY 321, a granulocyte-macrophage colony-stimulating factor/interleukin-3 fusion protein, on chemotherapy-induced multilineage myelosuppression in patients with sarcoma, *J Clin Oncol* 12(4):715, 1994.

Wahrenberger A: Pharmacologic immunosuppression: cure or curse? *Crit Care Nurs Q* 17(4):27, 1995.

Wilkes GM, Ingwersen K, Barton-Burke M: *Oncology nursing drug reference,* Boston, 1994, Jones and Bartlett.

Index

Page references followed by lowercase Roman f indicate illustrations. Page references followed by lowercase Roman t indicate material in tables. Page references followed by lowercase italic n indicate material in footnotes. Drugs are indexed by generic names and selected trade names. Trade names of various generic drugs can be found in several tables delineated at the index entry "Trade names of drugs."